Differential Learning in Physiotherapy

Wolfgang I. Schöllhorn
Agnė Slapšinskaitė-Dackevičienė
Editors

Differential Learning in Physiotherapy

How to Foster Self-organized Learning

Springer

Editors
Wolfgang I. Schöllhorn
Institute for Sport Science
Johannes Gutenberg-University
Mainz, Germany

Agnė Slapšinskaitė-Dackevičienė
Department of Sports Medicine, Faculty of Nursing, Medical Academy
Lithuanian University of Health Sciences
Kaunas, Lithuania

ISBN 978-3-031-98786-1 ISBN 978-3-031-98787-8 (eBook)
https://doi.org/10.1007/978-3-031-98787-8

This Springer imprint is published by the registered company Springer Nature Switzerland AG
The registered company address is: Gewerbestrasse 11, 6330 Cham, Switzerland

Back to the Roots—Rethinking Physiotherapy Through Differential Learning

Why another book on physiotherapy, you may ask? After all, shelves are already filled with textbooks, manuals, and guidelines covering the latest findings from medicine, physiology, biomechanics, and beyond. This book, however, takes a different path. It is not about presenting new medical breakthroughs, nor about summarizing established knowledge. Instead, it offers a new perspective—translating recent scientific findings into practical consequences for physiotherapy and training. It is a book not of recipes, but of questions—questions meant to provoke critical reflection, encourage experimentation, and ultimately rethink the foundations of the profession.

Physiotherapy has long relied on implicit assumptions about movement, learning, and recovery. Assumptions that were often taken for granted, shaped by tradition, clinical perspectives, and historical context. This book invites you to deconstruct these assumptions. Inspired by Stephen Brookfield's (Brookfield 1987) approach to critical thinking, rooted in Derrida's philosophy of deconstruction (Derrida 2021), it challenges readers to uncover the assumptions underlying their own practice, critically examine them, and explore new possibilities. This is not deconstruction for its own sake but a necessary process to reshape physiotherapy on firmer, more reflective foundations—or, at the very least, to deepen our understanding of why we do what we do.

This book returns to the original references—not out of nostalgia, but to reclaim creative connections and intentions of the pioneers often get lost when reduced to textbook summaries. By engaging with these original ideas, we create space for new interpretations and alternative ways of thinking. This is particularly relevant in the context of *Differential Learning* (DL), which challenges two fundamental assumptions in classical physiotherapy: the notion of an idealized, person- and time-independent movement model as the ultimate goal and the belief that repetition is the primary driver of therapeutic success.

DL offers an alternative, rooted in system theory, first- and second-order cybernetics, and neurophysiology, while borrowing inspiration from complexity science, artificial neural networks, and self-organization. This book presents the theoretical foundation of DL, critically linking it to these broader scientific frameworks. It then translates these foundations into practical consequences, showing how variability, error, and nonlinearity can become tools for promoting recovery, adaptation, and resilience.

But this is not a book that strives for completeness—that would contradict its very premise. Instead, it presents an evolving discourse, a collection of provocations, and a series of exploratory experiments. Some chapters rely heavily on data and studies that have tested the predictions of DL theory since its first publication. Rather than imposing definitive answers, they seek to create the initial disturbance—an intellectual spark—that inspires new questions, new experiments, and innovative approaches.

The structure of the book reflects this journey from theory to practice. After the initial theoretical deconstruction (Chap. 1) and reconstruction (Chap. 2), the chapters move into practical applications (Chap. 3)—showing how DL has been applied successfully across sports and rehabilitation fields, from aiding musicians' recovery (Chap. 4) to stroke recovery (Chap. 5), from ACL rehabilitation (Chap. 6) to retraining balance (Chap. 7). The book also applies the DL lens to contemporary trends like High-Intensity Interval Training (HIIT) (Chap. 8)—exploring how these approaches might need to be rethought if seen through the lens of variability, noise, and self-organization.

This book invites you to swim against the current, back to the roots—not to find comfort in tradition, but to rediscover the raw creativity that shaped physiotherapy in its early days. It aims not just to inspire you to treat, but to heal—by understanding movement not as a mechanical process, but as a deeply embodied, context-sensitive, continuously evolving phenomenon. In order to avoid confusion and to avoid complicating readability by listing many country-specific terms, we have agreed to use the term physiotherapy and have dispensed with the historically later differentiation into occupational, ergotherapy, physical therapy, etc.

Physiotherapy does not need more certainties; it needs more critical thinkers. This book hopes to contribute to that need—by offering questions, connections, provocations, and evidence, while leaving the final answers for you to discover.

We wish you lots of inspiration when reading the book.

Agnė Slapšinskaitė-Dackevičienė
Wolfgang I. Schöllhorn

References

Brookfield SD (1987) Developing critical thinkers: challenging adults to explore alternative ways of thinking and acting. Wiley.

Derrida J (2021) Deconstruction in a Nutshell – a conversation with Jacques Derrida, with a new introduction. Fordham University Press. https://doi.org/10.2307/j.ctv1198zt6

Contents

Part I

Foundations and Theory of Differential Learning

1 Basic Assumptions of Classical Approaches in Physiotherapy and Training Critically Reflected

Wolfgang I. Schöllhorn

1.1 Introduction

The two most common latent and therefore little scrutinized assumptions in classical physiotherapy, as well as in sports teaching and training, are:

(a) Generalized role models that are largely person- and time-independent.
(b) These models can only be achieved by numerous repetitions in the form of copying the supposedly correct model, accompanied by corrective instructions.

The first assumption of person- and time-independent models is most often observed when applying the same treatment to different people or when applying the same measure to the same person irrespective of time if they return after a year with similar symptoms. Although most patients are treated in one therapist-one patient setup and the patient is always in the foreground in practice, the interventions are usually based on the logic of the traditional group- and mean-oriented sciences like medicine and psychology, which still suffer from the envy of physics (Howell et al. 2014; Sokal 2016). This term refers to the fact that writing and working practices in "softer sciences," such as the humanities or social sciences, rely too much on confusing jargon and complicated mathematics to appear more "rigorous" than in heavily mathematical natural science subjects such as physics. This is mainly due to a lack of consideration of the fundamental structural differences in their object of research (Montévil 2019). Whereas in physics it is mainly nonliving objects, which change only on very long timescales, that are the subject of research, the life sciences deal with objects that change by themselves on a much shorter timescale and thus give time an irreversible direction (Prigogine 1980; Prigogine and Nicolis 1971). While we can expect the same behavior from a rigid body regardless of time and therefore more easily satisfy the criteria of reproducibility, this is rarely the case with living beings.

The second assumption, the belief in repetition as a panacea, is most commonly applied because physiotherapists and patients are used to similar methods in different areas of life related to learning, such as school and sports. If we look at (physio-) therapy somewhat more abstractly as a measure that leads to a different (healthy) state, parallels become visible to what we commonly associate with learning, the origins of which are more diverse and linked to a longer history.

W. I. Schöllhorn (✉)
Institute for Sport Science, Johannes Gutenberg-University, Mainz, Germany
e-mail: schoellw@uni-mainz.de

W. I. Schöllhorn, A. Slapšinskaitė-Dackevičienė (eds.), *Differential Learning in Physiotherapy*,
https://doi.org/10.1007/978-3-031-98787-8_1

1.2 Deconstructing the Assumption of an Ideal, Person-, and Time-Independent Movement Technique

1.2.1 Weak Individuality

The challenge of this assumption is to deconstruct (Derrida 2021) the "independent" aspect and to show the dependency of movements on individuality and on time. Related to individuality, two types can be distinguished, a weak and a strong one (Burdack et al. 2023). While the weak individuality is associated with its usage in everyday language, the strong individuality goes along with forensic criteria.

Rather, in the sense of everyday language, individual aspects of movement have long been discussed and supported by predominantly anecdotal evidence. For example, in a visual perception experiment in psychology, test subjects were able to recognize their friends from a selection of videos of six test subjects by their gait (Cutting and Kozlowski 1977). In sport science, movement individuality has long been used to describe unexplained deviations from a general trend or averaged values. Sometimes the term individuality was also used in the context of a false inference if no regularities could be observed in groups or if these were too heterogeneous (in downhill skiing (Brüggemann et al. 1992); in rowing (Körndle and Lippens 1988); in basketball (Button et al. 2000); and in running (Stergiou et al. 2001)). If there are theoretically, e.g., six different curves of the same parameter from six different subjects, the grouping of the results depends mainly on the resolution of the measurement and less on the individuality of the subject who was measured. The main problem is that the lack of a (usually linear) group characteristic leads directly to conclusions about the individuality of a movement. In a positive sense, this approach could be seen as an attempt to draw attention to the individuality of movements. However, if one considers the duration of this approach and the lack of consequences, the impression is reinforced that individuality was only lip service to maintain the prevailing group- and mean-value-oriented philosophy in science.

Initial attempts to assess a possible individuality of gait movements quantitatively were achieved by comparing intra- to inter-individual variations (Pedotti 1977; Winter 1984). For this purpose, several gait cycles of several persons are analyzed biomechanically, and then the variation of a series of selected gait parameters of a single person is compared with the variations between the persons. If the variation of the parameters within a person was smaller than the variation between the persons, then this was an indication of individuality. However, this remains a weak indicator, as variance distributions can still overlap. This means that some of an individual's movements may be more similar to those of another person than to their own average. In classical statistics, this corresponds to the alpha error. To maintain the usual mean-oriented approach, the average curve was given a tolerance zone of one standard deviation, and deviations within this zone were tolerated for diagnoses that did not require treatment. Later we will see that this zone of variance, at least in ground reaction forces during gait, is meanwhile further broken down into individual- and situation-specific zones of fatigue or emotions (Burdack et al. 2020; Janssen et al. 2008), suggesting the use of the term noise mainly as a term for the limits of understanding.

The importance of individuality in therapy and movement research was additionally supported by the demand for individual case analysis. Although individual case analysis had been used in psychotherapy since Ebbinghaus (1913), it was not until the 1960–1980s, with the foundational works of Huber (1977) and Barlow and Hersen (1984), that it experienced a revival. It was only in the 1990s that it received more extensive attention in research studies. Nevertheless, single-case observations, in which a wide variety of processes are described exclusively, are often confused with single-case studies, in which a question is systematically investigated according to a precise design (Backman et al. 1997; Barker et al. 2011; Morgan and Morgan 2008; Yang et al. 2023; Yin 1984). In contrast to multilevel analysis, in which several single-case studies are summarized within the framework of a multilevel meta-analysis, individual cases and individual case studies do not claim to provide generalized findings.

In a similar way, individuality of movements was used by Bernstein (1967), Latash (2021) in the context of the degrees of freedom problem ("... *the motor behavior of each individual will be different*") and Newell (1986) within the coordinative structure model ("...*as a consequence the optimal pattern of coordination and control for a given task will be individual specific. Sometimes, however, individuals interpret the imposed constraints differently*") (Kugler et al. 1980). In both cases, the individuality of movements was set and theoretically justified by differences and changes in anatomy during maturation based on various growth curves. While Bernstein only recognized the individuality of movements at a later stage of the learning process (Bernstein 1967; Latash 2021), Newell (1986) linked the individuality of movements with anthropometric changes and the resulting changes in biomechanical control during growth and later with the finding of optimal movement patterns through not further specified self-organization. Magill (1983), following Lewin (1935), considered the individual, environment, and task as context variables for movement or behavior and avoided the problem of the driver for the solution, whereas Kugler et al. (1980) and Newell (1986) clearly shifted, at least theoretically, the relationship from externally prescribed solutions to the idea of self-organizing ones and thus gave more responsibility to the self of the learning system (Lewis and Granic 1999). Thus, the upcoming term self-organization, introduced by Ashby (1947) and von Foerster (1960) in physics, was used in the context of an abstract and not further specified interaction between an organism, the environment, and the task. However, guiding the learner to an optimal movement solution through constraining conditions corresponds to a more than generous interpretation of self-organization, as it provides the learner with concrete information about the solution and ultimately only enables him to find an individual style of an externally determined movement technique. This interpretation of the term self-organization is used most often in the social sciences and limits self-organization to the spontaneous emergence of order that is understood as one condition for emergence and neglects the original boundary conditions for self-organization. In contrast to this simple description of a phenomenon, self-organization from a system-dynamics or physics point of view does not provide any concrete information about the solution but presupposes the supply of diffuse energy (Ashby 1947; Haken 1988; Prigogine and Nicolis 1971; von Foerster 1960). This was also a basis for distinguishing order and control parameters, as we will see in the chapter on system-dynamics (see Sect. 2.1). Guided self-organization has recently been proposed as a model for combining targeted control and self-organization (Ammar et al. 2024a; Ay et al. 2012; Prokopenko 2013), which is very similar to the model of muscle control in the context of motor control (Loeb 1995; Wagner and Blickhan 1999, 2003), as integrated from the beginning by the DL approach (Schöllhorn 1999). Self-stabilizing muscle properties do not require all parameters to be controlled from top-down, but it is sufficient if the muscle is brought into a certain zone from where it then stabilizes itself.

In summary, no concrete and new practical consequences for motor learning processes were derived in the articles of Kugler, Newell or Bernstein, despite the individuality set. The definition of the motor learning process as a kind of search strategy "*for learning the dynamic laws that control exploratory behavior*" (Newell et al. 1989) of the learner corresponds to the exploratory approach suggested earlier in sports pedagogy. Nonetheless, this approach emphasized the role of the learner and was in complete contrast to the prevailing idea of prescriptive, teacher-centered learning approaches in sports but lacked concrete practical deductions and neglected proposed solutions that had already come from sports pedagogy (Mosston 1966; Nichols 1994; Rovegno et al. 2001).

From an epistemological perspective, the individuality of movement and movement learning cannot be proven using these approaches. Instead, it is defined and set as a starting assumption. In addition, with these approaches, it is not possible to falsify a general model that is independent of individuals and time. Nevertheless, the theoretical discussions of these models contributed to advancing our understanding of the process of motor learning and adaptation.

1.2.2 Strong Individuality

From Metrics to Topology: From Time-Discrete to Time-Continuous Analysis
In contrast to the more colloquial understanding of individuality, forensics, as the application of science for crime, sets stricter criteria for individuality. Forensics demands a model for strong individuality in which the available material must stand up to legal scrutiny. This model now forms the basis of all machine learning (ML) approaches that deal with pattern recognition in the context of person identification based on biometric data (e.g., signature, fingerprint, footprint, ear shape, iris diagnosis, gait, etc.). This requires two criteria to be met: (1) uniqueness and (2) reliability. While the first expects a very low probability of finding a second identical carrier of the characteristics, the second ensures that the same characteristics of the same carrier are found at different points in time.

Both criteria are closely linked and highly dependent on the type of data analysis they are based on, whether it involves time-discrete or time-continuous process-oriented analysis (Schöllhorn et al. 2002a, b; Burdack et al. 2020). The difference can best be described by the situation where we see a person we know standing at a great distance, and the resolution of our eyes does not allow us to recognize the person. However, as soon as the person starts walking, we recognize the person by their gait characteristics. The first corresponds to time-discrete analysis, the second to time-continuous analysis. Since both types are used in physiotherapeutic diagnostics, they will be discussed briefly here.

For methodological reasons, movement analyses up until the 1980s were largely limited to the analysis of time-discrete parameters, such as minimum knee joint angle, ankle joint angle at the time of foot strike or takeoff, mean vertical force during a ground contact, etc. With time-discrete data, the analysis of learning and development was mainly restricted to changes in the metrics of a movement (e.g., stride length, gait velocity, etc.) and thus limited to the analysis of changes within a single topology (e.g., walking). The differentiation of a movement into its topology and metrics is particularly important because it guided the development of movement research in one direction for a long time. One effect was that the main focus was concentrated on research objects for which the possibility of quantification was available. By focusing on the metrics of a movement, research questions relating to different topologies, such as various classes of movements (e.g., running, jumping, throwing), modes of movements (e.g., springy or creepy running), and movement styles (e.g., individual expressions of the previous classes and modes) (Schöllhorn 1996, 1997a) were largely excluded. Accordingly, only fluctuations or variance in the metrics of single movement topologies were measured and analyzed. Interestingly, these topologies were considered unquantifiable by Bernstein and have thus misled generations of researchers (Bernstein 1967).

The decomposition of movement into metrics and topology goes back to the research of movement gestalts in the context of Gestalt psychology (Kern 1933; Lewin 1935; Voigt 1933). Topology, as the study of the position and arrangement of geometric shapes whose properties are preserved in the case of continuous deformations, was seen as a way of approaching the problem of movement shapes in the Gestalt-psychological sense of part and whole. From a psychological point of view, the sensations experienced when walking or manually following predetermined shapes, such as a sine curve or a zigzag line, were of central interest (Kern 1933; Voigt 1933). Figure 1.1 shows examples of different metrics and topologies for the visual area as well as their motor equivalents and their effects on the movement description. In the visual domain, the initial value of a joint variable cor-

Fig. 1.1 Systemic analogies of metrics (e.g., place, size) and Gestalt/topology in the visual and movement domain

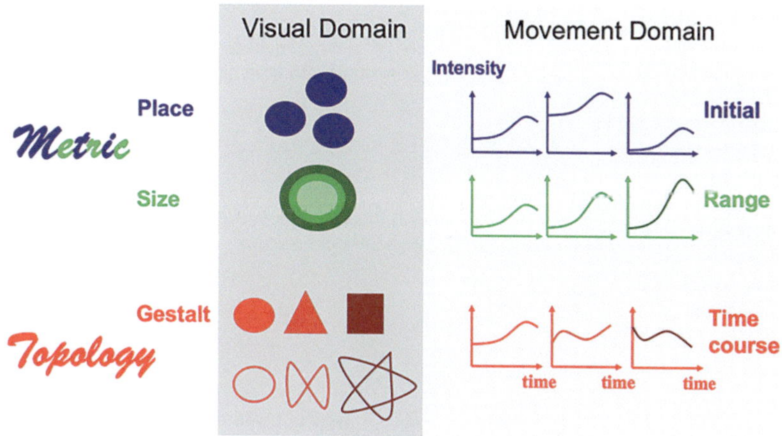

responds to the object location (top, bottom, left, right), the feature size corresponds to the object size (large, small), and the feature time-course corresponds to the object shape (i.e., circle, rectangle, triangle). In the metric, a shift in location in the visual domain would correspond to a change in the initial angle of a joint within the given range of motion, e.g., normal walking and walking with bent knee(s). A change in the object size in the visual area would correspond to an increase in the amplitude of a movement feature in the range of motion; for example, normal walking and walking with longer steps would lead to a larger amplitude of the hip angle. A change in the form or topology of the movement would, e.g., correspond to a change from running to jumping. While in the mathematical subject of geometry an additional distinction is made between the form and topology of an object, in the field of movement research both were summarized by Bernstein (1935, 1967) under the term movement topology, whereas Schmidt (1975) described them as invariants with constancy of form. Regardless of the designation, both were understood as qualities of movement that largely eluded quantification.

Later, we will discuss the same phenomenon in the development of motor learning approaches, where it is shown that both the variability-of-practice approach (Schmidt 1975) and the "*repetition without repetition*" (Bernstein 1967) exclusively referred to the topology of a single movement technique. The restriction to a single topology not only limited biomechanical studies to the investigation of single movement topologies but was also very sensitive to the filtering of the data (Schöllhorn 1996, 1997b). By applying the appropriate filter (strength), it was possible to influence the results accordingly, often filtering out individuality (Fink et al. 1998, 1999). This filtering technique proved valuable in identifying general and group-specific tendencies in the metrics of a single specific movement, such as amplitude or duration. But the quantification of a qualitative change in this movement that corresponds to the change of movement topology was hardly possible. This type of change is, however, typically associated with changes in coordination, as is common in motor learning during rehabilitation with qualitative changes (Fig. 1.2). Changing from walking with a stiff knee to walking with normally bent knees is a classical example of this kind of change. While, for example, in the two upper curves in Fig. 1.2, each time-discrete value finds some correspondence, this becomes problematic when changing from the second to the third curve in Fig. 1.2. With the process-oriented analysis of biomechanical data, this became possible (Schöllhorn 1993b, c, 1995, 1996). This approach focuses more on the comparison of the curve shapes than on the time-discrete amplitudes or initial values and therefore not only became a fruitful complement to the time-discrete approach but also opened the door for quantitative analyses of movement topologies (Schöllhorn 1997a).

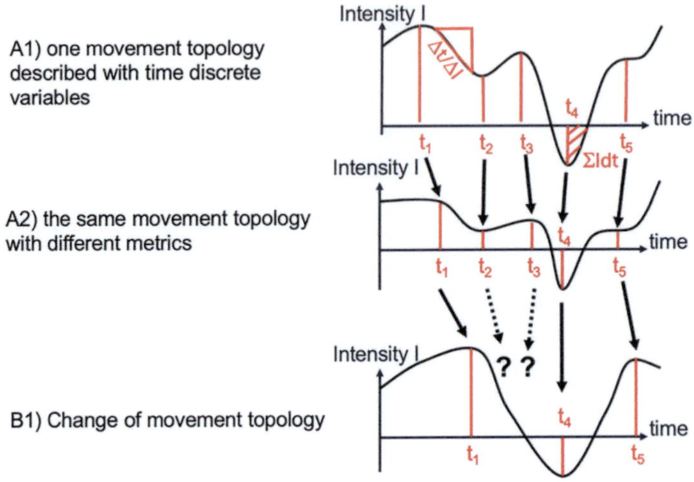

Fig. 1.2 Metric (A1–A2) and topological (B1) changes. Metric changes from A1 to A2 can be described utilizing time-discrete parameters. Topological changes from A to B are described with process-oriented parameters

A renewed proposal to use topology as a framework for describing motion was put forward by McGinnis and Newell (1982) but was not pursued further. Qualitative changes in handwriting or different walking and running speeds were sporadically described by means of changes in correlation coefficients between single joint angle time-courses (Newell 1989; Newell et al. 1989) or chain encoding models (Whiting and Zernicke 1982). However, in all cases, the analysis and diagnosis were limited to single modes or classes of movements and separated from each other. They were not connected to the system dynamics approach and its fluctuations during the phase transitions from one stable movement topology to another (Schöner et al. 1986) and were not further pursued because of the high sensitivity of the result to the sampling rate of the curves.

The first nonlinear machine learning approaches in the area of movement science were applied in high-performance sport in the 1990s, when training was also guided classically by general person- and time-independent models. By means of a Self-organizing map (Kohonen 1982), several biomechanically described trials of two world-class discus throwers within a training intervention project could be differentiated disjunctively (Bauer and Schöllhorn 1997). In these exploratory two single case studies, there was neither a pre-classification nor was the network monitored. The network simply separated the two subjects based on the similarity of the characteristics of 40 variable time-courses. Surprisingly, a successful learning intervention was also identified for one athlete by disjunctively separating the trials before and after the intervention. In the other athlete's trial series, the intervention was not successful in terms of increasing throwing distance, but the trials could be separated by training and competition sessions. Both findings already provided quantitative evidence for a dominance of individuality over a fine structure of situated variation. Interestingly, despite the repetitive and model-oriented training, the athletes developed a technique that was characteristic only of themselves. The development of an individual interpretation of a technique (despite model orientation and repetition) is therefore not a new phenomenon. It must be distinguished from self-organized learning in the scientific sense, where only diffuse energy is introduced into a system from outside, allowing it to find its own order (Polani et al. 2013). However, despite the high number of trials (reliability), the number of test subjects was too small to satisfy the forensic criterion of uniqueness. Nonetheless, assigning all trials to the right person satisfied the criteria of reliability and provided stronger evidence for the individuality of movement.

The quantification of movement topologies could also address a problem nearly as old as movement research itself (Woodworth and Thorndike 1901). This problem relates to the core research objective of specificity versus generality, which involves determining how much of a training or auxiliary exercise can be beneficially transferred to a target exercise.[1] In consequence, this also accompanies various motor learning models. While the variability-of-practice (VP) model (Schmidt 1975), for example, circumvents the problem of topologies by focusing on a single one (invariants) and only allows it to be stretched and compressed in terms of time and scope (variable parameters), the contextual interference (CI) learning model, or interleaved practice model, fosters the parallel learning of several movement forms in random sequence (Magill and Hall 1990) but completely neglects their relative similarity (Schöllhorn 2016). The VP and CI learning models will be discussed in more detail in the chapter on first-order cybernetic models (see Sect. 2.1).

The neglect of the relative similarity is somewhat astonishing because various studies had already shown reciprocal influences in the context of learning processes, mostly in the context of paradigms on pro- and re(tro)-active inhibition and facilitation (Meyer and Bucci 2016). Most importantly for therapy and training, if two exercises are too similar, mutual inhibition can occur, and if there is too little similarity, transfer can be negligible (Baldwin and Ford 1988; Nelson 1957). The same counts for the sequence of the exercises (Nelson 1957). Training A (e.g., tennis volley) before B (e.g., badminton volley) leads to other results than vice versa. Due to methodical reasons supported by problematic statements of recognized researchers (Bernstein 1967), the qualitative visual impression of the movements served as the basis for the similarity of different movement topologies for a long time. Single attempts by means of chain encoding for quantitative description of limb trajectories were not pursued further because they were either not sufficiently sensitive with regard to time scales (Whiting and Zernicke 1982) or were only very rough approximations at normative scale level within a single sport (e.g., tennis), which were also based on subjective visual assessments (Buszard et al. 2017). A deeper elaboration of this issue can be found under the topic of "*specificity and generality*" and in the context of "*similarity of exercise and transfer*" (Liu 1993; Osgood 1949; Proteau et al. 1992).

In contrast, the proposed process-oriented pattern recognition approach offered a more holistic (time- and variable-wise) and, in parallel, a more nuanced quantitative analysis by looking at all variable time-courses together and partitioning the patterns either by variables (e.g., anatomical) or by time or both.

Combining the partitioning by variables with the neurophysiological correlates of biomechanical variables (i.e., angles, angular velocities, angular acceleration, angular momentums, and forces) (Schöllhorn 1998) built the basis for the exemplary quantitative comparison of conditional sprint exercises with the sprint movement during the ground contact phase (see also the chapter on neuronal basis). Based on kinematic and dynamic time-course characteristics of the lower extremities, drop jumps, one-legged jumps, and hurdle jumps showed joint-specific differentiated similarities with the target movement (Liu 1993). While the limb movements showed reasonable similarity on the geometric level (joint angle time-courses), on the dynamic level (the angular momentums, eccentric and concentric forces), they were substantially different. These results directly raise the fundamental question of movement similarity and transferability: which type of similarity, and at what level of observation, has the greatest impact on transfer?

An application of the process-oriented pattern recognition approach to four different ski turning techniques (Schöllhorn et al. 2001a) and to three offense techniques in volleyball (Schöllhorn et al. 2001b) demonstrated its applicability for the quantification and classification of different movement topologies as well. In these cases, the techniques dominated. This was to be expected given the large effects of the different techniques

[1]Here, we focus on technical skill transfer. For an overview of the transfer problem related to other motor skills like strength, endurance, etc., see Issurin, V. B. (2013). Training Transfer: Scientific Background and Insights for Practical Application. *Sports Medicine*, *43*(8), 675–694. https://doi.org/10.1007/s40279-013-0049-6 2013

on the biomechanical signals that served as the basis for the recognition process.

Another study approached the problem of topological similarities in the context of sprint skills (Lippold et al. 2003). The study investigated the structural relationship between classical sprint drills (Sprint-ABC) and alternative sprint coordination exercises based on the theory of Differential Learning (Schöllhorn 1995), relying on biomechanical variable time-courses and by means of Artificial Neural Nets. The results showed that classical **sprint** drills lack structural similarity to the target skill (maximal sprint), whereas the DL-based exercises show greater proximity to sprint execution and a broader coverage of the motor solution space.

Instead of spatially bound dynamic and kinematic measuring devices, extensive research is now being carried out to transfer the methods and findings to data acquisition with wearable sensors (e.g., in mobile phones or clothes) to make them available more quickly and to use them for feedback interventions. One focus here is on the optimal number and placement of sensors (Hribernik et al. 2022). However, the parallel rapid development of shape-based pattern recognition is impressive due to its performance with its feedback-free video technology and without the preparation of the observed object.

1.2.2.1 Strong Evidence for Individuality by Using a Different Statistic

To give an idea of the scale of probabilities involved in the pattern recognition approach, we calculate the probability of correctly identifying all trials of one athlete from a set of trials conducted by multiple individuals as an example. This is just for reasons of comparison with the classic 5% threshold of the Fisher (Fisher and Russell 1922) and Neyman-Pearson (Neyman et al. 1933) statistic as the basis of the classic significance and effect size calculation and also suggesting an alternative approach (see also (Hopkins et al. 2009) and (Gigerenzer 2004)).

The statistics for pattern recognition were applied in a study that involved 8 trials of a discus specialist and 45 trials of a decathlete, both with very similar age, training experience, and anthropometry related to body height, body weight, arm span, width, etc. (Bauer and Schöllhorn 1997). Calculating the probability of randomly separating both athletes corresponds to a bowl filled with 8 red and 45 blue balls, with all 8 red balls drawn in a row. Drawing the first red ball has a probability of 8/53, the second red ball is 7/52, the third red ball is 6/51, and so on. This can also be calculated with the binomial coefficient $\binom{n}{k}$, where $n = 53$ and $k = 8$, and results in 886,322,710, which means the probability to separate all trials in the found way is 1/886,322,710, which is approximately 0.00000000113. Consequently, a high probability of two distinct individualities can be assumed here.

A similarly low probability was found in another study with a larger number of included subjects and selectively recorded over a time span of up to 4 years (Schöllhorn and Bauer 1998b). Thus, from 8 world-class male and 29 female javelin throwers, 51 kinematically described movements during the final throwing phase were analyzed, whereby eight throws by one female athlete were performed in competitions spread over 4 years, and six throws by another female athlete were performed over 3 years. Both athletes could be identified with 100% based on the kinematic time-course data of 250 ms of their throwing movement. Identifying eight throws of one athlete out of 51 recorded trials leads to a similar low probability of 1/636,763,050, which equals 0.00000000157. The identification of individual javelin throwers over a time span of 3 and 4 years based on 250 ms of a movement, despite performance (thrown distance) improvements, gave the first strong indication of the stability of individual movement patterns over time.

Meanwhile, the individuality of movements became further supported by studies on other whole-body movements like running (Hoitz et al. 2021; Horst et al. 2023; Jaitner et al. 2001b; Schöllhorn and Bauer 1997), shot put, discus, and javelin throwing (Horst et al. 2020; Schöllhorn and Bauer 1998b; Schöllhorn et al. 2014a, b), or karate kicking (Burdack et al. 2020). Most interestingly, apart from this exact athlete identification, none of the throws or running steps were identical, indicating a negligible probability of identical repetitions. Nonetheless, all variants were within the individuals' movement characteristics. In addition, the individuality of the movements could only be recognized if at least three kinematic variable time-courses were included in the pattern recognition. With fewer than three variables, no plausible order could be found (Fink et al. 1998; Jaitner et al. 2001b). This indicates a close connection between a more holistic view and the individuality of movement patterns. Individuality arises when several variables are taken into account.

As it was suspected at the time that the athletes may not have had enough repetitions to produce identical movements, similar studies were conducted in human gait, e.g., in young adults, where we could assume a corresponding higher number of repeated strides in their preferred style (Horst et al. 2016, 2017a; Janssen et al. 2008; Schöllhorn et al. 1999, 2002a). The same could be shown in professional musicians who practiced playing the flute for more than 30 years, up to 10 h a day (Albrecht et al. 2014). The results not only supported previous findings on intra- and inter-subject variability found in previous studies (Bates 1996; Devita and Skelly 1990; Winter 1984) but, due to the new process-oriented approach applied in parallel to multiple variables, also added corroboration to the hypothesis of strong individuality in everyday movements and movement executions during therapy.

In the meantime, the gait analyses have not only been carried out on samples with more test subjects per study to validate the criterion of uniqueness (Horst et al. 2021), but also for a period of up to 1 year (Horst et al. 2017b). All studies confirm the dominant role of individuality in walking movements regarding the two criteria of uniqueness and reliability. Most of the studies were based on the three-dimensional ground reaction forces generated during ground contact. A similar pattern was found when using kinematic (Jaitner et al. 2001b; Janssen et al. 2008, 2011; Schöllhorn and Bauer 1997, 1998a), in-shoe-pressure distribution (Schöllhorn et al. 2002b), or EMG data (Aeles et al. 2021; Jaitner et al. 1999, 2001a). If the individuality of movements is not only evident in sport but also in everyday movements such as walking, then we can also assume a high degree of individuality in the process of physiotherapy right from the start.

1.2.2.2 Individuality from the Beginning or Only at the End?

The data so far could give the impression that individuality can only be shown in movements that are associated with many repetitions, that is, that only develop at an advanced stage, but that the original assumption of person- and time-independent models should be retained beforehand to create a basis. To investigate this question, we analyzed the movement of beginners in weightlifting in a recent study and, at the same time, wanted to know to what extent this movement can be influenced by different learning approaches (Ammar et al. 2024b). To this end, all participants had to randomly perform a different exercise sequence with the barbell in the style of four different learning approaches at intervals of 1 week. After each exercise series, three weightlifting movements with the barbell were recorded without any instructions, and all curves were subjected to a pattern recognition procedure. The results showed relatively stable individual trajectories of the barbell with recognition rates of up to 80%, regardless of the exercise sequence performed beforehand. This result can also be interpreted as a strong indication of the individuality of movements, even in beginners, given that a prescribed movement was recognized solely based on the barbell trajectory and the ground reaction forces.

However, caution is now required when jumping to conclusions about individual learning behavior based on individual movement patterns. If we have individual movement patterns at the beginning and end of a learning process, this can still result from two different learning behaviors. If we assume that the movement patterns are individual at the beginning of a learning process and that everyone reacts to an intervention to the same extent, then the movement patterns would also be individual at the end of the learning process. Mathematically, this would correspond to an isomorphism. However, individual movement patterns can also result if everyone reacts differently to the same intervention. This can also lead to a violation of neighborhood conservation; that is, movement patterns that are close to each other at the beginning of the learning process no longer remain close to each other at the end of the learning process. Here, too, intervention studies provide initial indications, which will be discussed in the next chapter.

In sum, extensive studies highlight the individuality of movements, challenging the first of the two assumptions for successful physiotherapy. As a result, these findings diminish the likelihood of person- and time-independent models, which have traditionally been the focus of therapeutic approaches. Moreover, from a therapeutic and training science perspective, these findings raise numerous challenging questions, calling into question long-held assumptions and persistent conventional approaches.

Two pragmatic questions emerge from these findings: first, is it possible to train a patient or athlete to move beyond their own unique movement patterns? For instance, in security contexts, this raises the question of how effectively one can imitate the movements of others. This inquiry is closely tied to a second underlying assumption that challenges the role of repetition in training. Second, is it really necessary to alter a patient's or athlete's movement patterns to deviate from their individual characteristics? Both questions probe the amplitude required to achieve sustainable results and whether there exists a threshold where learning may be impeded by fear.

1.3 Deconstructing the Assumption of Repetition as the Ultimate Method

Having discussed the fundamental problems with the first traditional assumption for successful physiotherapy, let's look in more detail at the second assumption of achieving such a target through repetition.

1.3.1 Learning by Repetition: The Roots

A stroboscopic look at the history of repetition learning points to a close connection with obedience training in a military context. This close link was observed not only in ancient times but also in the context of sports until the end of the twentieth century. It was evident in the Western Hemisphere, including countries such as the UK, Portugal, Spain, and many Asian nations, due to the longstanding influence of the military and politics (Chapman et al. 2024). Historically, learning through repetition can be traced back at least to Plato (Böhm 2004), who saw repetition and contrast learning as the only means of learning, e.g., memorizing poetry. A similar influence in the same direction and more related to movement learning came from the military education in Sparta for preparing warriors. While Plato did not limit repetition learning to certain age groups, the second was mainly related to adult education (andragogy). A completely different reference to learning comes in the context of the education of children, where a pedagogue was to be distinguished from a teacher at school. Pedagogues (ἄγω(ágō), "*lead,*" and παῖς (país, genitive παιδός, paidos) "*boy, child*") in ancient Greece were slaves who were of no use for anything else and had to ensure that the sons of wealthy families (at that time, only boys were allowed) went to school safely. In school, the boys were playing, discussing with, and listening to the teachers, which is reflected in the Greek origin of school. School derives from Greek σχολή (scholē) (Greek), which meant "*leisure*" or "*that in which leisure is employed.*" According to the current state of research, we can therefore assume that the basic factors of effective learning were already known at that time and that, at least the education of children, in the modern understanding of pedagogy, was anything but linear. The teaching of children in its origins was always nonlinear. The ideals of the ancient Greeks also had a decisive influence on the education of warriors in ancient Rome, which is reflected in the quote "*Repetitio est mater studiorum*" (Repetition is the mother of studies) by the Roman poet

Horaz. In the Roman military, marching in groups and forming a turtle for defense took on even more importance and became an instrument of power and obedience. Marching with a uniform step length may be of advantage for military purposes, but it means that the tall ones have to step short at the front and the short ones long at the back, and only the middle ranks march at their optimum step length (Holt et al. 1991, 1995). The extent to which this leads to the development of an individually optimal or economic movement is doubtful.

In contrast, the original ideas of the Greek scholè experienced a renaissance with the Age of Enlightenment and the reform pedagogy movement with Rousseau's novel "Emile: On Education" in 1762 (Rousseau 1762). Despite the widespread and prevailing assumption at the time of the new born as blank slates without any ethics (Locke 1690), which had to be described by teachers and parents, ideas from Rousseau found relatively quick resonance in learner-centered teaching, in which physical activities played a major role (Basedow 1774; Pestalozzi 1781–1787). The focus shifted to developing one's own skills. These ideas also laid the groundwork for the introduction of the kindergarten system by Fröbel in 1826 (Froebel 1826), who recognized that an enriched environment is essential for healthy development. This concept later contributed to the re-establishment of Plato's labor schools (Dewey 1903; Kerschensteiner 1912), where discovery-based learning became a core element, as seen in Montessori and Steiner schools (Montessori 1909; Steiner 1907). More recently, experiential learning has been popularized by Kolb (1984), Metallidou, and Platsidou (2008).

While the traditional teaching mainly adopted methods from andragogy and military education, which were later additionally supported by the conditioning experiments with animals in the context of behaviorism that were completely under the control of the experimenter, the reform pedagogy clearly focused on a learner-centered education. This had been adopted in sports by the methodical series of exercises approach (Gaulhofer and Streicher 1924), first in gymnastics to allow the learner to begin with exercise according to their level of performance, and was later transferred to game-based teaching after the Second World War (Mahlo 1965; Mester 1959) to provide a more holistic approach for teaching games as an alternative to the prevailing technique-oriented approach of teaching games.

Repetition-based learning, as originated in andragogy, and the likewise repetition-based, behaviorist conditioning experiments with animals, also formed a basis for the search for neuronal mechanisms of learning. Animals were conditioned through numerous repetitions to certain behaviors, and then the changes in the neuronal connections were analyzed. Frequently, this is reversed in a kind of naturalistic fallacy, in which normative statements (repetition is necessary for learning) are legitimized by descriptive ones (neuronal effectivity after repetition improves), and it is claimed that many repetitions are needed to modify the neuronal system correspondingly, however, without having tested any alternative. Spontaneous learning, as occurs when touching a hot stove or learning to ride a bicycle or to swim, was largely excluded from the experiments due to methodological problems associated with replication criteria. A similar methodical problem arises when a single event, like a world record in sport, is to be proven with the help of inferential statistics.

Furthermore, this also resulted in the at-first-glance tempting ideas of learning through the repetition of simultaneous presentation of conditioned and unconditioned stimuli (see Pavlov's experiment on saliva production in dogs). A closer look reveals a much more differentiated picture. Rather unknown is the great dependence of the learning effects in these conditioning experiments on the exact relative timing of the conditioned (CS) and unconditioned (UCS) stimuli. Only if the UCS is offered quite a precise short time after the CS will the UCS be conditioned (Fig. 1.3). If the time delay between both is too long, the effect is weakened and can disappear; if the UCS is offered shortly before the CS, conditioning can even be blocked for the future (Domjan 2003). This high sensitivity of the conditioning process to the time difference between

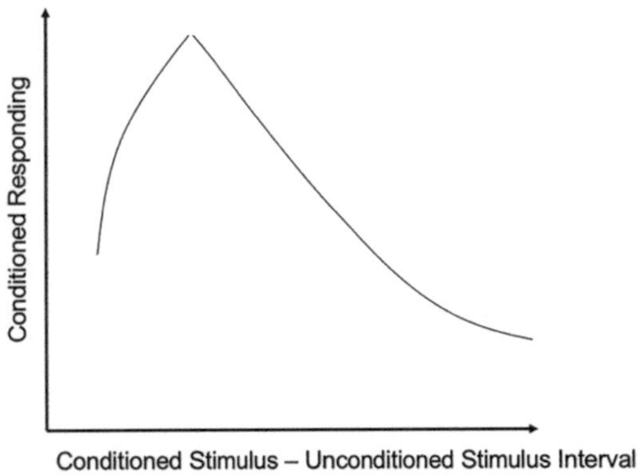

Fig. 1.3 Idealized curve of traditional effects of the CS-US interval on the vigor of Pavlovian conditioned responding. (Modified after (Domjan 2003))

CS and UCS makes its application in real learning processes very critical, especially in repetitive learning.

A similar situation is found on the neuronal counterpart that is associated with Hebb's abbreviated learning rule, "*Neurons wire together if they fire together*" (Hebb 1949; Löwel and Singer 1992). Originally Hebb stated that "*… when an axon of cell A is near enough to excite a cell B and repeatedly or persistently takes part in firing it, some growth process or metabolic change takes place in one or both cells such that A's efficiency, as one of the cells firing B, is increased*" (Hebb 1949). In the search for the neuronal mechanisms, von der Malsburg (1981) suggested the "correlation theory of brain function" for sensory integration. Due to the dependence of the firing rate on amplitude, frequency, and phase (Singer 1993), as well as different threshold values of the neurons, this also turns out to be far more complicated than assumed initially and is still known as the unsolved "binding problem" (Caporale and Dan 2008). For example, presynaptic afferents are enhanced by high-frequency stimulation (HFS) on the one hand and by the simultaneous occurrence of low-frequency stimulation (LFS) paired with large postsynaptic depolarization (long-term potentiation (LTP)) on the other. In contrast, long-term depression is triggered by LFS, either alone or paired with a small postsynaptic depolarization (Caporale and Dan 2008). In consequence, the investigation of the temporal dependence of LTP and LTD revealed a similar sensitivity to conditioning: LTP was generated when the weak input preceded the strong input by less than 20 ms, and reversing the order led to LTD (Levy and Steward 1983). More recent studies have described the critical window on the order of tens of milliseconds (Bi and Poo 1998; Debanne et al. 1998; Magee and Johnston 1997). Evidence for this effect on the wiring of neurons at further distances is still pending. In addition, this model is mapping only events that are happening in parallel (e.g., visual perception of objects); movements of different joints are only partially parallel; many elements of complex movements are both parallel and sequential and therefore have never been the object of this model's suggestion. Although the events may occur sequentially in the periphery or proximally and distally, they may arrive there in parallel due to the different signaling distances to the cortical structures. For example, if a foot is stimulated first and shortly afterwards a hand is stimulated, both stimuli can still reach the brain simultaneously, assuming the same conduction velocity of the neurons, due to the different distance to the brain. The same applies in the other direction. For this reason, purely sequential tasks such as typing, speaking, or writing must be distinguished from others, which are usually described as parallel. Nonetheless, drawing pedagogical conclusions from these unresolved issues still appears to be premature.

1.3.2 No New Practical Consequences Despite Ancient Knowledge About Trial-to-Trial Variation

Against the background of the pedagogical and historical assumptions, repetition learning is traditionally associated with the creation of "neuronal highways" through as many repetitions as possible. This should allow the movements to be carried out relatively automatically and reliably in a wide variety of situations in the future; that is, they can be reproduced with a high probability. Philosophical wisdom from the Greek Heraclitus, such as "*You never step into the same river twice,*" or from the Chinese Lao Tze, "*The only constant is variation,*" and the more recent quote, specifically related to movements, "*Repetition without repetition*" (Bernstein 1935, 1967), were often quoted in sport psychology until the beginning of the twenty-first century without linking their implications for any practical consequences on movement learning. Mainly, those quotes were used for excuses, in case of deviations from the expected behavior. Recently, Bernstein's quote has been experiencing a rediscovery and reinterpretation in some new master theories (Renshaw and Chow 2019) based on findings that will be discussed in a later chapter. This very far-fetched reinterpretation again verifies the misjudgment of the long-standing problem of the restriction to the variation of the movement metric and neglect of the variation of the movement topology. Such reinterpretations primarily serve to distract from the actual origin of the change in understanding, which is linked to the adoption of central ideas of DL since the beginning of the century.

In motor research, the problem of non-repeatability was treated very generally and linked to the novelty problem, which went hand in hand with the question of the origin of the numerous motor programs (Schmidt 1975). The accompanying question was, if every movement is different, where do the constantly new programs come from? Furthermore, the fact that every movement repetition showed small deviations was not compatible with a one-to-one storage of motor programs due to capacity reasons of the CNS. Within the framework of schema theory (Schmidt 1975), these long-observed variances in the metrics of a movement were assigned as variable parameters (e.g., absolute forces, absolute duration, range of movement, etc.), which in the variability-of-practice model should serve to stabilize single and already automized, generalized motor programs (GMPs) that were operationalized in the form of invariants through their blocked variation. These invariants or topologies summarize groups of movements with the same relative timing and the same relative forces.[2]

Contrary to many statements, with the schema model, the novelty problem was merely minimally reduced but not solved, as an infinitely large number divided by an integer number (of GMPs) still remains an infinitely large number (Schöllhorn 2016). While Bernstein (1935, 1967) considered the quantification of movement topologies to be impossible in principle, Schmidt (1975) defined them by different generalized motor programs (GMPs) that had to be acquired or stabilized separately. However, both Schmidt and Bernstein saw the repetition of the same topology as the basis for successful learning, Schmidt explicitly with the repetition of the invariants, Bernstein implicitly through his studies of selected movement forms within the same topology (e.g., the hammer blow). While Schmidt's model suggested at least the intentional variation of the metrics for stabilizing a movement, Bernstein and coworkers did not indicate any new learning approach. Bernstein's "*repetition without repetition*" therefore referred exclusively to the variance of metrics and actually repeated a subset of Heraclitus' quote. Nonetheless, Bernstein acknowledged the importance of understanding the role of movement topologies. Until the end of the twentieth century, variation in topology as an active intervention was therefore no subject of research in sport psychology, even though it was used in the practice of sports pedagogy, physical education, and physiotherapy to teach the acquisition of more complex forms of movement. Interestingly, already in the 1970s/1980s in Physiotherapy, the balance abilities for falling prevention were

[2]A similar idea could be found beforehand in apparatus gymnastics (Schmidt was a nationally ranked gymnast in college https://senate.universityofcalifornia.edu/_files/inmemoriam/html/RichardAllenSchmidt.html), which in the middle of the last century was worldwide characterized by the gymnastic educational system of the former Eastern Bloc (Borrmann [1956], [1964]). Here, similar gymnastics elements were combined on different gymnastics apparatus as part of a basic training program, e.g., support swing elements on the side horse, parallel bars, floor or hang swing elements on the rings, high bar, or uneven bars, to make the training process more effective.

treated by various tasks and exercises on various surfaces with different softness, most probably unaware of the learning models offered by sport psychology. Newell (1991) raised awareness of these problems in the field of motor development, which were referred to as qualitative changes in movements. Nevertheless, there were rarely, if at all, new consequences in therapy, training, or learning practice derived from scientific findings from Bernstein's "*repetition without repetition*" from 1935 until the end of the twentieth century.

An earlier suggestion in relation to different topologies could have been derived from the contextual interference (CI) learning model (Battig 1979; Shea and Morgan 1979) when the variability-of-practice (VP) model (Schmidt 1975) was included and the different effects of variation within and between generalized motor programs (GMPs) were investigated (Wulf and Lee 1993). In incidental CI learning, the repetitions of a task to be learned were interrupted by additional tasks (Battig 1966, 1979; Shea and Morgan 1979). Despite short-term disadvantages during the acquisition phase with randomized exercise sequences in comparison to blocked exercise sequences, in the long term, it led to advantages in the subsequent learning or memory phase. Thus, all tasks were precisely prescribed, and incorrect or deviating movements had to be repeated to achieve the same number of correct repetitions as the comparison group (Shea and Zimny 1983). Similar to the traditional learning models, the basis was the orientation toward a person- and time-independent model, which had to be achieved through many repetitions and corrections. The information that was induced by the exercise was considered the same for everyone. However, systematic learning effects for CI learning have so far only been shown for movements with a small number of degrees of freedom (sDGF) (Ammar et al. 2023; Barreiros et al. 2007; Brady 2004), whereby the name given to interference effects has so far shown inconsistent findings (Ammar et al. 2024d). In movements with sDGF, the learning effects were greater when the tasks to be learned had different GMPs or topologies. If the movements share the same topology but differ in the metrics, the effects tend to diminish or even vanish (Wulf and Shea 2002). Yet, it is striking that most studies have largely overlooked the critical question of how similar or dissimilar these topologies actually are. This oversight raises serious methodological concerns, suggesting that our understanding of movement transfer may be fundamentally flawed (Apidogo et al. 2023; Schöllhorn 2016).[3]

In addition, the repetition-based therapeutic interventions are, similar to the majority of studies, traditionally relying on studies that are not only based on averages, from which no derivation to a single patient or athlete is possible (Osgood 1949), but also are carrying characteristics that make a transfer to practice even more problematic. Besides statistical problems (Gigerenzer 2004, 2018), in the majority, only models are used where single variables are manipulated in experimental studies to find possible cause-and-effect relationships. Thus, either the external boundary conditions are kept constant to investigate the influence of a single psychological (i.e., emotions, stress, etc.) or physiological (neuronal or metabolism fatigue, etc.) intervention on the learner on the one side, or on the other side, single external boundary conditions are manipulated (i.e., climbing stairs, walking on inclined or declined surfaces, endurance training in various environments, strength training, etc.) to identify specific responses of the individual to these single stimuli. As much as this approach fulfills the criteria of scientific logic,

[3]Without explicit mention, the finger experiment by Haken and coworkers (Haken, H., Kelso, J. A., & Bunz, H. (1985). A theoretical model of phase transitions in human hand movements. *Biol Cybern*, *51*(5), 347–356. https://doi.org/10.1007/bf00336922), with the qualitative changes of the relative phases in cyclic movements with increasing movement frequency or the changes of the relative timing in discrete movements with increasing movement speed, provided latent indications of the behavior of specific topologies (in-phase and anti-phase; the experiment will be discussed in more detail in the system dynamic chapter). Despite the qualitative phase shift in the motor area, in the visual area this corresponds to a rotation of a triangle by 180°, whereby the tip of the triangle is turned downwards. A real qualitative change that would correspond to the shift from a circle to a triangle or to a square would correspond to a shift in curves from sine wave to sawtooth wave or rectangular characteristics.

the simplifications of the models are still too strong compared to reality, in which single variables rarely change without interacting with numerous other variables. The same applies to the handling of the criterion of the reproducibility of measurement results, which is still strongly oriented toward its origins in physics. To satisfy this criterion, an arbitrary threshold value is set, below which the test quality criterion of (retest) reliability is no longer considered to be fulfilled (Abe et al. 2018). For this purpose, even in biomechanics, which is closest to physics in sport sciences, correspondingly large numbers of repetitions are required. In biomechanics, for requested reliability in EMG studies, ten repetitions have been recommended (Gollhofer et al. 1990; Horstmann et al. 1988), and in gait studies, at least eight (Bates et al. 1983a) to ten (Hamill and McNiven 1990) repetitions are demanded for corresponding reliability in kinematic and kinetic data. The fluctuations during these repetitions were considered statistical and measurement errors and interpreted as functional variability. It is suspected that the content of the intervention was often subordinated to the test criterion of reproducibility in the form of repetitions.

1.3.3 Fluctuations Not Only in Movement Metrics But Also in Movement Topology

There has been a long tradition of scientific interest in fluctuations and trial-to-trial changes (Cattell 1957; Henry 1959; Thouless 1936; Woodrow 1932). However, due to methodical limitations, their quantification was restricted to the fluctuations of time-discrete values. Once the process-oriented methodology for identification of single persons based on their movements provided an approach for the quantitative analysis of movement topologies, the next step was to investigate the common behavior of metrics and topology (Fig. 1.4) as well as their mutual dependencies during a learning process of a sport movement in more detail (Schöllhorn 1995, 1996, 1998). For this purpose, discus throws by a specialist and a decathlete, both members of the German national

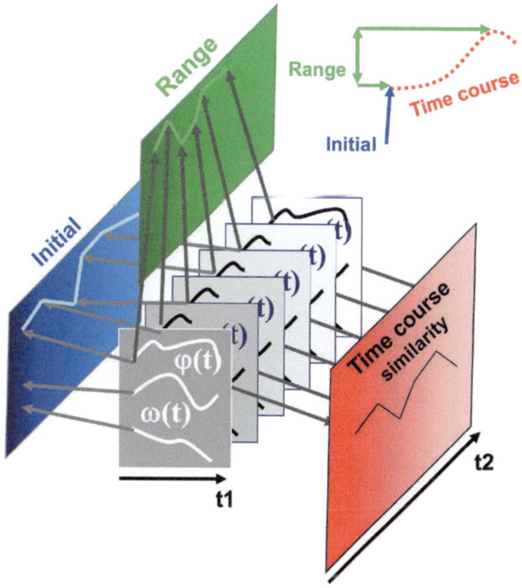

Fig. 1.4 Design for comparing time-courses of metric (Initial and Range) variables with topological (time-course-curve shape) variables during a learning process. Note that the time scales for the learning time-course t2 differ from the time scale t1 of movement execution. (Schöllhorn 1997a, b)

teams at that time, were analyzed as part of a learning project on augmented feedback intervention (Mendoza and Schöllhorn 1990, 1993; Schöllhorn 1993a, 1998). Both athletes had already acquired a stable throwing pattern at an international performance level through extensive repetition and model-oriented training beforehand. Eight throws by the discus specialist were analyzed at competitions over a period of 1 year (Schöllhorn 1993b), and 45 throws by the decathlete in training and at competitions over a period of six months were analyzed biomechanically (Schöllhorn 1995; Schöllhorn 1996, 1998). Not only were the throwing arm or landing leg biomechanically analyzed, as was often required by top coaches, but the entire (more holistic) movement was biomechanically described based on the joint angles and their velocities by means of a 14-segment body model (Schöllhorn 1993c). Because most of the discus velocity is produced during the final double-supported throwing phase, only this phase was analyzed.

To get a rough impression of the process-oriented analysis approach, it is explained here

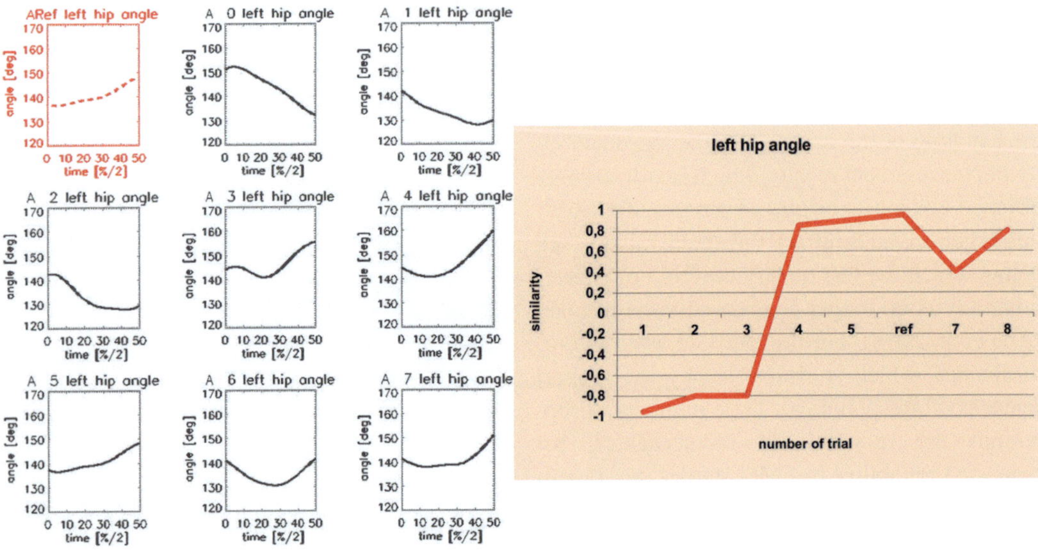

Fig. 1.5 Qualitative changes of the left hip angle joint time-courses of eight trials. (The reference time-course ARef and A5 are identical)

using the time-course of the left hip angle as an example. For this purpose, the hip-angle-time-course of the best is selected as a reference, and the others are compared with it for similarity.[4] We could also choose the first throwing test as the starting point (from where the system develops) or the last one as the end point (where the system has developed to), but we chose the trial with the highest release speed of the discus as the reference movement. Figure 1.5 shows all eight hip-angle-time curves of the specialist. The first hip angle curve VR comes from the best with the highest takeoff speed and is identical to trial V5. Here, the similarity of all curves relative to VR is still defined in simplified linear terms as a scalar product, which most people still know from school as the angle between two vectors and corresponds to the cosine, that is, can assume values between −1 and + 1, analogous to a correlation of two data series. Later, nonlinear methods with slightly improved recognition rates were used (Bauer and Schöllhorn 1997). If we compare the reference curve ARef with the second curve A0, we can see their opposite behavior. While the reference throw A Ref shows an increase in the hip angle and thus describes an increasing hip extension, the hip angle decreases in the first throw A0, and the athlete pulls the hip back toward the release. Similar reverse behavior can be observed in all three first attempts, A0–A2, which are reflected in negative similarity values. Only with the fourth attempt, A3, could a change in the direction of the reference throw be observed; the right hip is extended toward the release. Only the seventh attempt, A6, shows a slightly different course, in which the angle initially becomes smaller but is then extended slightly, delayed until the release. As all the last five throws, A3–A7, show a positive similarity value close to 1, it can be said that the learning process was successful over time. Between the third A2 and fourth A3 recordings, a 1-week training intervention with biomechanical feedback learning (Farfel 1962) on trunk twisting before the double-supported throwing phase was carried out (Mendoza 1993; Mendoza and Schöllhorn 1990, 1991; Schöllhorn 1995).

[4]This procedure was chosen in analogy to physical measurement methods in which a quantity is always compared with a unit reference quantity. For example, the physical quality "length" of an object is always specified in multiples of the distance that light travels in a certain time, given in m (meter), or the physical quality "time" in multiples of the oscillation period of a transition between the two hyperfine structure levels of the ground state of the atom Cesium 133, given in s (seconds).

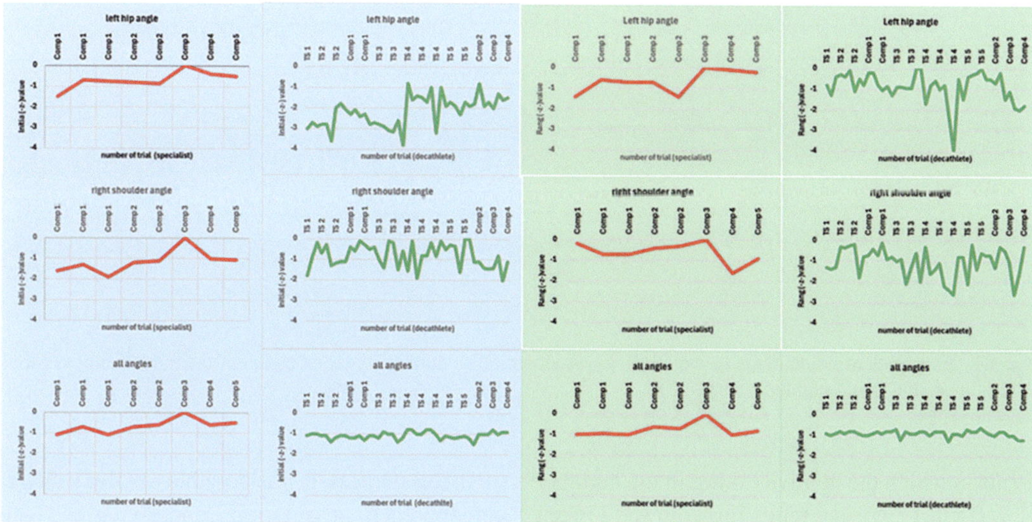

Fig. 1.6 Examples of fluctuations of metric (initial (left, blue background) and range (right, green background)) variables during 1 year of competition and training sessions (discus specialist: red; decathlete: green)

The initial values and ranges of the respective variables were chosen as parameters for the metrics of the movement, and the corresponding time-course features for the topology (Fig. 1.6). These characteristics were chosen in analogy to their system-theoretical correspondences in the visual domain (Fig. 1.2), which will be discussed in more detail in the chapter on neurological foundations.

Although the process-oriented approach was initially realized with primarily linear statistical methods, such as the P-technique of factor analysis (Cattell 1945; Schöllhorn 1993b), cluster analysis, and orthogonal reference functions (Schöllhorn 1995, 1996), it provided a solution for quantifying the topology of movements and its variance.

In the decathlete's curves, the movement topology allowed for the identification of different throwing strategies in the individual training sessions and competitions (Bauer and Schöllhorn 1997), but no enduring change over time. Neither the learning process nor the training sessions were recognizable based on the movement metric variables. Despite the many repetitions that both throwers had completed by the beginning of the study, identical repetitions could not be identified for either the metrics or topology characteristics (Fig. 1.7). Surprisingly, all categories of variables showed fluctuations, despite the repetitive and model-oriented training up to that point, but only the topology showed a plausible structure that could be assigned to a learning process (Schöllhorn 1996). The fluctuations in the data thus appeared to apply not only to the movement metrics but also to the movement topology. This suggests that our movement system for effective learning varies not only in metrics, e.g., larger, smaller, slower, or faster, even when supposedly repeating the same movement (a single topology), but also varies the internal rhythmicity. This finding also demonstrated the possibility of analyzing movements with a large number of degrees of freedom (lDGF), as they occur in methodical exercise series in sports pedagogy, and opened the door to approaching numerous other issues, especially in the context of motor learning processes.

Interestingly, a movement topology or movement class seemed to be repeated more consistently than movement metrics. However, corresponding scales for variances need to be considered to allow the exact comparison. A similar situation could be observed earlier in experi-

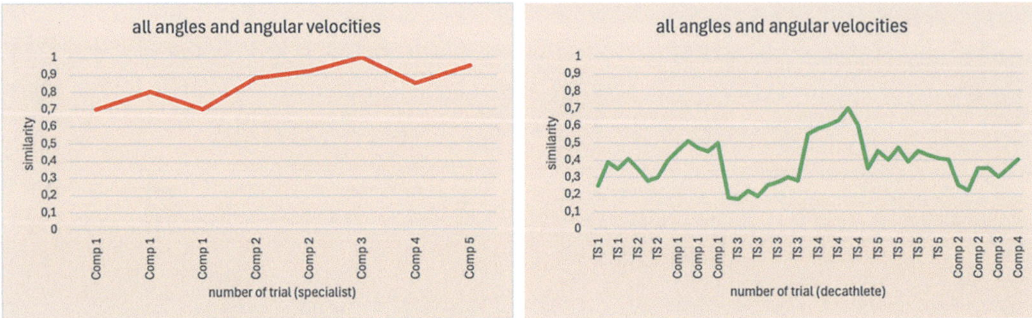

Fig. 1.7 Examples of fluctuations in the topology of all variables during 1 year of competition and training sessions (discus specialist red; decathlete: green)

ments in which the relative timing in the hammer blow (Drill 1933), in typing (Terzuolo and Viviani 1980), or in piano playing (Michon 1974) could have been understood as fluctuations in topology, but at that time the focus was on the constant part, the invariants, and fluctuations of the relative timing tended to be neglected or considered as measurement errors. Similar to the earlier described filtering in data processing, the information not considered relevant to a given theory was removed, a kind of adjusting the data to one's own expectations. Especially after the Second World War, with the upcoming Computers and Cybernetics, the tendency was rather to show analogies between them and human motor control. In this context, programs as analogies to invariants were a welcome but also misleading metaphor. Both also fit very well with the political mood during the Cold War to make the assembly line work more effectively and to demonstrate the superiority of the political systems. Practically, assembly line work was carried into physiotherapy and training practice. Qualitative changes in the invariants within the fraωework of a learning process were not considered and were only described verbally (on a nominal scale). The suspicion, therefore, arises that, unfortunately, the methodology of therapy and learning was adapted to the technology available at the time, rather than the other way around. People would rather have solutions and were looking for problems to which the solutions could be applied, instead of setting the problems as the focus of interest.

In this context, it was possible to offer a different approach to questions underlying the gap between the variability used in therapeutic or sports pedagogical practice and the variability discussed in sports psychology research. These questions were related to the extent to which the metrics and topology of movements exist from the beginning, or whether they are independent of each other, and how they develop during ontogenesis or learning processes.

For the joint analysis of the development of movement metrics and topology in the discus learning process, the specialist's throw with the highest release speed was also selected as a reference for the metric variables. Hereby, it is irrelevant whether a similarity or distance measure is used; both can be mathematically converted into one another by appropriate scaling. This step allowed us to correlate the changes in the respective characteristic categories with each other on the time-course of learning. Both athletes showed several significant correlations between all category time-courses (Fig. 1.8), but the number of correlations between the "Initial" and "time-course" feature categories was significantly lower for the specialist than for the decathlete. A significant correlation can be interpreted here as a dependency of the movement time-course on the initial conditions, as these lie before the time-course. As the specialist had fewer of these, he appeared to be more advanced in the learning process than the decathlete, as he had widely decoupled his movement time-courses from the initial conditions.

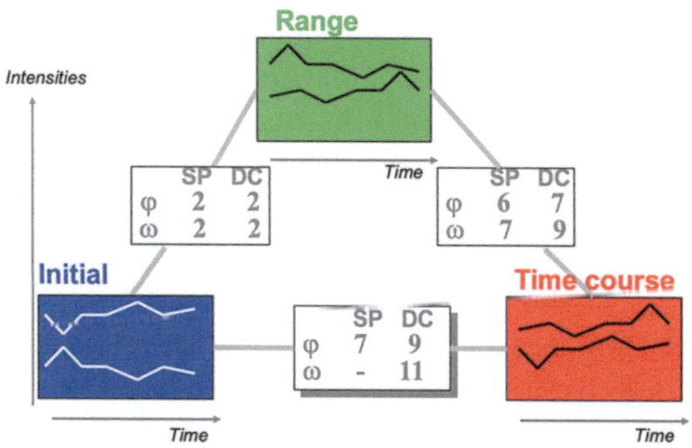

Fig. 1.8 Number of significant correlations between metric (initial and range) and topological (time-course) variables during the learning processes of a discus specialist (SP) and a decathlete (DC) φ: angular variables; ω: angular velocity variables

In everyday life or in children's learning processes, dependencies of the time-course on the initial condition can often be observed. Once a small child has learned the first steps of walking, the instruction to look upwards or to walk with raised arms (changing the initial condition of the shoulder angle) is already enough to disrupt controlled walking. Something similar can be observed, for example, when learning to drive a car, turning the head to the left also very often moves the steering wheel to the left with the hands. In these beginning stages of motor learning, the two categories seem not yet to be decoupled. Only during the time-course of the learning process do they become decoupled, but only by varying both categories (movement topology and metrics) in appropriate combinations. The situation is similar with the visual system: if only a triangle is ever offered as a stimulus, in different sizes, the system will not be able to recognize a circle or a rectangle. The findings therefore indicated the need for a targeted variation of metrics and topologies to be able to form these categories in the first place and to be able to control these categories independently of each other (Hubel and Wiesel 1962; Wiesel and Hubel 1963). The same applies to a new topology to be learned. Its execution will only be stable when variations of the topology and the metrics are decoupled by corresponding variations. Future research will show to what extent a primary variation of metrics is more likely to be applied for stabilization, whereas primary variations of topology are more likely to be preferred for refinement and the variation of both for acquiring new movements. The focus on the variation of metrics in all the learning models that primarily investigated the stabilization of already skilled movements suggests this suspicion (Schöllhorn et al. 2022).

For a qualitative change in the coordination of movement, the variation of the movement topology was therefore obvious. Clearly, the variations in topology went beyond the "*repetition without repetition*" in Bernstein's metrics and Schmidt's variable parameters. This research on the variation of the decomposed aspects of movement already pointed to massive problems with the repetitive approach and prepared the ground for more variation in therapy and sports training, as it was then realized in differential learning and became widespread with numerous other names. In contrast to numerous theoretical discussions and opinion papers available before the turn of the century, these consequences were underpinned by solid measurement data.

Some Epistemological Considerations

Since some of the more recent discussions and opinion papers tended to make hasty generalizations, a few essential epistemological backgrounds should be discussed here. Being able to perform a learned movement identically or similarly again at a later point in time latently assumes that the identical or similar conditions will then prevail. While the first is typically associated with weak causality, the second is strong causality, as many more conditions are required to map similar causes to similar effects (Argyris et al. 1994). At the latest since the emergence of the uncertainty principle and quantum theory in physics (Heisenberg 1927), weak causality in connection with Laplace's demon has only been regarded as a historical model with no serious significance in today's scientific context. Gödel's incompleteness theorem pointed in the same direction. While uncertainty theory restricted the simultaneous measurement accuracy of position and momentum, thus making predictability impossible due to the effects of variations occurring below the measurement threshold at the atomic level with increasing time, Gödel showed that in sufficiently powerful, consistent formal systems there are always statements that are true but undecidable, that is, they can neither be proved nor disproved.

The idea of depicting an object of investigation in a representative way is also subject to a similar error of reasoning. With his concept of representativeness and the associated assumption of a probabilistic nature of the environment in which organisms act, Brunswik (1955) moves away from the deterministic stimulus-response assignment of classical behaviorism, but with probabilistic (Brunswik 1939) remains with the basic idea of high repetition numbers, albeit with minimum scatter (seeing the same object from different perspectives and different distances). However, how exactly it is determined whether an experiment is representative of real environments remains open. The same applies to more recent suggestions to transfer the concept to therapy and everyday life or training and competition. How the concept of representativeness based on high repetition numbers is to be unified with self-organization or emergence in one theory also remains puzzling. It also remains unclear how his model for decision-making processes in simple, clearly defined environments can be transferred to more complex, dynamic environments, such as social interactions or multidimensional problems. As a supporter of positivism (Tolman 1956), Brunswick reduced the complexity of reality to measurable empirical facts, while subjective experiences were excluded because they could not be measured. With the exclusive focus on the measurable variations of the stimuli, individual differences of the perceivers were also disregarded.

The Duhem Quine thesis (Afriat 2004; Duhem 1954; Quine 1953) at the latest should have made it clear that no system of theories can be definitively verified or falsified, as a new element can always be added that was excluded from previous observations, meaning that identical conditions for comparison are no longer given. This was one condition for the development of general model theory (Stachowiak 1973) on the basis of pragmatist philosophy (Dewey 1920; Peirce 1883).

This has profound implications for physiotherapy and training, as it suggests that we cannot draw definitive conclusions about the specific consequences of any intervention. Instead, we are often left to anticipate outcomes based solely on probabilities. This uncertainty challenges the very foundation of our treatment approaches, compelling us to reconsider how we assess and apply therapeutic interventions as physiotherapists. Alternatively, the model of nonlinear causality, which links small causes with large effects and large causes with small effects, has therefore become more widespread in recent times, especially in therapy and training, where increasingly more various responses are observed on the same intervention (Bates et al. 1983b; Bouchard et al. 1999). Especially for living systems, this model for causality became attractive and is frequently described with the somewhat exaggerated metaphor of the butterfly strike, which could lead to storms in Europe if carried out in South America.

In the traditional logic of physiotherapy, as in sports training, repetitions should serve to lay a deep "track," as minor deviations or disturbances are to be expected in future situations, and they should not disturb the learned movement. The often-used metaphor for this is the track-like wear and tear in the cobbled streets of ancient Rome caused by carriages, which are difficult to get out of once you have entered them. This metaphor is very similar to the definition of stability in physics, where a system is considered stable when the system goes back to its original state after a disturbance. Interestingly, the problem of learning new movements when the traces of a learned movement are too deep due to monotonous repetitions of the same can also be observed in the context of motor learning: Repetitive learning seems to have a detrimental effect on the learning of new movements (Kast and Leukel 2016).

Although these epistemological considerations may sound sophisticated and removed from practice, they contain essential insights for physiotherapists, teachers, and coaches: Reality in general and human behavior in particular can only be predicted to a very limited extent because there will always be an aspect that has not yet been considered. This applies equally to the therapy, learning, and training process. Even science will never be able to cover all aspects. The smallest unnoticed aspect can prevent success, but it can also make it possible. All interventions will always depend on the sensitive observation skills and experience of the therapists, teachers, and trainers, but also on their openness and willingness to experiment. Every patient, pupil, or athlete will be a new experiment full of new aspects to discover.

In conclusion, the path forward in motor learning, therapy, and sports training lies in recognizing the limitations of traditional approaches and adopting a more dynamic and integrated framework. By systematically varying movement topologies and metrics, we can enhance our understanding of motor learning processes and ultimately improve practice outcomes. The time has come to re-evaluate our strategies, to cultivate learning environments that reflect the complexity of human movement and embrace the inherent variability that defines it. Everyday observations of people walking or running in various moods suggest that these interventions could potentially alter process-oriented characteristics of movement, which could then be accurately assessed using newly developed analytical methods.

1.3.4 Fluctuations Due to Specific Situations

One obvious question following these findings was to identify possible conditions for these fluctuations in movement topology. A first candidate for this was the influence of emotions on our movement behavior. The extent to which emotions can be shown in the direct execution of movements was the subject of the study by Janssen et al. (2008), in which the test subjects were asked to demonstrate four different emotions while walking across a force plate several times. In addition to the recognition of the individuals based on the ground reaction forces, the results also showed up to 100 percent recognition of the emotions shown, but interestingly, only within the individuals. This means that the emotions could only be differentiated within the individual after the individual had been recognized. An analogous study in which the test subjects listened to three types of music before crossing the force plate led to the same findings. Interestingly, in both studies, the individual was dominant in the gait pattern, and only when the individual was recognized, in addition to a situational fine structure of the emotions and music types, was it assignable. The individual situational adaptations through emotions and/or music were all confirmed by later studies (Janssen 2017; Michalak et al. 2009). Interestingly related to the assumption of being able to achieve a given model, in none of the studies were we able to identify two identical movement patterns, although all trials of individuals clustered together. However, it seemed as if the emotions and the music provided an individual fine structure within the often-stated tolerance zone of one standard deviation around an average, so the fluctuations around this were not completely random. In consequence, both cause specific fluctuations and therefore can be used for therapy and training to guide the learning process in a certain direction.

This sparked curiosity about possible even more sensitive influences on our movement behavior. Numerous studies on the dependence of psycho-physiological parameters on circadian rhythms (Minors 1981; Müller 2004; Vitaterna et al. 2001) and thus the dependence of our movement coordination on time in general provided indications of a possible factor. Therefore, our interest shifted to how human movements behave without explicit intervention: do they oscillate around a central value, or does the system drift away continuously? The former would correspond to the traditional average-oriented model and the attempt to "Tame the chance" (Hacking 1990) and the latter to the arrow of time in the sense of Heraclitus' and Lao Tze's quotes. This approach could also be of interest for diagnosis by analyzing the frequency content of these fluctuations.

During the earlier deconstruction of the person- and time-dependent model assumption, it became apparent that no two identical movement patterns were found. This still could have been attributed to the findings of earlier studies based on discrete-time data (Bates et al. 1983a; Winter 1984). In addition, the fluctuations were assumed to be largely random in time. Hausdorff and colleagues challenged this assumption by providing evidence for a long-term cyclicity of self-determined walking over an hour based on entropy measures (for quantifying disorder in time series) applied to step cadences (Hausdorff et al. 1995; Hausdorff et al. 1996), thus supporting the assumption that automated cyclical movements such as walking would return to a point that has already been taken once and in line with the traditionally average-oriented model with a tolerance range, just with some time delay. On one hand, this assumption is problematic because the same stride cadence can be achieved with an infinite number of body positions, which is reflected in the idea of motor equivalence (Lashley 1930; Raibert 1978; Wing 2000). Therefore, the whole system's state could drift away despite keeping a constant step cadence. On the other hand, the simplification of the high-dimensional gait movement to the one-dimensional step cadence depends largely on the spatial resolution of the scaling and the presuppositions for applying entropy calculations. Related to the first, entropy calculations require long data series and stationarity, which largely excludes the analysis of constantly drifting away signals. Related to the scaling, if the cadence varies by 0.2 s, for example, and a resolution of 0.002 s, 100 numbers are available for the random arrangement. This is associated with a problem of the concept of randomness in stochastics. In everyday use, randomness refers exclusively to the distribution and unpredictability of single numbers, which is referred to as primary randomness (Spencer-Brown 1953, 1957). Thus, randomness is commonly assumed to be much more disordered than mathematically expected (see (Schöllhorn 2016)). In the case of cyclicality, however, the frequent neglect of secondary randomness is of greater importance (Spencer-Brown 1953, 1957; Stern 2011). To avoid situational shifts in the uniform distribution, appropriately large samples are selected. To guarantee randomness in these large sets of numbers, the sequences of numbers contained therein must also occur with corresponding frequency and uniform distribution. This theoretically applies to any length of number sequences. However, if the number sequences must occur several times in the large data set to meet the random criteria, a certain cyclicality should be detectable due to secondary randomness alone. In consequence, the eventual coming back to a central value could be simply due to the concept of stochasticity (Spencer-Brown 1957) and the measurement resolution.

For a first experiment on the temporal dependence of process-oriented movement patterns, ten professional and semi-professional flutists played the same passage of a flute concerto by Mozart (KV 314) three times on three different days (Albrecht et al. 2014). Giving the same piece to different musicians is comparable to the specification of a generalized technique model for movements. The whole-body and finger movements were recorded and biomechanically analyzed. Despite time normalization to compensate for different playing tempi, each flutist was recognized 100% based on the kinematics of the finger movements and 94% based on the ground reaction forces of the body movements. The assignment of the movements to the three playing days was about chance level, but again without identical movement patterns.

Due to the possible influence of emotions, which could have been caused by the music itself or the desire to improve on previous performances and could have interacted with the circadian rhythms, another design was used to minimize these interactions. For this purpose, the ground reaction forces and kinematic data of the lower extremities of six women and two men during walking across force platforms were recorded at the same time of day on eight days over a 2-week period (Horst et al. 2016). The test subjects were only asked to look straight ahead at a neutral smiley so that they did not aim at the measuring plates, thereby changing their posture, and to minimize the possible influences of emotions, comparison with previous movements, etc., as

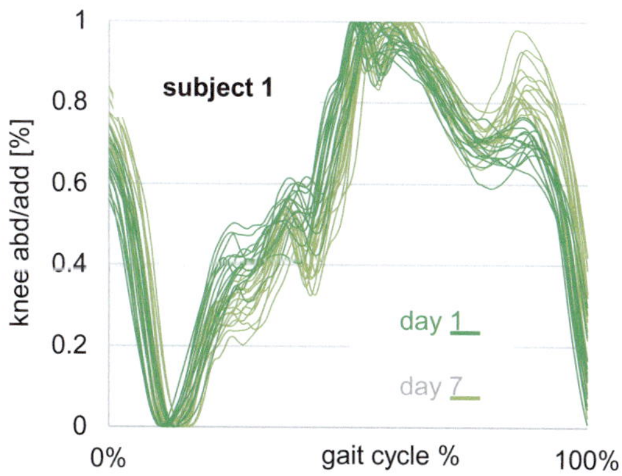

Fig. 1.9 Exemplary 2 × 15 knee angle time-courses from a single subject on two different days

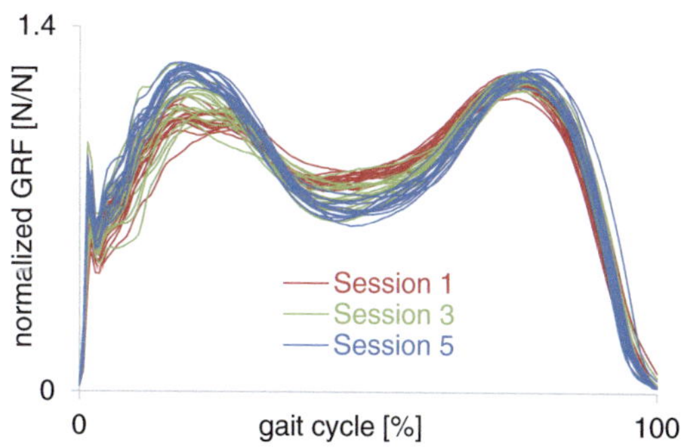

Fig. 1.10 Exemplary ground reaction force of a single subject 3× 15 gaits during the same day with break durations between 10 and 150 min

discussed earlier. Again, all participants were clearly identified based on biomechanical process-oriented data by means of support vector machines (SVMs). In addition, there was a 95% daily recognition within individuals (with a guess probability of 12% = 1/8). Figure 1.9 shows exemplarily clear changes of the variable time-courses within days. And again, no identical gait patterns were identified. This was an additional indication that even automated movements such as walking are subject to constant drift, but so far only within individual characteristics.

These findings led even deeper into the problems regarding the behavior of the drift at different time scales, specifically, how fast and how sustained these drifts are. In a first experiment on a shorter time scale (Horst et al. 2017a), the same biomechanical parameters as in the previous experiment were measured during 15 double steps per session, but in 6 sessions on the same day with time intervals between 10 and 150 min. Based on the time-courses of the kinematic data and with the help of a different ML algorithm (kernel-based discriminant regression analysis), an 88% differentiation of the sessions was already achieved for the 10-min breaks between the recordings, which increased to 99% with a 40-min break and to 100% after a 90-min break, showing examples of the curves of a subject for three sessions (Fig. 1.10). The curves show clear differences in the individual sessions and indicate again a fine structure of the individual gait patterns within the tolerance zone that is usually specified and considered random. It seems as if our neuromusculoskeletal system is subject to constant changes of its own accord, and this was already indicated in the above-mentioned study on the differentiation of the discus thrower's training sessions (Bauer and Schöllhorn 1997) that had a fundamental influence on the idea of the DL approach.

Looking for a drift or persistence on a longer time scale of 7–16 months, (Horst et al. 2017b) the ground reaction forces of ten trials were recorded from 128 subjects at two measurement points and analyzed using Support Vector Machines (SVM). Out of a total of 1280 gait trials, only two trials were incorrectly assigned, which corresponds to a recognition rate for the individual of 99.8%. If the SVMs were only trained with the data from one measurement day and tested with the data from the second measurement day, the recognition rate was still 88%. Both findings together indicate that the movement patterns drift further away with increasing time distance; that is, the probability of two identical movement patterns decreases increasingly. Whether this can also be seen in ages where the physical conditions are changing faster, for example, in childhood, adolescence, or the elderly, will be shown in future research. If it turns out that the type and amount of intervention depend not only on the person but also on the time, then the extent of drifting away could provide an indication of the appropriate time.

Since none of these and several other studies on running (Burdack et al. 2020; Hoitz et al. 2021; Horst et al. 2021) have succeeded in finding two identical movement patterns, and the timescales related findings point to a rather increasing drift over time, we can assume with a very high probability that the next movement to be performed, even after thousands of repetitions, will contain something new that has never appeared before in the same context. Consequently, in light of this evidence, the second latent assumption of a time-independent model for successful physiotherapeutic repetition-based interventions becomes untenable. This raises a provocative question for physiotherapists: if every movement is inherently unique, how can we truly expect our patients to replicate a "perfect" movement pattern, and are we limiting their potential by adhering too rigidly to conventional repetition-based methods?

The problem in therapy and training again seems to be closely connected with our latent assumptions. If we traditionally assume a learning system that only changes because of interventions but otherwise remains relatively constant over time, then it seems plausible to start with greater variety and then gradually reduce it toward repeating the assumed role model or target movement as performance levels increase or become more stable (Fig. 1.11). However, if we challenge this assumption according to recent findings (or verify quantitatively old knowledge of aging), that people are constantly changing even without external influences, then larger and ongoing variations are advantageous from the outset to keep pace with the changes in the system.

This leads to the suspicion that the theories provided by science were most often adjusted to the measurement methods that were available at the respective time. If we assume, in the simplest case, a linear change for the drift, then the decreasing variation intervention based on traditional ideas would very soon show no overlap, no resonance, with the changed system (Fig. 1.11). This is directly observable throughout childhood and adolescence, during which growth rates between 4 and 15 cm per year until the 18th year of life can occur (Nejedly 2020; Westphal 1995). If a child grows by this amount, the extremities also increase to a comparable extent, which biomechanically leads to a corresponding change in the muscular levers and momentums of inertia that necessitates an adequate constant adjustment of neuronal control. A learned activation pattern that a child has learned at the beginning of a year will no longer function at the end of the year, as all the forces and momentums have changed. However, similar changes appear to occur not only in childhood and adolescence but also in adulthood, on even shorter time scales, as these studies show. From this perspective, the often-stated optimal learning age of approx. 10–12 years (Janacsek et al. 2012) also appears to be more dependent on the learning method than on age. During this period, the growth rate reaches a first minimum (Brandt and Reinken 1988; Thompson and Moreno 2018), which, in conjunction with the lowest variability through repetition, leads to an increased learning rate. Before and after this period, the growth rates increase again until adulthood, which is accompanied by a loss in stability of movement patterns and can presumably only be compensated for with increased variability of the exercises. It seems that repetition-based motor learning during the school years is primarily due to the constant anatomical changes that introduce noise into the system. The same would apply to the increasing physical changes with age: With increasing age, the variations of exercises should increase. With advancing age, the tissue loses stiffness and the anatomical changes increase. To compensate for these changes, exercise must therefore be more variable to have enough noise for the necessary adaptation.

These constantly persisting changes in living systems (e.g., patient, athlete) not only call into question the assumption that a target movement can be achieved through repetition but ultimately also lead to problems in the development of a biomechanically, individually optimized movement technique. In addition to the creation of differential equations, this is based on the determination of **boundary conditions**, which

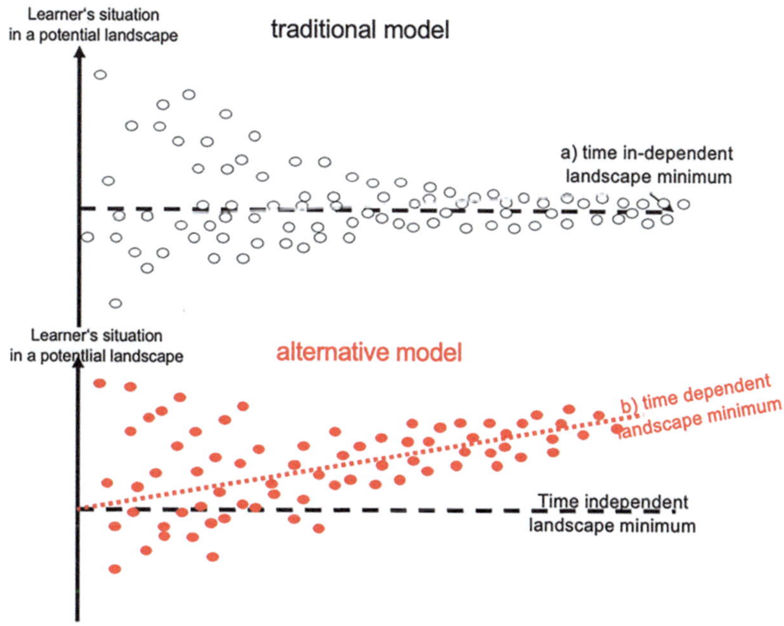

Fig. 1.11 Assumptions of time (in)dependent potential landscape minimum. (**a**) time-independent landscape minimum; (**b**) time-dependent landscape minimum

are usually measured on the moving individual (e.g., maximum contraction speed of individual muscles, relative timing of these contractions, volitional characteristics, e.g., for maximum voluntary contraction, etc.). And there precisely arise the logical problems. If the original to be modeled executes a movement for measurement purposes, then this execution of the movement already changes the system itself and thus creates conditions that no longer correspond to those previously measured, which restricts the corresponding accuracy in predictions. The same seems to happen even with corresponding recovery phases. Whether this is influenced by the basic energy consumption of our system (e.g., brain, heart, breathing), by thoughts, circadian rhythms, etc., will be a challenge for future studies. The process of biomechanically modeling movement techniques can therefore only ever be a rough approximation with corresponding tolerance limits.

The Machine Learning (ML) methods developed in the context of movement pattern recognition, as described earlier, meanwhile provide various approaches to investigate these problems and contribute to the understanding of complex dependencies in the field of coordination learning in a different manner.

In summary, the newly developed tools in the field of process-oriented pattern recognition allowed a new approach in which the fluctuations in the movement metrics and topology were no longer understood as measurement errors but as a realization on par with all others (Schöllhorn and Bauer 1998a, b, c; Schöner et al. 1986). In practical terms, the findings indicate that to be aware of preparing the patient and athletes for situations that do not happen in the therapy or training session, it may tend to not only prepare them for certain skills but also to train their adaptability (Schöllhorn 1999).

1.4 Caution in Drawing Conclusions from Individual Movements to Individual Therapy or Individual Training

At first glance, one might conclude that while the individuality of movements creates varying starting conditions for therapies and other interventions, we should simply introduce more variation into our approaches and continue following traditional/classical methods. This train of thought was already at the core of the methodical exercise series in sport (Gaulhofer and Streicher 1924) in the context of the reform pedagogical philosophy of learner-centered teaching. It also serves as the structural skeleton for most traditional therapeutic and rehabilitation measures. Here, only the difficulty of the initial exercise is adjusted to the ability level of the patient/learner, but subsequently, all go through the same exercise sequences with increasing similarity to the role model movement.

On the other hand, the overwhelming and ever-increasing evidence regarding individual movement patterns has frequently led to premature conclusions about personalized therapies or unique learning behaviors. Before reaching such conclusions, several additional factors must be clarified. Theoretically, individual movement patterns could arise simply because they were present from the outset, with everyone responding similarly to various interventions. This would correspond to a neighborhood-preserving mapping; that is, similar movement patterns at the beginning of an intervention are still similar to the same extent after the intervention. Concerns about a predetermined life are unjustified here, as there are still an infinite number of different interventions. In addition, the studies on the individuality of movements have primarily concentrated on movements that are highly automated and have reached the final stages of the learning process due to extensive repetition. As a result, it remains unclear to what extent these movements developed from individual characteristics at the outset or whether they were shaped through personalized intervention processes when similar movement patterns were initially present.

Initial indications of individual movement characteristics from the outset are provided by a recent study on absolute beginners learning a snatch movement in weightlifting. Despite different learning approaches during the first training session, the movements of the barbell were largely attributable to individual athletes (Ammar et al. 2024c). However, it is still unclear to what extent the initial individual characteristics are retained at an advanced stage. Even if they were the same, individual paths could theoretically still lead there.

A fundamental problem with this reasoning is that the individuality of movement and response to an intervention are two completely different things. A sphere and a cube (different initial conditions) placed on an inclined plane (gravitational effect) show different reactions. Doing squats with a weight of 100 kg is normal for a heavyweight weightlifter but too much for a juvenile dancer. The dependence of the response on the initial conditions is, to a large extent, part of the adaptive stress/strain model in occupational physiology (Rohmert 1984). Models on the high sensitivity of initial conditions in acute processes have been suggested in the area of strength (Sust 1996, 2009) and endurance research (Brooks 1985; Mader and Heck 1986; Wackerhage et al. 2022). In the area of coordination, this would correspond to motor control models such as the equilibrium point hypothesis (Feldman and Levin 2009). All these models serve to describe a state but not the process in the context of learning interventions or developmental aspects. They only allow statements about momentary behavior when certain conditions are met, but these models were not developed for how these conditions are to be achieved or changed. While classic intervention studies approach this problem classically by comparing group-oriented mean values before and after, there are a few alternative proposals in the field of sports shoes (Bates et al. 1983b) and energy metabolism (Bouchard et al. 1999; Bouchard and Rankinen 2001) that suggest individuality in these areas. In the first area, differences in the progression curves of biomechanical parameters when running with different sports shoes and barefoot reflect only spontaneous adaptation. The lack of commonalities between the curve characteristics suggests acute individual reactions and indicates weak individuality. It would have been interesting to see whether these curves change and to what extent they change when the shoes are worn for a longer time. In the second area, the interventions normally take place over several weeks and use different relative changes of discrete metabolic parameters to draw conclusions about the possible individuality of the reactions. However, the comparability of the initial conditions is only determined based on a few parameters, and any coordinative changes that occur during this duration of interventions are neglected for methodological reasons.

Although everyday interventions in the form of shoes with different heel heights, different cushioning properties or medical measures such as orthopedic insoles and orthoses only have a marginal influence in physiotherapy and must be clearly distinguished from active movement interventions, studies with them are often used to gain a first understanding of specific adaptive behavior in the context of motor coordination.

As part of a study on the biomechanical influence of four different heel heights (1.4–8.1 cm) on gait behavior in women, neural networks not only provided indications of height-dependent individual and group trends but also of individual adaptation behavior based on time-continuous data (Schöllhorn et al. 2002a). Up to 5.4 cm the gait patterns within the individuals remained quite similar, whereas the 8.1 cm grouped all gait patterns into an extra group. The increase to 8.1 cm heel height fundamentally changed the gait pattern in the entire group compared to the heel heights up to 5.4 cm and provided the highest recognition rate for the individuals there. This can be seen as further evidence that extreme situations bring out the truly individual characteristics. A comparison of the relative similarities of the individuals below and above 5.4 cm heel height also revealed relative shifts between the individuals, which corresponds to a destruction of neighborhood conservation. For example, if subjects A and B, as well as E and F, were most similar to each other up to a heel height of 5.4 cm, subjects A and F, as well as B and E, could be more similar under the 8.1 cm condition. This indicates that there are interventions that have similar effects for many people up to a certain point, but if this point is exceeded, fundamentally different reactions occur. Whether neighborhood preservation will form a criterion for creating functional groups has to be shown in future research. Similar phenomena can be observed in competitive sport with classic overtraining, in which there is persistent stagnation or even a drop in performance despite an increase in training volume or intensity. Up to a certain point, the performance is increasing for all, but beyond this point, some will suffer from the symptoms of overtraining. In occupational physiology, this can be associated with the burnout syndrome, where the straw breaks the camel's back (Saultz 2020), which happens earlier with reduced variability. Lower variability corresponds to increased stiffness, which can be beneficial in the short term, but in the longer term is more likely to lead to breakage, e.g., injury or illness, in a dynamic environment. These insights highlight the importance of tailoring interventions to patients. Just as heel heights affect gait behavior, treatment modalities can produce similar outcomes until a tipping point is reached, after which individualized responses may arise. Recognizing this concept can enhance therapeutic strategies, underscoring the need for continuous assessment and adaptability, especially in cases of patient stagnation or regression, akin to overtraining in sports. This understanding helps physiotherapists determine when a change in approach is necessary to meet each patient's unique needs effectively.

Another largely overlooked issue regarding individual learning behavior, in the sense of strong individuality, arises when interventions are performed not with mechanical support but as movement-based interventions for long-term learning, as commonly used in physiotherapy. To this end, it is necessary to examine the extent to which only the respective person exhibits their specific learning behavior, and, on the other hand, the associated learning process would also have to be the same for each learning process in the future. Investigating this concerns a fundamental methodological problem on the one hand, and on the other, it opens a hitherto overlooked potential resource for effective learning in therapy and training. In personalized treatment, the exercise history is usually considered (e.g., which sports or which exercises have been done and for how long), but the learning methods used are very rarely evaluated, as one typically assumes repetition learning and methodical exercise series, which are supported to some extent by cognitive information. To what extent the decrease in learning progress with increasing skill level could be caused by using the same methods over and over again is still unknown territory. It would be surprising if the responsiveness in terms of intervention methods did not also decrease. This would mean that the methods should also be subject to a certain variation to achieve optimal therapy and learning.

In physiotherapy, this problem could also affect the situation where a patient may come to therapy with the same or similar diagnosis a few weeks or months later. Is it then more effective to use the same exercises again, or is it better to use different ones or simply in a different sequence with different breaks in between, etc.?

From a scientific point of view, this is associated with the reliability criterion of strong individuality, that is, in the context of individuality of learning, connected with the following problem. If a movement has been learned once, it will be learned faster the second time (Haith and Krakauer 2014) due to the body's memory. Even if the learned movement is completely forgotten, the learning will be different from the first time (Coltman et al. 2019).

One way to approach this problem, at least for a large part, would be to examine the learning behavior for different movements that go along with the need for quantifying the similarity of movements. Beyond the simple similarity of movements and based on the previous findings related to emotion, fatigue, and music recognition in walking people, the decomposition of general and individual characteristics in a movement signal is the next candidate for a deeper understanding of motor learning.

Most recently, the first studies approached this problem by looking for individual characteristics across various movement topologies. Indications for individual characteristics of decathletes across three throwing techniques were found by means of ML algorithms (SVMs) (Horst et al. 2020; Schöllhorn et al. 2014a, b). By neglecting the movement of the throwing arm, the shot put, discus, and javelin throwing movements, athlete-specific commonalities in all three throwing disciplines could be identified. Although research is still needed to determine the percentages and their changes during a learning process, the findings already indicate that a transfer takes place between the throwing disciplines, which points to an economization of training. This, in turn, supports the idea of training general throwing fundamentals on the one hand, and on the other, it can be assumed that training one throwing discipline will also influence the others.

In the second study, the ground reaction forces during walking, running, and handwriting also revealed individual characteristics across disciplines by means of ML algorithms (cycle GANNs) (Burdack et al. 2023). While the first case involved three sports movements, three everyday movements were analyzed here, which can be assumed to have significantly more stable movement patterns due to more repetitions. Although only the integral reaction forces on the ground or at the tip of the writing pen served as the basis for the analysis, and the two cyclical movements (walking and running) are controlled more strongly at the spinal cord level than the writing movement, individual characteristics could be recognized across the movement topologies. Although these are more pronounced within the locomotor movements, they can also be observed in the more cognitively controlled writing movement. This suggests a nuanced approach to exploring the reciprocal influence of movement and individual characteristics, particularly regarding therapeutic issues. For instance, can altering a writing pattern change a person's gait, or do modifications in individual characteristics need to occur first to facilitate changes in both?

1.5 Summary and Conclusion

Overall, this chapter challenges two dominant assumptions in classical physiotherapy and sports training: that person- and time-independent movement models can be universally applied and that repetition and correction lead to optimal learning. Drawing from biomechanics, systems theory, and philosophical perspectives, the text argues that **every individual demonstrates unique movement patterns** from the very beginning, shaped by their biological, psychological, and contextual factors. Traditional statistical approaches tend to mask this individuality, leading to generalized interventions that may not be effective for everyone. The chapter proposes a shift toward **process-oriented and topological analyses**, which better capture the dynamics of movement over time. It also critiques the overreliance on repetition, tracing its roots to outdated industrial and educational models. Ultimately, the chapter advocates for a **more personalized, variability-oriented approach to learning and rehabilitation**, where individual differences are not viewed as errors but as essential elements of effective and adaptive motor development.

Questions

1. What are the two main assumptions in classical physiotherapy and training that the chapter critiques?
2. How does the concept of individuality in movement differ between "weak" and "strong" forms?
3. Why do traditional statistical methods struggle to capture true individuality in motor behavior?
4. How does process-oriented analysis offer a more detailed view of movement variation than discrete-time approaches?
5. What historical or cultural influences have shaped the belief in repetition as a foundation for learning?
6. How do concepts like movement topology and movement metrics help explain qualitative changes in motor learning?
   A. Both concepts only measure amplitude changes, so they cannot reveal qualitative differences.
   B. Topology captures changes in the *shape* or class of a movement, whereas metrics track size- or time-based adjustments; separating them makes true coordination shifts visible.
   C. They are two ways of averaging group data to minimize variance.
   D. Using them removes the need for time-continuous analysis.
   E. They show that metrics are irrelevant for learning.
7. Why might individuality in movement appear even at the beginning of the learning process?
   A. Group instruction quickly forces learners to diverge from each other.
   B. Pattern-recognition studies of absolute beginners show stable, person-specific trajectories before much practice, implying anatomical-neuromotor uniqueness from the outset.
   C. Early measurements are dominated by random error masquerading as individuality.
   D. Novices share identical topologies, so individuality cannot be detected until later.
   E. Equipment differences, not learners, create the first movement variations.
8. What challenges arise when trying to generalize therapeutic interventions based on group averages?
   A. Large between-person variability and tipping-point effects mean a protocol that helps the "average" can overshoot, stall, or backfire in many individuals.
   B. Group averages guarantee that every patient will respond identically.
   C. Averages reduce statistical power, making any intervention appear ineffective.
   D. They eliminate ethical approval requirements, so studies become harder to publish.
   E. Group data automatically account for all interaction effects among variables.
9. How do epistemological concepts like uncertainty and nonlinearity affect how we interpret therapy outcomes?
   A. They indicate that classical physics provides an exact template for rehabilitation.
   B. They prove that, with enough variables, perfect prediction of therapy success is possible.
   C. They show causality in living systems is always linear and time-reversible.
   D. They justify ignoring individual differences because randomness cancels them out.
   E. They remind us that outcomes are probabilistic and sensitive to small, often unmeasured factors, so predictions from any model remain tentative.

10. How might a shift from repetition-based models to variability-based approaches change therapy or coaching practices?
    A. Treatment sessions would become shorter because variability removes the need for feedback.
    B. Therapists would ask patients to stop practicing once a movement feels comfortable.
    C. Coaches would focus exclusively on copying expert models with greater precision.
    D. Practitioners would deliberately vary both metrics and topologies, treating individual differences as resources, thereby fostering adaptability instead of chasing a single "ideal" repetition.
    E. Exercises would rely solely on machine-paced drills to enforce uniformity.

References

Abe TD, Buckner SL, Jessee MB, Mattocks KT, Mouser JG, Bell ZW, Loenneke JP (2018) Short term (24 hours) and long term (1 year) assessments of reliability in older adults: can one replace the other? J Aging Res Clin Pract 7(3). https://doi.org/10.14283/jarcp.2018.15

Aeles J, Horst F, Lapuschkin S, Lacourpaille L, Hug F (2021) Revealing the unique features of each individual's muscle activation signatures. J R Soc Interface 18(174):20200770. https://doi.org/10.1098/rsif.2020.0770

Afriat A (2004) Duhem, Quine and the other dogma. preprint. https://philsci-archive.pitt.edu/3967/

Albrecht S, Janssen D, Quarz E, Newell KM, Schöllhorn WI (2014) Individuality of movements in music – finger and body movements during playing of the flute. Hum Mov Sci 35:131–144. https://doi.org/10.1016/j.humov.2014.03.010

Ammar A, Trabelsi K, Boujelbane MA, Boukhris O, Glenn JM, Chtourou H, Schöllhorn WI (2023) The myth of contextual interference learning benefit in sports practice: a systematic review and meta-analysis. Educ Res Rev 39:100537. https://doi.org/10.1016/j.edurev.2023.100537

Ammar A, Boujelbane MA, Simak M, Fraile-Fuente I, Rizz N, Washif J, Zmijewski P, Jahrami H, Schöllhorn WI (2024a) Unveiling the acute neurophysiological responses to strength training: an exploratory study on novices performing weightlifting bouts with different motor learning models. Biol Sport. https://doi.org/10.5114/biolsport.2024.133481

Ammar A, Salem A, Simak M, Horst F, Schöllhorn WI (2024b) Acute effects of motor learning models on technical efficiency in strength-coordination exercises: a comparative analysis of Olympic snatch biomechanics in beginners. Biol Sport:151–161. https://doi.org/10.5114/biolsport.2025.141662

Ammar A, Simak ML, Salem A, Horst F, Schöllhorn WI (2024c) Unveiling individuality in the early phase of motor learning: a machine learning approach for analysing weightlifting technique in novices. Front Bioeng Biotechnol 12:1426058. https://doi.org/10.3389/fbioe.2024.1426058

Ammar A, Trabelsi K, Boujelbane MA, Salem A, Boukhris O, Glenn JM, Zmijewski P, Jahrami HA, Chtourou H, Schöllhorn WI (2024d) The effects of contextual interference learning on the acquisition and relatively permanent gains in skilled performance: a critical systematic review with multilevel meta-analysis. Educ Psychol Rev 36(2):57. https://doi.org/10.1007/s10648-024-09892-z

Apidogo JB, Ammar A, Salem A, Burdack J, Schöllhorn WI (2023) Resonance effects in variable practice for handball, basketball, and volleyball skills: a study on contextual interference and differential learning. Sports (Basel) 12(1). https://doi.org/10.3390/sports12010005

Argyris JH, Faust G, Haase M (1994) Die Erforschung des Chaos. Heidelberg. Springer

Ashby WR (1947) Principles of the self-organizing dynamic system. J Gen Psychol 37(2):125–128. https://doi.org/10.1080/00221309.1947.9918144

Ay N, Der R, Prokopenko M (2012) Guided self-organization: perception–action loops of embodied systems. Theory Biosci 131(3):125–127. https://doi.org/10.1007/s12064-011-0140-1

Backman CL, Harris SR, Chisholm JA, Monette AD (1997) Single-subject research in rehabilitation: a review of studies using AB, withdrawal, multiple baseline, and alternating treatments designs. Arch Phys Med Rehabil 78(10):1145–1153. https://doi.org/10.1016/s0003-9993(97)90142-8

Baldwin TT, Ford JK (1988) Transfer of training: a review and directions for future research. Pers Psychol 41(1):63–105. https://doi.org/10.1111/j.1744-6570.1988.tb00632.x

Barker J, McCarthy P, Jones M, Moran A (2011) Single-case research methods in sport and exercise psychology. Taylor & Francis, London

Barlow DH, Hersen M (1984) Single case experimental designs: strategies for studying behavior change. Pergamon Press, New York

Barreiros J, Figueiredo T, Godinho M (2007) The contextual interference effect in applied settings. Eur Phys Educ Rev 13(2):195–208. https://doi.org/10.1177/1356336x07076876

Basedow JB (1774) Das in Dessau errichtet Philantropinum. Crusius

Bates BT (1996) Single-subject methodology: an alternative approach. Med Sci Sports Exerc 28(5):631–638. https://doi.org/10.1097/00005768-199605000-00016

Bates BT, Devita P, Kinoshita H (1983a) The effect of intra-individual variability on sample size. In: Nigg B, Kerr B (eds) Biomechanical aspects of sport shoes and playing surfaces. University of Calgary Press, pp 191–198

Bates BT, Osternig LR, Sawhill JA, James SL (1983b) An assessment of subject variability, subject-shoe interaction, and the evaluation of running shoes using ground reaction force data. J Biomech 16(3):181–191. https://doi.org/10.1016/0021-9290(83)90125-2

Battig WF (1966) Facilitation and interference. In: Bilodeau EA (ed) Acquisition of skill. Academic Press, New York, pp 215–244

Battig WF (1979) Are the important "individual differences" between or within individuals? J Res Pers 13(4):546–558. https://doi.org/10.1016/0092-6566(79)90015-1

Bauer HU, Schöllhorn WI (1997) Self-organizing maps for the analysis of complex movement patterns. Neural Process Lett 5(3):193–199. https://doi.org/10.1023/a:1009646811510

Bernstein N (1935) The problem of the interrelation of co-ordination and localization (in Russian). Arch Biol Sci 38:1–35

Bernstein N (1967) The co-ordination and regulation of movements, 1st edn. Pergamon Press, New York

Bi GQ, Poo MM (1998) Synaptic modifications in cultured hippocampal neurons: dependence on spike timing, synaptic strength, and postsynaptic cell type. J Neurosci 18(24):10464–10472. https://doi.org/10.1523/jneurosci.18-24-10464.1998

Böhm W (2004) Geschichte der Pädagogik: von Platon bis zur Gegenwart. Beck. München

Borrmann G (1956) Über die Entwicklung der Bewegungsfertigkeiten im Gerätturnen: ein Betrag zur Erforschung der Technik und der im Bildungsvorgang des Unterrichts auftretenden Bewegungsfehler und ihrer Ursache. PhDThesis. Deutsche Hochschule für Körperkultur. Leipzig. Germany.

Borrmann, G. (1964) Theorie des Turnens. Deutsche Hochschule für Körperkultur. Leipzig.

Bouchard C, Rankinen T (2001) Individual differences in response to regular physical activity. Med Sci Sports Exerc 33(6) https://journals.lww.com/acsm-msse/fulltext/2001/06001/individual_differences_in_response_to_regular.13.aspx

Bouchard C, An P, Rice T, Skinner JS, Wilmore JH, Gagnon J, Pérusse L, Leon AS, Rao DC (1999) Familial aggregation of VO(2max) response to exercise training: results from the HERITAGE Family Study. J Appl Physiol (1985) 87(3):1003–1008. https://doi.org/10.1152/jappl.1999.87.3.1003

Brady F (2004) Contextual interference: a meta-analytic study. Percept Mot Skills 99(1):116–126. https://doi.org/10.2466/pms.99.1.116-126

Brandt I, Reinken L (1988) The growth rate of healthy children in the first 16 years: Bonn-Dortmund longitudinal developmental study. Klin Padiatr 200(6):451–456. https://doi.org/10.1055/s--2008-1033752. (Die Wachstumsgeschwindigkeit gesunder Kinder in den ersten 16 Lebensjahren: Longitudinale Entwicklungsstudie Bonn-Dortmund)

Brooks GA (1985) Anaerobic threshold: review of the concept and directions for future research. Med Sci Sports Exerc 17(1):22–34

Brüggemann GP, Gattermann E, Göhner U, Janda H, Lampe L, Mester J (1992) Individualisierung der Skitechnik – Grundlage für gesundes, sicheres und freudvolles Skilaufen

Brunswik E (1939) Probability as a determiner of rat behavior. J Exp Psychol 25(2):175–197. https://doi.org/10.1037/h0061204.

Brunswik E (1955) Representative design and probabilistic theory in a functional psychology. Psychol Rev 62(3):193–217. https://doi.org/10.1037/h0047470

Burdack J, Horst F, Aragonés D, Eekhoff A, Schöllhorn WI (2020) Fatigue-related and timescale-dependent changes in individual movement patterns identified using support vector machine. Front Psychol 11:551548. https://doi.org/10.3389/fpsyg.2020.551548

Burdack J, Giesselbach S, Simak ML, Ndiaye ML, Marquardt C, Schöllhorn WI (2023) Identifying underlying individuality across running, walking, and handwriting patterns with conditional cycle-consistent generative adversarial networks. Front Bioeng Biotechnol 11:1204115. https://doi.org/10.3389/fbioe.2023.1204115

Buszard T, Reid M, Krause L, Kovalchik S, Farrow D (2017) Quantifying contextual interference and its effect on skill transfer in skilled youth tennis players. Front Psychol 8:1931. https://doi.org/10.3389/fpsyg.2017.01931

Button C, Davids K, Bennett SJ, Taylor MA (2000) Mechanical perturbation of the wrist during one-handed catching. Acta Psychol 105(1):9–30. https://doi.org/10.1016/S0001-6918(00)00044-5

Caporale N, Dan Y (2008) Spike timing-dependent plasticity: a Hebbian learning rule. Annu Rev Neurosci 31:25–46. https://doi.org/10.1146/annurev.neuro.31.060407.125639

Cattell RB (1945) The description of personality: principles and findings in a factor analysis. Am J Psychol 58:69–90. https://doi.org/10.2307/1417576

Cattell RB (1957) Personality and motivation structure and measurement. World Book, New York

Chapman R, Cope E, Richardson D, Littlewood M, Cronin C (2024) How did we get here; a historical and social exploration of the construction of English FA coach education. Sport Educ Soc 29(9):1133–1152. https://doi.org/10.1080/13573322.2023.2256754

Coltman SK, Cashaback JGA, Gribble PL (2019) Both fast and slow learning processes contribute to savings following sensorimotor adaptation. J Neurophysiol 121(4):1575–1583. https://doi.org/10.1152/jn.00794.2018

Cutting JE, Kozlowski LT (1977) Recognizing friends by their walk: Gait perception without familiarity cues. Bull Psychon Soc 9(5):353–356. https://doi.org/10.3758/BF03337021

Debanne D, Gähwiler BH, Thompson SM (1998) Long-term synaptic plasticity between pairs of individual CA3 pyramidal cells in rat hippocampal slice cultures. J Physiol 507(Pt 1):237–247. https://doi.org/10.1111/j.1469-7793.1998.237bu.x

Derrida J (2021) Deconstruction in a nutshell a conversation with jacques derrida, with a new introduction. Fordham University Press. https://doi.org/10.2307/j.ctv1198zt6

Devita P, Skelly WA (1990) Intrasubject variability of lower extremity joint moments of force during the stance phase of running. Hum Mov Sci 9(2):99–115. https://doi.org/10.1016/0167-9457(90)90022-6

Dewey J (1903) Democracy and education; the elementary school teacher, vol IV. The University of Chicago Press

Dewey J (1920) Reconstruction in philosophy. Henry Holt

Domjan M (2003) The Prinicples of learning and behavior, 5th edn. Wadasworth, Belmont

Drill R (1933) Untersuchungen über den Hammerschlag: ein Beitrag zur Analyse der menschlichen Arbeitsbewegungen. Beck. München

Duhem PMM (1954) The aim and structure of physical theory. Princeton University Press, Princeton

Ebbinghaus H (1913) Memory: a contribution to experimental psychology. Ann Neurosci 20(4):155–156. https://doi.org/10.5214/ans.0972.7531.200408

Farfel VS (1962) Wege zur Vervollkommnung der sportlichen Technik (Das methodische Prinzip der Schnellinformation). Teorija i praktika fiziskoj kultury 5:23–28

Feldman AG, Levin MF (2009) The equilibrium-point hypothesis–past, present and future. Adv Exp Med Biol 629:699–726. https://doi.org/10.1007/978-0-387-77064-2_38

Fink C, Preiß R, Schöllhorn WI (1998) How to find the optimal cutoff frequency for filtering kinematic data XVI. In: International symposium on biomechanics in sports Konstanz, Germany

Fink, C., Schöllhorn, WI., Jaitner, T. (1999) A more pragmatic criterion for filtering data. In: W. Herzog, A. Jinha (Hrsg.), Proceedings Of The XVII ISB Congress (S. 565). Calgary

Fisher RA, Russell EJ (1922) On the mathematical foundations of theoretical statistics. Philoso Trans R Soc Lond Ser A 222(594–604):309–368. https://doi.org/10.1098/rsta.1922.0009

Froebel FWA (1826) Die Menschenerziehung, die Erziehungs- Unterrichts- und Lehrkunst, angestrebt in der allgemeinen deutschen Erziehungsanstalt zu Keilhau. (Human education, the art of education, instruction and teaching, pursued in the general German educational institution at Keilhau) Wiebrad

Gaulhofer K, Streicher M (1924) Grundzüge des Österreichischen Schulturnens. Deutscher Verlag für Jugend und Volk. Wien

Gigerenzer G (2004) Mindless statistics. J Socio-Econ 33(5):587–606. https://doi.org/10.1016/j.socec.2004.09.033

Gigerenzer G (2018) Statistical rituals: the replication delusion and how we got there. Adv Methods Pract Psychol Sci 1(2):198–218. https://doi.org/10.1177/2515245918771329

Gollhofer A, Horstmann GA, Schmidtbleicher D, Schönthal D (1990) Reproducibility of electromyographic patterns in stretch-shortening type contractions. Eur J Appl Physiol Occup Physiol 60(1):7–14. https://doi.org/10.1007/bf00572179

Hacking I (1990) The taming of chance. Cambridge University Press, Cambridge

Haith AM, Krakauer JW (2014) Motor learning: the great rate debate. Curr Biol 24(10):R386–R388. https://doi.org/10.1016/j.cub.2014.03.077

Haken H (1988) Information and self-organization: macroscopic approach to complex systems. Springer, Berlin

Haken H, Kelso JA, Bunz H (1985) A theoretical model of phase transitions in human hand movements. Biol Cybern 51(5):347–356. https://doi.org/10.1007/bf00336922

Hamill J, McNiven SL (1990) Reliability of selected ground reaction force parameters during walking. Hum Mov Sci 9(2):117–131. https://doi.org/10.1016/0167-9457(90)90023-7

Hausdorff JM, Peng CK, Ladin Z, Wei JY, Goldberger AL (1995) Is walking a random walk? Evidence for long-range correlations in stride interval of human gait. J Appl Physiol (1985) 78(1):349–358. https://doi.org/10.1152/jappl.1995.78.1.349

Hausdorff JM, Purdon PL, Peng CK, Ladin Z, Wei JY, Goldberger AL (1996) Fractal dynamics of human gait: stability of long-range correlations in stride interval fluctuations. J Appl Physiol (1985) 80(5):1448–1457. https://doi.org/10.1152/jappl.1996.80.5.1448

Hebb DO (1949) The organization of behavior; a neuropsychological theory. Wiley, London

Heisenberg W (1927) Über den anschaulichen Inhalt der quantentheoretischen Kinematik und Mechanik. Z Phys 43(3):172–198. https://doi.org/10.1007/BF01397280

Henry FM (1959) Reliability, measurement error, and intra-individual difference. Res Q Am Assoc Health Phys Educ Recreat 30(1):21–24. https://doi.org/10.1080/10671188.1959.10613003

Hoitz F, von Tscharner V, Baltich J, Nigg BM (2021) Individuality decoded by running patterns: movement characteristics that determine the uniqueness of human running. PLoS One 16(4):e0249657. https://doi.org/10.1371/journal.pone.0249657

Holt KG, Hamill J, Andres RO (1991) Predicting the minimal energy costs of human walking. Med Sci Sports Exerc 23(4):491–498

Holt KG, Jeng SF, Ratcliffe R, Hamill J (1995) Energetic cost and stability during human walking at the preferred stride frequency. J Mot Behav 27(2):164–178. https://doi.org/10.1080/00222895.1995.9941708

Hopkins WG, Marshall SW, Batterham AM, Hanin J (2009) Progressive statistics for studies in sports medicine and exercise science. Med Sci Sports Exerc 41(1):3–13. https://doi.org/10.1249/MSS.0b013e31818cb278

Horst F, Kramer F, Schäfer B, Eekhoff A, Hegen P, Nigg BM, Schöllhorn WI (2016) Daily changes of individual gait patterns identified by means of support vector machines. Gait Posture 49:309–314. https://doi.org/10.1016/j.gaitpost.2016.07.073

Horst F, Eekhoff A, Newell KM, Schöllhorn WI (2017a) Intra-individual gait patterns across different timescales as revealed by means of a supervised learning model using kernel-based discriminant regression. PLoS One 12(6):e0179738. https://doi.org/10.1371/journal.pone.0179738

Horst F, Mildner M, Schöllhorn WI (2017b) One-year persistence of individual gait patterns identified in a follow-up study – a call for individualised diagnose and therapy. Gait Posture 58:476–480. https://doi.org/10.1016/j.gaitpost.2017.09.003

Horst F, Janssen D, Beckmann H, Schöllhorn WI (2020) Can individual movement characteristics across different throwing disciplines be identified in high-performance decathletes? Front Psychol 11:2262. https://doi.org/10.3389/fpsyg.2020.02262

Horst F, Slijepcevic D, Simak M, Schöllhorn WI (2021) Gutenberg Gait database, a ground reaction force database of level overground walking in healthy individuals. Sci Data 8(1):232. https://doi.org/10.1038/s41597-021-01014-6

Horst F, Slijepcevic D, Simak M, Horsak B, Schöllhorn WI, Zeppelzauer M (2023) Modeling biological individuality using machine learning: a study on human gait. Comput Struct Biotechnol J 21:3414–3423. https://doi.org/10.1016/j.csbj.2023.06.009

Horstmann GA, Gollhofer A, Dietz V (1988) Reproducibility and adaptation of the EMG responses of the lower leg following perturbations of upright stance. Electroencephalogr Clin Neurophysiol 70(5):447–452. https://doi.org/10.1016/0013-4694(88)90022-3

Howell JL, Collisson B, King KM (2014) Physics envy: psychologists' perceptions of psychology and agreement about core concepts. Teach Psychol 41:4. https://doi.org/10.1177/0098628314549705

Hribernik M, Umek A, Tomažič S, Kos A (2022) Review of real-time biomechanical feedback systems in sport and rehabilitation. Sensors 22(8):3006. https://www.mdpi.com/1424-8220/22/8/3006

Hubel DH, Wiesel TN (1962) Receptive fields, binocular interaction and functional architecture in the cat's visual cortex. J Physiol 160(1):106–154. https://doi.org/10.1113/jphysiol.1962.sp006837

Huber H (1977) Single case analysis. Behav Anal Modif 1:1–15

Issurin VB (2013) Training transfer: scientific background and insights for practical application. Sports Med 43(8):675–694. https://doi.org/10.1007/s40279-013-0049-6

Jaitner T, Schöllhorn WI, Ernst H, Mendoza L (1999) Individual changes of EMG patterns in learning a ballistic movment. In: The XVII Congress of International Scoiety on Biomechanics, Calagary, Canada

Jaitner T, Ernst H, Mendoza L, Schöllhorn WI (2001a) Changes of EMG patterns during motor learning of ballistic movements. In: XVIIIth Conference of the International Society on Biomechanics, Zürich, Switzerland

Jaitner T, Mendoza L, Schöllhorn WI (2001b) Analysis of the long jump technique in the transition from approach to takeoff based on time-continuous kinematic data. Eur J Sport Sci 5:1–12

Janacsek K, Fiser J, Nemeth D (2012) The best time to acquire new skills: age-related differences in implicit sequence learning across the human lifespan. Dev Sci 15(4):496–505. https://doi.org/10.1111/j.1467-7687.2012.01150.x

Janssen D (2017) Analyse und Klassifikation der Effekte unterschiedlicher Emotionsinduktionsmethoden auf das menschliche Gangmuster sowie den Übergang zwischen Gehen und Laufen, vol 9. Kovacs

Janssen D, Schöllhorn WI, Lubienetzki J, Fölling K, Kokenge H, Davids K (2008) Recognition of emotions in Gait patterns by means of artificial neural nets. J Nonverbal Behav 32(2):79–92. https://doi.org/10.1007/s10919-007-0045-3

Janssen D, Schöllhorn WI, Newell KM, Jäger JM, Rost F, Vehof K (2011) Diagnosing fatigue in gait patterns by support vector machines and self-organizing maps. Hum Mov Sci 30(5):966–975. https://doi.org/10.1016/j.humov.2010.08.010

Kast V, Leukel C (2016) Motor experts care about consistency and are reluctant to change motor outcome. PLoS One 11(8):e0161798. https://doi.org/10.1371/journal.pone.0161798

Kern G (1933) Motorische Umreißung optischer Gestalten. Neue Psychologische Studien 9:65–104

Kerschensteiner G (1912) Begriff der Arbeitsschule n der Pädagogik. Teubner. Leipzig

Kohonen T (1982) Self-organized formation of topologically correct feature maps. Biol Cybern 43(1):59–69. https://doi.org/10.1007/BF00337288

Kolb DA (1984) Experiential learning: experience as the source of learning and development. Pearson Education

Körndle H, Lippens V (1988) Do rowers have a particular 'footwriting'? In: Biomecahnics in sport, London

Kugler PN, Scott Kelso JA, Turvey MT (1980) 1 On the Concept of Coordinative Structures as Dissipative Structures: I. Theoretical Lines of Convergence**This work was supported by NIH grants HD 01994, NS 13617 and AM 25814. In: Stelmach GE, Requin J (eds) Advances in psychology, vol 1. North-Holland, pp 3–47. https://doi.org/10.1016/S0166-4115(08)61936-6

Lashley KS (1930) Basic neural mechanisms in behavior. Psychol Rev 37(1):1–24. https://doi.org/10.1037/h0074134

Latash ML (2021) Bernstein's construction of movements. Routledge, London

Levy WB, Steward O (1983) Temporal contiguity requirements for long-term associative potentiation/depression in the hippocampus. Neuroscience 8(4):791–797. https://doi.org/10.1016/0306-4522(83)90010-6

Lewin K (1935) A dynamic theory of personality – selected papers. Lewin Press

Lewis MD, Granic I (1999) Who put the self in self-organization? A clarification of terms and concepts for developmental psychopathology. Dev Psychopathol 11(2):365–374. https://doi.org/10.1017/s0954579499002102

Lippold T, Schöllhorn WI, Perl J, Bohn C, Schaper T, Hillebrand T (2003) Differenzielles Training im leichathletischen Sprint – Strukturierung von Sprintkoordinationsübungen mit Simulation und Optimierung eines Trainingsprozesses (BISP Jahrbuch 2003, Issue

Liu Y (1993) Kinematik, Dynamik und Simulation des leichtathletischen Sprints: Dissertationsschrift. Peter Lang

Locke J (1690) An essay concerning human understanding. Thomas Basset

Loeb, EE (1995) Control implications of musculoskeletal mechanics, In: Proceedings of 17th International Conference of the Engineering in Medicine and Biology Society, Montreal, QC, Canada, 1393–1394 vol. 2, https://doi.org/10.1109/IEMBS.1995.579743

Löwel S, Singer W (1992) Selection of intrinsic horizontal connections in the visual cortex by correlated neuronal activity. Science 255(5041):209–212. https://doi.org/10.1126/science.1372754

Mader A, Heck H (1986) A theory of the metabolic origin of "anaerobic threshold". Int J Sports Med 07(S01):45–65. https://doi.org/10.1055/s-2008-1025802

Magee JC, Johnston D (1997) A synaptically controlled, associative signal for Hebbian plasticity in hippocampal neurons. Science 275(5297):209–213. https://doi.org/10.1126/science.275.5297.209

Magill RA (1983) Insights into memory and control in motor behavior through the study of context effects: a discussion of Mathews et al. and Shea and Zimny. In: Magill RA (ed) Memory and control of action, vol 12. North-Holland, pp 367–376. https://doi.org/10.1016/S0166-4115(08)61999-8

Magill RA, Hall KG (1990) A review of the contextual interference effect in motor skill acquisition. Hum Mov Sci 9(3–5):241–289. https://doi.org/10.1016/0167-9457(90)90005-X

Mahlo F (1965) Theoretische Probleme der taktischen Ausbildung in den Sportspielen. Theor Prax Korperkult 14(9):809–815

McGinnis PM, Newell KM (1982) Topological dynamics: a framework for describing movement and its constraints. Hum Mov Sci 1(4):289–305. https://doi.org/10.1016/0167-9457(82)90017-3

Mendoza L (1993) Biomechanisch gestützte Techniksteuerung im Hochleistungssport. Sportbuch Strauß. Cologne.

Mendoza L, Schöllhorn WI (1990) Technical training in the field of high performance athletes with a biomechanical feedback system. In: Brüggemann GP, Rühl JK (eds) Techniques in athletics. Sport Buch Strauß, pp 412–419

Mendoza L, Schöllhorn WI (1991) Die Ansteuerung räumlihcer Merkmale der Diskuswurftechnik im Hochleistungsbereich mit Hilfe eines biomechanischen Schnellinformationssystems. Leistungssport 3:5

Mendoza L, Schöllhorn W (1993) Training of the sprint start technique with biomechanical feedback. J Sports Sci 11(1):25–29. https://doi.org/10.1080/02640419308729959

Mester L (1959) Gemeinschaftserziehung und Mannschaftsspiel. Das Spiel: Kongress für Leibeserziehung, 3–5 Oktober 1958 Osnabrück, Germany

Metallidou P, Platsidou M (2008) Kolb's Learning Style Inventory-1985: validity issues and relations with metacognitive knowledge about problem-solving strategies. Learn Individ Differ 18(1):114–119. https://doi.org/10.1016/j.lindif.2007.11.001

Meyer HC, Bucci DJ (2016) Neural and behavioral mechanisms of proactive and reactive inhibition. Learn Mem 23(10):504–514. https://doi.org/10.1101/lm.040501.115

Michalak J, Troje NF, Fischer J, Vollmar P, Heidenreich T, Schulte D (2009) Embodiment of sadness and depression–gait patterns associated with dysphoric mood. Psychosom Med 71(5):580–587. https://doi.org/10.1097/PSY.0b013e3181a2515c

Michon JA (1974) Programs and "programs" for sequential patterns in motor behavior. Brain Res 71(2):413–424. https://doi.org/10.1016/0006-8993(74)90985-8

Minors DSWJM (1981) Circadiane rhythms and the human. Wright PSG

Montessori M (1909) Selbsttätige Erziehung im frühen Kindesalter. Nach den Grundsätzen der wissenschaftlichen Pädagogik methodisch dargelegt. Julius Hoffmann. Stuttgart

Montévil M (2019) Measurement in biology is methodized by theory. Biol Philos 34(3):35. https://doi.org/10.1007/s10539-019-9687-x

Morgan DL, Morgan RK (2008) Single-case research methods for the behavioral and health sciences. Sage, London

Mosston M (1966) Teaching physical education: from command to discovery. C. E. Merrill Books, Columbus

Müller W (2004) Biorhythmik I: Circadiane Rhythmen und innere Uhren. In: Tier- und Humanphysiologie: Eine Einführung. Springer, Berlin/Heidelberg, pp 273–284. https://doi.org/10.1007/978-3-662-10555-9_13

Nejedly N (2020) Normal and abnormal growth in the pediatric patient. Curr Probl Pediatr Adolesc Health Care 50(3):100771. https://doi.org/10.1016/j.cppeds.2020.100771
Nelson DO (1957) Studies of Transfer of Learning in Gross Motor Skills. Res Q Am Assoc Health Phys Educ Recreat 28(4):364–373. https://doi.org/10.1080/10671188.1957.10612945
Newell KM (1986) Constraints on the development of coordination. In: Wade MG, Whiting HTA (eds) Motor development in children: aspects of coordination and control. Martinus Nijhoff, pp 341–360
Newell KM (1989) On task and theory specificity. J Mot Behav 21(1):92–96. https://doi.org/10.1080/00222895.1989.10735467
Newell KM (1991) Motor skill acquisition. Annu Rev Psychol 42:213–237. https://doi.org/10.1146/annurev.ps.42.020191.001241
Newell KM, Kugler PN, Van Emmerik REA, McDonald PV (1989) Search strategies and the acquisition of coordination. In: Wallace SA (ed) Advances in psychology, vol 61. North-Holland, pp 85–122. https://doi.org/10.1016/S0166-4115(08)60019-9
Neyman J, Pearson ES, Pearson K (1933) IX. On the problem of the most efficient tests of statistical hypotheses. Philos Trans R Soc Lond Ser A 231(694–706):289–337. https://doi.org/10.1098/rsta.1933.0009
Nichols B (1994) Moving and learning: the elementary school physical education experience. McGraw-Hill Inc., New York
Osgood CE (1949) The similarity paradox in human learning: a resolution. Psychol Rev 56(3):132–143. https://doi.org/10.1037/h0057488
Pedotti A (1977) A study of motor coordination and neuromuscular activities in human locomotion. Biol Cybern 26(1):53–62. https://doi.org/10.1007/bf00363992
Peirce CS (1883) Studies in logic. Little, Brown
Pestalozzi JH (1781–1787) Lienhard und Gertrud. Ein Buch für das Volk (Vol. 1–4). Georg Jakob Decker
Polani D, Prokopenko M, Yaeger LS (2013) Information and self-organization of behavior. Adv Complex Syst 16(02n03):1303001. https://doi.org/10.1142/s021952591303001x
Prigogine I (1980) From being to becoming: time and complexity in the physical sciences. W. H. Freeman
Prigogine I, Nicolis G (1971) Biological order, structure and instabilities. Q Rev Biophys 4(2):107–148. https://doi.org/10.1017/s0033583500000615
Prokopenko M (2013) Guided self-organization: inception. Springer, Berlin/Heidelberg
Proteau L, Marteniuk RG, Lévesque L (1992) A sensorimotor basis for motor learning: evidence indicating specificity of practice. Q J Exp Psychol Sect A 44(3):557–575. https://doi.org/10.1080/14640749208401298
Quine WVO (1953) From a logical point of view. Harvard University Press
Raibert MH (1978) A model for sensorimotor control and learning. Biol Cybern 29(1):29–36. https://doi.org/10.1007/BF00365233
Renshaw I, Chow JY (2019) A constraint-led approach to sport and physical education pedagogy. Phys Educ Sport Pedagog 24(2):103–116. https://doi.org/10.1080/17408989.2018.1552676
Rohmert W (1984) Das Belastungs- Beanspruchungs-Konzept. Zeitschirft für Arbeitswissenschaft 38:193–200
Rousseau JJ (1762) Emile, Ou De L' Education. Menard Et Desenne, Fils, Paris
Rovegno I, Nevett ME, Babiarz M (2001) Chapter 5: learning and teaching invasion-game tactics in 4th grade: introduction and theoretical perspective. J Teach Phys Educ 20:341–351
Saultz J (2020) Burnout. Fam Med 52(1):5–7. https://doi.org/10.22454/FamMed.2020.598170
Schmidt RA (1975) A schema theory of discrete motor skill learning. Psychol Rev 82:225–260. https://doi.org/10.1037/h0076770
Schöllhorn WI (1993a) Biomechanisch gestütztes Techniktraining im Diskuswurf. Leistungssport, 23 (2), 55–58
Schöllhorn WI (1993b) Biomechanische Einzelfallanalyse im Diskuswurf. In: Prozess- und produktorientierte Technikanalyse mechanischer Energieformen, vol 19. Harri Deutsch Verlag. Frankfurt
Schöllhorn WI (1993c) Process-oriented analysis of movement patterns. In: XIVth Congress of International Society of Biomechanics, Paris
Schöllhorn WI (1995) Time course oriented analysis of biomechanical movement patterns by means of orthogonal reference functions. In: XVth Congress of the international society of biomechanics, Jväskylä
Schöllhorn WI (1996) Topology and metrics of a ballistic grossmotor movement during a learning process. In: First conference on bernsteins traditions in motor control, University Park, PA, USA
Schöllhorn WI (1997a) Erkennung von Zustands- und Bewegungsmustern während eines Lernprozesses mit Hilfe eines generalisierten Ordnungsparameters. In: Bös K, Schmidtbleicher D, Müller A (eds) Sport im Lebenslauf. Czwalina, pp 302–306
Schöllhorn WI (1997b) Komplexe Bewegungskoordination systemdynamisch betrachtet (Complex movement coordination from a system dynamic perspective). In: Hirtz P, NSF (eds),Bewegungskoordination und sportliche Leistung integrativ betrachtet – 2. Bernstein-Konferenz. Czwalina, pp 66–75
Schöllhorn WI (1998) Systemdynamische Betrachtung komplexer Bewegungsmuster im Lernprozeß: Prozeßorientierte Strukturierung der Entwicklung eines Bewegungsablaufs (Dynamic system approach for the learning process of complex movement patterns). Peter Lang GmbH. Frankfurt
Schöllhorn WI (1999) Individualität – ein vernachlässigter Parameter. Leistungssport, 29 (2), 5–12

Schöllhorn WI (2016) Invited commentary: differential learning is different from contextual interference learning. Hum Mov Sci 47:240–245. https://doi.org/10.1016/j.humov.2015.11.018

Schöllhorn WI, Bauer H-U (1997) Linear – nonlinear classification of complex time cours patterns. In: 2nd Congress of European College of Sport Science Copenhagen

Schöllhorn WI, Bauer H-U (1998a) Assessment of running patterns using neural networks. In: Mester J, Perl J (eds) Sport und Informatik. Sport Buch Strauss, pp 169–176

Schöllhorn WI, Bauer HU (1998b) Identifying individual movement styles in high performance sports by means of self- organizing Kohonen maps In: 16 International symposium on biomechanics in sports, Konstanz. https://ojs.ub.uni-konstanz.de/cpa/article/view/1556

Schöllhorn WI, Bauer HU (1998c) Erkennung von individuellen Laufmustern mit Hilfe von neuronalen Netzen Informatik im Sport. Computer Science in Sport. In: Bericht ueber das Internationale Symposium vom 12–14. Juni 1997 in Koeln, Cologne. https://www.bisp-surf.de/Record/PU199809304244

Schöllhorn WI, Stefanyshyn D, Nigg BM, Liu W (1999) Recognition of individual walking patterns by means of artificial neural nets. International Meeting of the European Society for Movement Analysis in Adults and Children, September 23–25, 1999, Heidelberg, Germany Scientific Programme. Gait & Posture. 10, 49–91. https://doi.org/10.1016/S0966-6362(99)90392-2

Schöllhorn WI, Müller E, Lindinger S, Raschner C, Schwameder H (2001a) Individuality and Generality in ski turning techniques. In: Müller E, Schwameder H, Raschner C, Lindinger S, Kornexl E (eds) Second international Congress on science and skiing II. Dr. Kovac, pp 69–83

Schöllhorn WI, Römer J, Jaitner T (2001b) Comparing three volleyball spiking techniques by means of a process oriented pattern recognition approach. In: XVIIIth Congress of the International Society of Biomechanics Zürich, Switzerland

Schöllhorn WI, Nigg BM, Stefanyshyn DJ, Liu W (2002a) Identification of individual walking patterns using time discrete and time continuous data sets. Gait Posture 15(2):180–186. https://doi.org/10.1016/s0966-6362(01)00193-x

Schöllhorn WI, Schaper H, Kimmeskamp S, Milani T (2002b) Inter- and Intra-individual differentiation of dynamic foot pressure patterns by means of artificial neural nets. Gait Posture 16. S172. https://doi.org/10.1016/S0966-6362(02)00097-8

Schöllhorn WI, Beckmann H, Janssen D (2014a) Identification of transdisciplinary individual movement patterns. In: 19th annual ECSS Congress Amsterdam

Schöllhorn WI, Janssen D, Beckmann H (2014b) Identification of transdisciplinary individual movement pattern. In: 19th Annual Congress of the European College of Sport Science (ECSS), Amsterdam

Schöllhorn WI, Rizzi N, Slapšinskaitė-Dackevičienė A, Leite N (2022) Always pay attention to which model of motor learning you are using. Int J Environ Res Public Health 19(2). https://doi.org/10.3390/ijerph19020711

Schöner G, Haken H, Kelso JA (1986) A stochastic theory of phase transitions in human hand movement. Biol Cybern 53(4):247–257. https://doi.org/10.1007/bf00336995

Shea JB, Morgan RL (1979) Contextual interference effects on the acquisition, retention, and transfer of a motor skill. J Exp Psychol Hum Learn Mem 5(2):179–187. https://doi.org/10.1037/0278-7393.5.2.179

Shea C, Zimny ST (1983) Context effects in memory and learning moivement information. In: Magill RA (ed) Memory and CONTROL OF Action. North Holland, pp 345–366

Singer W (1993) Synchronization of cortical activity and its putative role in information processing and learning. Annu Rev Physiol 55:349–374. https://doi.org/10.1146/annurev.ph.55.030193.002025

Sokal AD (2016) Physics envy in psychology: a cautonary tale. New York University Press, New York

Spencer-Brown G (1953) Statistical significance in psychical research. Nature 172(4369):154–156. https://doi.org/10.1038/172154a0

Spencer-Brown G (1957) Probability and scientific inference. Longmans Green

Stachowiak H (1973) Allgemeine Modell theorie (General model theory). Springer

Steiner R (1907) Die Erziehung des Kindes: vom Gesichtspunkte der Geisteswissenschaft Rudolf Steiner Verlag

Stergiou N, Jensen JL, Bates BT, Scholten SD, Tzetzis G (2001) A dynamical systems investigation of lower extremity coordination during running over obstacles. Clin Biomech 16(3):213–221. https://doi.org/10.1016/S0268-0033(00)00090-5

Stern JM (2011) Spencer-brown vs. probability and statistics: entropy's testimony on subjective and objective randomness. Information 2(2):277–301. https://www.mdpi.com/2078-2489/2/2/277

Sust M (1996) Modulares deterministisches Modell menschlicher Bewegungen. In: Ballreich RBW (ed) Grundalgen der Biomechanik des Sports. Enke, pp 196–218

Sust M (2009) Hillsche Gleichung und die Sportwissenschaft – 70 Jahre Hillsche Gleichung. Spectrum der Sportwissenschaft 21(1):38–67

Terzuolo CA, Viviani P (1980) Determinants and characteristics of motor patterns used for typing. Neuroscience 5(6):1085–1103. https://doi.org/10.1016/0306-4522(80)90188-8

Thompson LA, Moreno MA (2018) Growth and growth charts in children. JAMA Pediatr 172(6):604–604. https://doi.org/10.1001/jamapediatrics.2018.0601

Thouless RH (1936) Test unreliability and function fluctuation. Br J Psychol 26:325–343. https://doi.org/10.1111/j.2044-8295.1936.tb00802.x

Tolman EC (1956) Egon Brunswik: 1903-1955. Am J Psychol 69(2):315–324. http://www.jstor.org/stable/1418173

Vitaterna MH, Takahashi JS, Turek FW (2001) Overview of circadian rhythms. Alcohol Res Health 25(2):85–93

Voigt R (1933) Über den Aufbau von Bewegungsgestalten. Neue Psychologische Studien 9:1–32

von der Malsburg C (1981) The correlation theory of brain function (Internal Report 81–2 Issue)

von Foerster H (1960) On self-organizing systems and their environments. In: Yovitz MC, Cameron S (eds) Self-organizing systems. Pergamon Press, pp 31–50

Wackerhage H, Gehlert S, Schulz H, Weber S, Ring-Dimitriou S, Heine O (2022) Lactate thresholds and the simulation of human energy metabolism: contributions by the Cologne sports medicine group in the 1970s and 1980s. Front Physiol 13:899670. https://doi.org/10.3389/fphys.2022.899670

Wagner H, Blickhan R (1999) Stabilizing function of skeletal muscles: an analytical investigation. J Theor Biol 199(2):163–179. https://doi.org/10.1006/jtbi.1999.0949

Wagner H, Blickhan R (2003) Stabilizing function of antagonistic neuromusculoskeletal systems: an analytical investigation. Biol Cybern 89(1):71–79. https://doi.org/10.1007/s00422-003-0403-0

Westphal O (1995) Normal growth and growth disorders in children. Acta Odontol Scand 53(3):174–178. https://doi.org/10.3109/00016359509005968

Whiting WC, Zernicke RF (1982) Correlation of movement patterns via pattern recognition. J Mot Behav 14(2):135–142. https://doi.org/10.1080/00222895.1982.10735268

Wiesel TN, Hubel DH (1963) Effects of visual deprivation on morphology and physiology of cells in the cats lateral geniculate body. J Neurophysiol 26:978–993. https://doi.org/10.1152/jn.1963.26.6.978

Wing AM (2000) Motor control: Mechanisms of motor equivalence in handwriting. Curr Biol 10(6):R245–R248. https://doi.org/10.1016/S0960-9822(00)00375-4

Winter DA (1984) Kinematic and kinetic patterns in human gait: variability and compensating effects. Hum Mov Sci 3(1):51–76. https://doi.org/10.1016/0167-9457(84)90005-8

Woodrow H (1932) Quotidian variability. Psychol Rev 39(3):245–256. https://doi.org/10.1037/h0073076

Woodworth RS, Thorndike EL (1901) The influence of improvement in one mental function upon the efficiency of other functions. (I). Psychol Rev 8(3):247–261

Wulf G, Lee TD (1993) Contextual interference in movements of the same class: differential effects on program and parameter learning. J Mot Behav 25(4):254–263. https://doi.org/10.1080/00222895.1993.9941646

Wulf G, Shea CH (2002) Principles derived from the study of simple skills do not generalize to complex skill learning. Psychon Bull Rev 9(2):185–211. https://doi.org/10.3758/bf03196276

Yang L, Armijo-Olivo S, Gross DP (2023) Single-case experimental design in rehabilitation: basic concepts, advantages, and challenges. Am J Phys Med Rehabil 102(5):454–460. https://doi.org/10.1097/phm.0000000000002215

Yin RK (1984) Case Study research: design and methods. Sage. London

Theoretical Bases of Differential Learning

2

Wolfgang I. Schöllhorn
and Agnė Slapšinskaitė-Dackevičienė

2.1 Introduction

After the basic assumptions of classical therapy and training had been deconstructed, the search for alternative models was required. It was helpful to look outside the box into areas of knowledge that deal with the transformation of systems. Here, too, it was important to go back to the origins and not rely on secondary interpretations.

Besides the practical experience collected as a high-performing athlete in different sports disciplines on national and international levels and as a high-performing coach and consultant of international top athletes, the theory of differential learning (DL) was influenced by several science disciplines. At the forefront are Bertalanffy's general system theory (GST), Wiener's cybernetics, Shannon and Weaver's signaling theory, von Foerster's cybernetic pedagogy or second-order cybernetics, neurophysiology, and reform pedagogy, as well as the knowledge of artificial neural networks (ANNs). A rough outline of the areas and their influence on DL is presented below.

2.2 Systems Theory and Cybernetics

After the deconstruction of the two basic assumptions of classical Physiotherapy (PT) and traditional training, it was necessary to look for alternatives that also correspond to the supposedly contradictory observations and experiences in everyday training and therapy. These should provide a different perspective on the problems of individuality and non-repeatability (low probability of identical repetitions). In addition, they should have neurophysiological equivalents to be able to integrate findings from this area, and they should be in accordance with the already existing models in sports pedagogy. Coming from biomechanics and physics, all approaches should not be limited to qualitative verbal models but rather should be supported by quantitative data.

An approach for the search for a different way of dealing with individuality is provided, on the one hand, by the reference to the minimum number of variables required and, on the other hand, by the differences between time-continuous and time-discrete analyses. In the first case, individuality could only be identified based on time courses of several biomechanical variables; in the

W. I. Schöllhorn (✉)
Institute for Sport Science, Johannes Gutenberg-University, Mainz, Germany
e-mail: schoellw@uni-mainz.de

A. Slapšinskaitė-Dackevičienė
Department of Sports Medicine, Faculty of Nursing, Medical Academy, Lithuanian University of Health Sciences, Kaunas, Lithuania

Faculty of Public Health, Health Research Institute, Medical Academy, Lithuanian University of Health Sciences, Kaunas, Lithuania
e-mail: agne.slapsinskaite-dackeviciene@lsmu.lt

W. I. Schöllhorn, A. Slapšinskaitė-Dackevičienė (eds.), *Differential Learning in Physiotherapy*,
https://doi.org/10.1007/978-3-031-98787-8_2

second case, pattern recognition based on time-continuous data was superior to recognition based on time-discrete data (Fink et al. 1999; Schöllhorn and Bauer 1998a, b, c; Schöllhorn et al. 2002). In both cases, the differences can be assigned to the same topic, a more holistic (several variables and time-continuous) view compared to a more atomistic (single variables and time-discrete) one.

The topic of holistic vs. atomistic observation or analysis has been a subject of science since Plato and is often associated with his quote, "*The whole is more than the sum of the parts.*" In modern times, this topic of whole and parts has been given a more differentiated, critical approach through works in evolutionary biology (Smuts 1926) and Gestalt psychology of perception (Köhler 1917; Lewin 1935; Wertheimer 1912) and subsequently with the general systems theory (GST) (von Bertalanffy 1935, 1950, 1951a, b, c, 1953), system dynamics (Forrester 1961), cybernetics (Wiener 1948), and information theory (Shannon and Weaver 1949).

Inspired by biology, the original systems theory has focused more on the structure and complexity of living systems and their transdisciplinary commonalities, whereas cybernetics has concentrated more on how systems function. Thus, cybernetics extended the early work in information theory on human communication language to messages for controlling machines and societies (Smith 1974). One branch of system theory, the original system dynamics approach, applied electrical engineering concepts to the understanding of the functioning of business and social organizations (Forrester 1961). GST and cybernetics have been developed mainly in parallel with a high degree of abstraction. The abstract level, on the one hand, was, and is, necessary to be able to transfer the developed models to many fields but, on the other hand, is associated with the disadvantage of frequently misusing the terminology to imply many things, as everyone can then interpret what suits them without having to be specific (e.g., Sokal hoax (Sokal 2000; Sokal and Bricmont 1999)). A similar problem concerns the discrediting of research areas, e.g., by some sport psychologists, who generalized findings that were based on their very first approaches and models, for whose purpose they were not developed (see General Model Theory (Schöllhorn et al. 2022; Stachowiak 1973)).

2.3 Cybernetics and Movement Science

Wiener's, Shannon's, and Weaver's approaches to cybernetics and signal theory were intended to be developed to find an abstract and general language for systems with analogous problems (Shannon and Weaver 1949; Wiener 1948). The feedback loop model had a major role in regulating machines. Despite references to the first applications of a feedback loop model by the Greek inventor and mathematician Ctesibius for the construction of the most accurate clock, up to the invention of the pendulum clock by the Dutch physicist Huygens in the seventeenth century (Nocks 2007), it was only the elaborations in the context of cybernetics that initiated extensive developments in this area. The feedback loop model was subsequently used in numerous areas, e.g., in the test-operate-test-exit (TOTE) model (Miller et al. 1960). Their analysis of the information content of a signal with an exclusively external observer, which explicitly did not deal with its meaning and relevance, was extended in the 1970s by von Foerster from "first-order cybernetics" to "second-order cybernetics" or "cybernetics of cybernetics" (von Foerster 1974), through which the internal observer or interpreter of the signal receiver was given an at least equally important role. Nonetheless, the original first-order cybernetics was applied more often in the field of movement research and, unfortunately, remained largely limited to this.

First-order cybernetics can be distinguished from second-order cybernetics based on seven arbitrarily selected aspects (Table 2.1).

2.3.1 Applications of First-Order Cybernetics in Motor Learning Research

According to the criteria in Table 2.1, the models discussed briefly below can be assigned to first-

Table 2.1 Differences between first-order and second-order cybernetics

	First-order cybernetics	Second-order cybernetics
Observer position	External and objective	Part of the system
System understanding	Focus on homeostasis and system equilibrium	Focus on change and self-organization
Controllability	Controllable through targeted stimuli	Recognition of the complexity and limited controllability of systems
Causality	Weak and strong linear causality	Nonlinear and circular causality
Concept of reality	Belief in objective, observer-independent reality	Emphasis on the subjective construction of reality
Therapeutic attitude	Therapist as an expert with control over the system	Therapist as a part of the system in a cooperative approach
Temporal classification	Dominated from the 1950s to the late 1970s	Development from the late 1970s

order cybernetics: the stochastic learning models of Estes and Brunswik (Brunswik 1939; Estes 1950), the models of technique training in sports science (Harre 1971), and the program-oriented models of sports psychology (Keele 1968; Schmidt 1975; Shea and Morgan 1979). Until the end of the last century, these were the dominant models in sports science and subjects of coach education. Together with selected models from sports pedagogy, they formed the starting point for the search for alternative models that could lead to other practical consequences. To avoid old knowledge being redeveloped under a different name and to be able to do something really new, you have to be familiar with the approaches that are used today and reflect on them correspondingly. A schema of the motor learning approaches that were most often used in sport practice is displayed in Fig. 2.1.

The approaches shown in Fig. 2.1 might give the impression that they are universal motor learning approaches that can be applied to all types of movements and at different stages of learning. However, a closer analysis based on scientific theories reveals that the learning models are linked to very specific assumptions (Fig. 2.2) (Schöllhorn et al. 2022). Some models were only intended for learning new movements, such as discovery learning, methodical exercise, and game series (Basedow 1774; Dewey 1903; Gaulhofer and Streicher 1924; Kerschensteiner 1912; Mahlo 1965). Others focused exclusively on the stabilization of already skilled movements, such as variability of practice (Schmidt 1975) and contextual interference learning (Shea and Morgan 1979). In contrast, the studies on proactive and retroactive inhibition focused on a shorter timescale of immediate interactions within a learning sequence (Osgood 1949; Smirnov 1973). Spacing, on the other hand, focused exclusively on the influence of pauses between learning units (Bjork and Allen 1970). The area of application of differential learning is discussed in more detail in Chap. 3.

2.3.1.1 The Statistical Learning Model

This model has been suggested by Estes (1950)) and is grounded in the idea that learning involves the formation of associations between stimuli and responses based on probabilistic principles. Over time, the probability of making a particular response to a given stimulus is adjusted based on the history of reinforcement learning. This model is classified as first-order cybernetics since learning is also based on feedback from the environment to update the probabilities of the stimulus (S)–response (R) relationship but widely neglects the perceiver's characteristics. Unlike traditional behaviorist models, which often assume fixed S–R relationships, Estes introduced variability into the learning process. Similarly, Brunswik's concept of representativeness relies on probabilistic reasoning to explain behavior (Brunswik 1939, 1955). Unlike strict behaviorists who reject internal processes outright, Brunswik acknowledged their existence but insisted that they should be studied in the tradition of behaviorism indirectly and empirically by analyzing how organisms use environmental cues. He avoided speculative models of the mind (common in early cognitive psy-

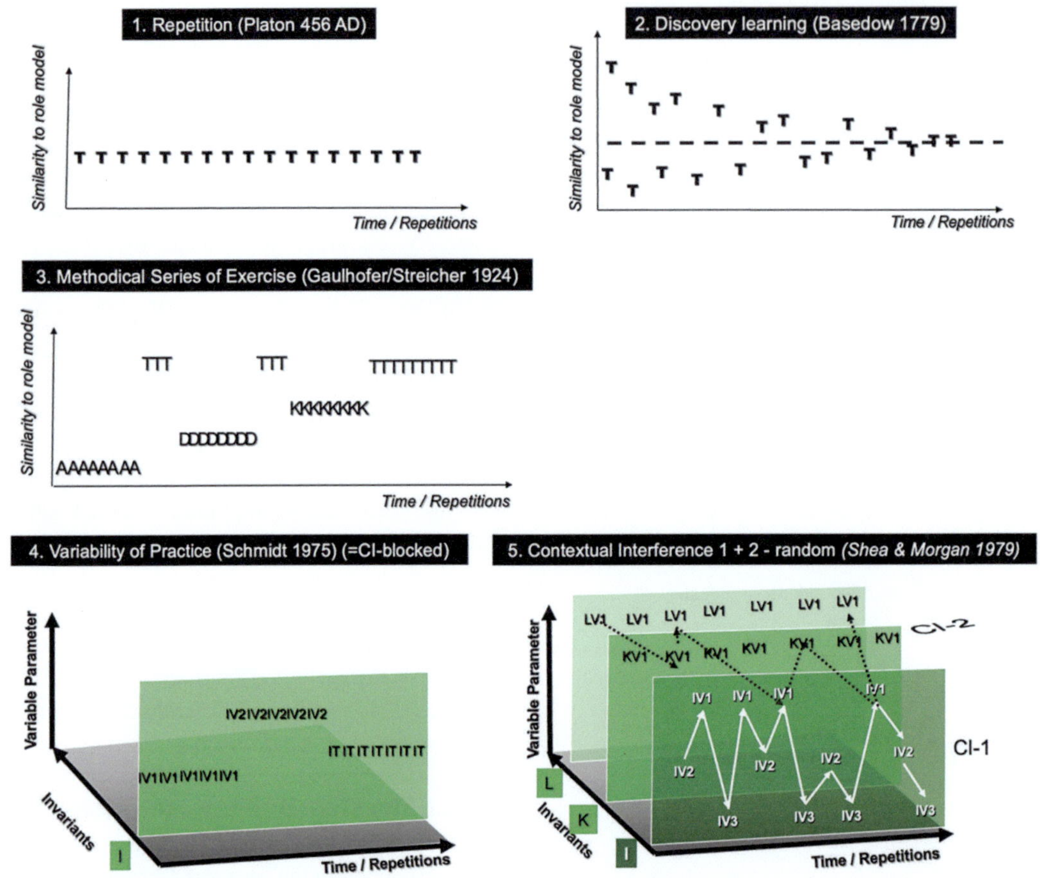

Fig. 2.1 Schemata of five motor learning models. CI: contextual interference, CI-1: contextual interference switching between variable parameters within the same invariant, CI-2: contextual interference switching between different invariants with different generalized motor programs (GMPs), IVi: invariant I with variable parameter Vi, KVi: invariant K with variable parameter Vi, LVi: invariant L with variable parameter Vi, T: target movement, and A, D, K: various exercises with increasing similarity to the target movement T

chology) and, instead, focused on how internal processes could be inferred from behavior in realistic, ecologically valid contexts. Estes models how learning adjusts to response probabilities based on reinforcement, while Brunswik analyzes how organisms use probabilistic cues to make decisions in an uncertain environment. By relying on probabilities, both models support the notion that learning requires many similar trials to uncover the underlying statistical relationships.

Significantly, reasoning based on probabilities requires memory and internal processing in the form of comparing new stimuli with the probability distribution of past events. It is difficult to reconcile both with the model of direct perception in conjunction with Gibson's affordance concept, which excludes internal processing. Interestingly, Gibson's background was in clinical psychology, where the individual was at the center, and he had a great enthusiasm for behaviorism and its methods to find more universal laws (Lobo et al. 2018). To avoid the usual overemphasis on external stimuli as pursued in behaviorism, he proposed the inseparability of the perceiver and the object of perception, which has recently drifted in the direction Gibson wanted to avoid through the shift toward invitations (Withagen et al. 2012). In addition, there are phenomena such as the spontaneous emergence of complex behaviors or patterns from simpler interactions, some-

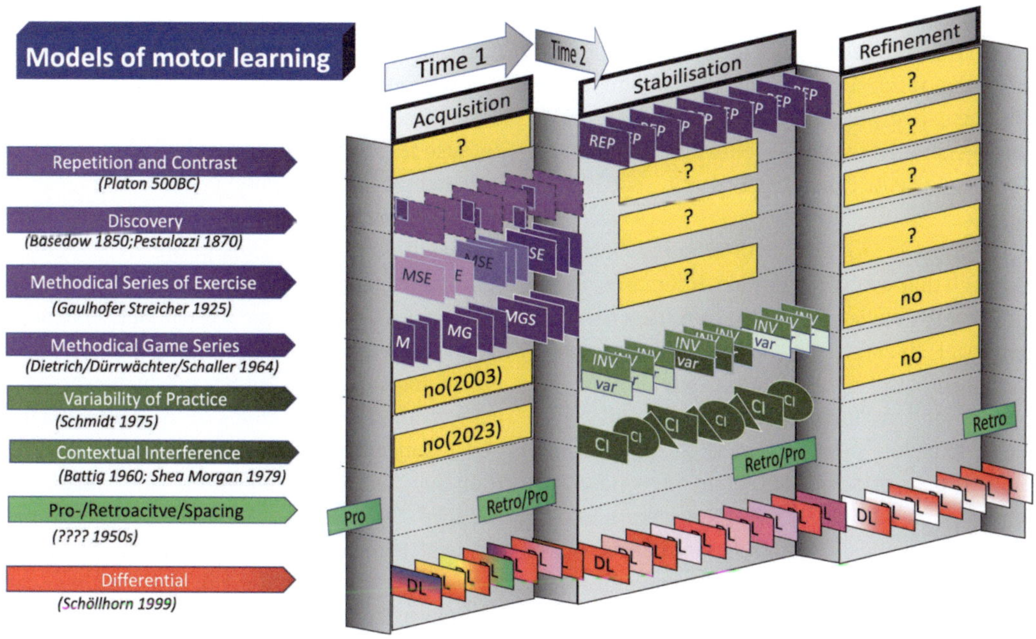

Fig. 2.2 Various motor learning models and their original purposes. Question marks correspond to missing research, and "no" corresponds to evidence based on selected studies

times in a surprisingly short time or without exhaustive trial-and-error learning, that could not be modeled with this probabilistic approach. Although internal processes were accepted, the exclusive investigation of behavior based on external stimuli in the tradition of behaviorism treated internal processes as a black box (Tolman and Brunswik 1935). The response R was exclusively modeled as a function of the stimuli S: R = f(S) (Estes 1950; Estes et al. 1959). Using the same probabilistic model, as proposed by Shannon and Weaver for modeling information, and neglecting the influence of the perceiving person, as already proposed by Lewin with B = f(E,P) (B: behavior, E: environment, and P: person), this model can also be assigned to first-order cybernetics. Although the knowledge gained primarily from animal experiments still neglected the active influence of the perceiving individual, which had already been introduced by Wundt's (Wundt 1874) apperception, it was only later permanently anchored in constructivism. In practical terms, the confrontation of variable stimuli for learning was a confirmation of the statements made in connection with the introduction of kindergartens, according to which healthy child development requires an enriched environment (Froebel 1826). Neurophysiological changes due to enriched environments, even in different ages, meanwhile, supported these phenomena (Dinse 2004; Godde et al. 2002).

One of the sport-related exceptions was the integration of Estes' findings for the justification of distributed practice and its advantages for learning by forgetting (Bjork 1994; Dinse 2004; Estes and Burke 1953).The growing difficulty in retrieving information as the time since the learning event increases not only reinforces the importance of distributed practice (Ebbinghaus 1913) but also inspires the concept of desirable difficulties for enhanced memory consolidation (Bjork 1994). With increasing time between the learning intervention and the posttest, memory tests became more difficult but led to greater learning effects in the long term. If the intervals passed a threshold and became too long, the effect was reversed. The associated optimal trend in difficulty served to generalize the phenomenon to the desirable difficulties. Although these were reformulated shortly afterward within the framework of a challenge point model (Guadagnoli and Lee 2004), both fell short of the original model of subjective information within the framework of cybernetic pedagogy in terms of their differentiation, generality, and theoretical underpinnings (Jumarie 1990; Pask 1975, 1992; von Cube 1965).

In contrast to the error-oriented learning approach that was still common at the time, deviations in the statistical model were described as numerical deviations in a value-neutral way. Mathematically, nonevaluative handling in the form of random fluctuations in the stimuli originating from the environment (Estes and Burke 1953) was considered neither in physiotherapy nor in sports training. Interestingly, the findings of Estes' statistical learning model (Estes 1950, 1955) were only given little consideration in these fields of research as well, although they anticipated some aspects that were later used again (Suppes 1992) in the context of the system dynamic model, with the addition of the random fluctuations (Schöner et al. 1986) of individual movements for the optimization of a learning process for perception.

2.3.1.2 Models from Training Theory and Training Science

The training theory of sports has its origins in the former Soviet Union and was shaped by the prevailing political system, in close connection with the Cold War (Harre 1971; Matveev 1964, 1981). Training theory is often also defined as "master theory," as it differs from training science due to its prescientific character. Training theory, which was primarily oriented toward high-performance sports and focused on Olympic medals, was structurally atomistic and normative. The atomistic approach assumed that complex athletic performance could be reduced to the smallest, fundamental units in a hierarchical model. The normative approach largely described how something should be and how to behave according to statistical average-oriented norms. This approach corresponds to the prescriptive approach in the field of physical education and psychomotor research in the Anglo-Saxon language area (Newell 1986) but in difference was supported by statistically determined norm values of the corresponding performance levels.

The constituent areas of holistic performance development included not only condition training but also technique and tactics training, as well as social and emotional content. The tactic area was the least developed, primarily for methodological reasons. Initially, problems in the area of classic technique diagnosis and technique control had the greatest influence on the DL model. Technique diagnosis was based on the biomechanical profiling of individual top athletes, which was compared with the mean values of the corresponding performance classes (Ballreich 1969, 1970, 1972; Ballreich and Baumann 1983; Bothmichel and Nehmer 1967; Gutewort et al. 1973). The biomechanical technique analysis or profiling, as the basis for the subsequent control process, was carried out using selected discrete-time characteristics, which allow changes within a topology but encounter problems when the topology changes during therapy or training. To partially compensate for this problem, the movements were divided into shorter phases. Individual performance profiles were regularly used for the training of top athletes and have been carried out extensively in the context of training science since the 1960s.

The subsequent and preparatory performance control (therapy and training) followed the logic of model-based learning within a control loop strongly influenced by the Russian physiologist Anokhin's concept of feedback (Anokhin 1935). The basic approach of control-loop learning based on discrete-time characteristics has been retained to this day, neglecting possible individuality both in the learning process and in the target value specification. The individual norm-oriented approach was transferred to physiotherapy very soon. The target values were and are derived from the mean values of the highest or the next highest performance or learning level class. In line with a limited scientific understanding of large samples (Choi and Nandram 2021; Gigerenzer 2004; Kaplan et al, 2014), only a few individual case studies of high-performing athletes (e.g., world record throw in javelin (Gregor and Pink 1985)) or a time series of individual cases (Schöllhorn 1993a, b) were published.

A versatile and comprehensive coordination training program, which consisted of a different number of specific coordinative skills depending on the author (Blume 1978; Fleishman 1954; Hirtz 1976, 1988; Rubinstein 1968), was considered the norm and long-term prerequisite for the technical perfection process of a top athlete. This was based on the idea of the ability–skill concept, to which a broader effect was ascribed in the case of abilities (e.g., throwing ability, jumping ability, and balancing ability) and a more specific effect in the case of skills (e.g., javelin-throwing skill and high jump skill). The largest number of motor abilities was identified by (Fleishman 1954) based on the results of having factor-analyzed 200 everyday and sport motoric tests. In the search for possible underlying general or "super" abilities comparable to the g-factor in intelligence research (Spearman 1904), the abilities to control, adapt, and motorically learn were suggested (Blume 1978). Interestingly, in both East and West Germany, the demand for versatile and varied exercise design—especially in school sports—was seen as an essential prerequisite for a successful athletic career. This approach followed the German tradition of the idealistic view of humanity from the Romantic period in the eighteenth century, emphasizing the need to develop adaptability and learning ability (Hirtz 1976, 1988; Paschen 1961). However, studies on a possible transfer of general abilities to specific skills have not yet led to any clear findings because of the high heterogeneity of study designs and various operational definitions of the abilities (Brachman et al. 2017; Kümmel et al. 2016; Lesinski et al. 2015). In contrast to motor abilities, which cannot be learned but can be trained, the more recent proposals for physical literacy in the United Kingdom of the post anti-sport Thatcher era (Whitehead 2001, 2007) and basic motor qualifications (Kurz et al. 2008) or basic motor competencies (Herrmann et al. 2015) in German-speaking countries are considered trainable but are more of a normative political requirement for sociocultural reasons in general than analysis of learning processes. Strangely, despite the varied and extensive efforts and requests since the 2000s, 80% of adolescents and 28% of adults do not reach the recommended levels of physical activity for health-related benefits (Hohberg et al. 2022; King et al. 2002).

While the classic models define a basic motor skill operationally, either theoretically derived or based on factor analyses, whose results depend on chosen exercises, and derive a mostly repetitive intervention from this and examine its effect on a specific skill, more recent approaches in artificial intelligence propose an alternative approach (Burdack et al. 2023; Horst et al. 2020). Pattern recognition algorithms are used to identify underlying commonalities of different movements (e.g., walking, running, and handwritings or shot put, discus, and javelin throws) at an individual level to make training more individualized and effective.

The different performance levels depending on the training process led, depending on the author, to an arbitrary subdivision of the continuous learning process into two (technique acquisition and technique optimization (Martin et al. 1991)), three (coarse, fine, and finest forms (Meinel 1960) and cognitive, associative, and autonomous stages (Fitts and Posner 1967)), and five (acquisition, refinement, consolidation, application, and variable disposition (Letzelter 1978)) learning phases, to which corresponding therapy, learning, and training contents were attributed. Not infrequently, the phase designations correspond more to normative activity regulations that reflect the current political education and teaching models than to a process that could also be observed in independent-from-external-control, individual, self-organized learning. Common to all phase-oriented models was the problem of precise phase delineation, which was closely linked to the problem of quantifying movement topologies. An alternative model was proposed more recently, with the two-phase model relying on the system dynamics of the amount of fluctuations with stabilization and adaptation (Tani et al. 2014).

Overall, the models originating from training theory and training science were closely linked to normative master doctrines, which were hierarchically structured and lacked alternative experimental studies on skill and ability acquisition.

Irrespective of this, the diversity of master teachings reflected a spectrum of creativity that provided a comprehensive basis for the hypotheses to be tested. With regard to motor learning, the main aim was to clarify the contradictions between sporting success through group-oriented, hierarchically and externally controlled models (Matveev 1964, 1981) and the models of individuality, versatility, and adaptability (Hirtz 1976, 1988; Paschen 1961).

2.3.1.3 Models from Sport Psychology

The Closed-Loop Model

The central element of early cybernetics was the control loop, most frequently explained using the example of the thermostat, with which a desired room temperature is specified. If the temperature falls below this, the room is heated; otherwise, it is not. In the field of motor control research, the control loop was used in the modeling of tendon reflexes, among other things (Wagner 1954). The closed-loop model in sport psychology was developed as an alternative to the open-loop model, in which each movement was assigned to a motor program (Keele 1968; Lashley 1951). The open-loop model mainly served to describe the phenomenon of overshooting movement that is observable in patients with an impaired cerebellum. In movement-oriented psychology, the closed-loop model was the prototype for modeling motor control processes (Milsum 1966). A first approach resulted in the test-operate-test-exit (TOTE) model (Miller et al. 1960) by means of an inner control loop while integrating cognitive–psychological processes. The control-loop model was also the inspiration for the closed-loop model of motor control for slow movements (Adams 1968), which, similar to the reafference model (von Holst and Mittelstaedt 1950), uses a copy of the movement plan in order to compare the movement result with it via a feedback loop and thus successively minimize the Ist-Sollwert (actual set point value) difference. So, cybernetics primarily offered an abstract model that was generalized from technical applications, and subsequently, various fields looked for possible applications. However, while the model had practical consequences for the construction of devices in technology, in other cases, it was mainly used to describe known phenomena in movement science.

Similarly, a transfer of the same model to an external control loop formed the basis for extensive research on motor learning, which became known mainly in the Anglo-Saxon-speaking world in the context of research on knowledge of result (KR) and knowledge of performance (KP) (Adams et al. 1975; Adams 1987) while in the Russian- and German-speaking communities it had already gained prominence under the concept of objective supplementary information. (Farfel 1977; Mendoza 1993). While in the inner control loop, the learners approach a predetermined target value based on feedback from their own sensory system and are therefore dependent on their own sensitivity, in the outer control loop, feedback is given by the therapist, trainer, teacher, or measuring devices. The latter is enjoying increasing popularity due to recent developments in the field of wearable sensors (De Fazio et al. 2023).

In addition to the danger of making learners dependent on too frequent external feedback (Wulf et al. 1993) or steering them in the wrong direction and ignoring their own sensory perception over time (Buekers et al. 1992), the multitude of aspects (e.g., information content, modality, precision, timing, and frequency) of information transfer during a learning process offers a wide range of possibilities for influence and experimentation, which have so far been largely neglected in research into individual characteristics. Besides this, a clear distinction must be made between research on augmented feedback and research on emotional feedback, which distinguishes between positive, negative, neutral, descriptive, prescriptive, corrective, affective, and comparative feedback (Silverman et al. 1992).

2.3.1.4 Positive Effects of Augmented Feedback Only with Repetitive Learning

In the research on augmented feedback, a rough distinction is made between two approaches. On the one hand, there is knowledge of result (KR), in which the learner only receives information about the result of the movement, and on the other hand, knowledge of performance (KP), in which information about the execution of the movement process is provided. While in the first case, there are a large number of studies with a positive influence on movements with a small number of degrees of freedom (sDGF) (for a review of these publications, see (Adams 1987)), such findings are much rarer in the second area. Notable exceptions include the work of Mendoza and Schöllhorn 1990, and 1993; as well as Smith and colleagues (1997). Generalizations to applications in physiotherapy that are problematic in terms of scientific theory emphasized the importance of repetition (Lee et al. 1991; Winstein 1991), albeit with a reference to a quote from (Bartlett 1932): "*When I make a stroke I do not, as a matter of fact, produce something absolutely new, and I never repeat something old.*" A most recent review on the comparison of KR and KP research indicates more advantages for motor learning when it is supported by prescriptive KP than by KR (Oppici et al. 2024). In this context of repetitions, in physiotherapy and training, it may also be more advantageous to provide information about the movement process and what is to be done instead of providing only the movement result.

With regard to DL, which, in its most extreme form, does not provide augmented feedback for several reasons, it is important to note that all studies on KR research were conducted with positive findings only in connection with and in comparison to repetitive learning (Adams 1987; Lauber et al. 2013). Doubts about a consistently positive effect of augmented feedback arose, above all, in practical application studies (Lee and Magill 1983; Salmoni et al. 1984; Silverman et al. 1992; Winstein 1991). In addition, the effects of KR seem to be dependent on age (Liu et al. 2013); children responded differently to feedback than adults. In this context, it is also still unclear whether the effects of KR learning on age depend on the learning history of the elderly, who have learned mainly through repetition. The same question arises in relation to the learning of infants, who learn most of their activities without augmented KR feedback. Both have, however, in common the fact that their bodies are subject to above-average rates of change. For babies, the explorative approach with increased noise seems to solve the problem, whereas the repetition approach, despite KR, does not seem to be supportive in the elderly.

Studies on the effect of ironic processes and erroneous feedback point to other problems, especially when feedback is combined with subsequent corrective instructions. In an ironic process, e.g., when receiving the instruction "*Don't think of a pink elephant,*" thought control can paradoxically lead to unintended outcomes, particularly when mental resources are strained. This effect has been shown in golf putting (e.g., "*Don't overshoot the glow spot*" (Wegner et al. 1998)), gaze behavior in penalty situations (e.g., "*Don't look beside the goalkeeper*" (Bakker et al. 2006; Binsch et al. 2010)), holding a pendulum (*Don't swing in x-axis direction* (Wegner et al. 1998)), and relaxation (e.g., "*I'd like you to continue to relax while …*" (Wegner et al. 1997)). We have similar conditions when exercises are corrected in the therapy or training process, and the errors are commented on by saying that they should not be done. The use of negation in the context of corrective instructions is a largely unexplored area, although there is clear evidence from psychological research of its detrimental effects (Wegner 1997). A similar detrimental effect of feedback is observable when giving erroneous feedback (Buekers et al. 1992). After 150 or 75 trials in two studies on an anticipation task, subjects performed according to the erroneous KR information, thereby ignoring their own sensory feedback, even after a 1-month or 1-week interval (Buekers et al. 1992).

Most recent studies provide evidence that external feedback is not necessary if the system has sufficient variation (Ramírez-Ruiz et al. 2024). This theory is supported by studies where no additive effect could be found by combining random contextual interference and augmented feedback (Wu et al. 2011). To what extent the lack of augmented feedback is the secret of effective learning in the youngest children during the first 2 years is open to speculation. Interestingly, toddlers learn the most and the fastest during this period, when they understand the least spoken language from others and are therefore unable to implement augmented feedback. Indications of possibilities for variation and possible sequencing within a longer developmental process are suggested and discussed in connection with the neurophysiological aspects. Despite numerous criticisms on the necessity and effectiveness of augmented feedback (Buekers et al. 1992; Lee et al. 1993; Silverman et al. 1992), the approach seems to be attractive to many therapists and coaches because it gives them the feeling of having control over the learning progress or at least being able to influence it.

Besides these critical and uncertain properties of feedback research, due to three other reasons, DL, in its most extreme form, relied on constantly creating situations that allow the learner to experience the effects directly and dispense with external feedback. First, learning should be a genuine, self-organizing process, where the learner will find their own solution, because the coach or therapist rarely knows what is best for the learner. This was supported by the second reason that exactly this phenomenon is observable when children are learning during the first 2 years of life, when they are not able to understand instructions from the parents, or when we learn to ride a bicycle. Parents are rarely seen teaching their children how to crawl or how to walk. No one could satisfactorily describe how to do it, and if they could, whether the description is an adequate guide is another problem. We need several trials with a few falls, and suddenly, we will make it, without having been told with how much force we must extend our knees in which direction. The same is the case with holding the head up and keeping it for 1 min in toddlers. One day they fail, and the next day, they are already adjusted to it and are able to keep it. The third reason is related to the anatomy and physiology of the brain. The understanding and processing of language happens in completely different areas and levels from the control of movement. Transferring cognitive knowledge in the form of language into ability is a very special process and does not appear to be absolutely necessary for abilities or skills. Children learn many movements before they begin to speak. On the other hand, language, with its sequential character, seems to be very limited in its ability to adequately describe complex movements with their highly parallel character and tends to slow down learning. Simply compare how long you would need to describe a walking step with the duration of executing one. This problem is also associated with implicit and explicit learning (Beek 2000).

2.3.1.5 The Variability of Practice Model by Schmidt (1975)

R. A. Schmidt, who was mentored by J. Adams, further developed the closed-loop model by modifying the two memory units and primarily by further differentiating the motor programs into invariant generalized motor programs that are combined with variable parameters by means of schemata. The variability of practice (VP) model, which was derived from the schema theory (Schmidt 1975), also contains the main characteristics of a closed-loop model. In addition, in this model, groups of movements are assigned common generalized motor programs (GMPs) (e.g., in the form of relative forces or relative timing) that are linked to variable parameters (e.g., absolute forces, absolute times, etc.) for the specific execution of the movement. The VP model recommends keeping the invariants (I) or GMPs constant and practicing a blocked variation of the variable parameters ($V_1V_1V_1V_2V_2V_2V_3V_3V_3$...). The invariant corresponds to a single-movement topology that is to be kept constant; only the metrics in the form of variable parameters should be varied in a blocked form. Both the closed-loop model of learning and the schema-based model originally served exclusively to stabilize an already mastered movement and therefore primarily represent more differentiated models for achieving the subgoals of the older model of the Methodical Series of Exercise (MSE) (Gaulhofer and Streicher 1924). The MSE model was an application of reform pedagogical learning principles to the learning of complex new movements. This learner-centered form of skill acquisition adapted the initial exercises to the learner's individual ability and skill level. From there, learners were able to gradually progress toward the target technique with various exercises. In contrast to this, the teacher-centered form of skill acquisition was the same for everyone and was prescribed by the teacher or trainer, regardless of the skill level.

2.3.1.6 The Variability of Practice Model Becomes Restricted to Movements Without Gravitational Influence

Initially, Schmidt claimed that the schema theory model was universally valid for all movements. However, he later had do admit that his model could not be applied to movements involving gravitational and inertial forces—such as everyday or sports movements—but only to relatively slow fine motor movements in the horizontal plane (most of which were executed on a table), where movements are primarily dominated by muscle forces (Schmidt 2003). Constantly changing gravitational and inertial forces lead to a continuous modification of the assumed invariants, such as the relative muscle forces and their relative timing (Schneider and Zernicke 1989; Schneider et al. 1989; Schöllhorn 1998). Notwithstanding the numerous unfulfilled claims, the schema theory model inspired numerous movement researchers (Lee et al. 2016). One of its findings anticipated what is now standard in artificial neural net research and was also used by the DL approach. The inter- and extrapolation aspect of DL comes from two studies that compared the VP approach with the repetition approach (Catalano and Kleiner 1984; Kerr and Booth 1978; Schmidt and Bjork 1992). When the transfer test was conducted within a practiced range (interpolation) (Fig. 2.3), the performance and performance gains were comparable to or better than the practiced range. However, when the transfer test was outside the practiced range (extrapolation)—(Fig. 2.3), they were significantly worse compared to the practiced range. The same can be observed when training artificial neural networks (Haykin 1994). Somehow, this aspect was not mentioned explicitly in the research on the VP model. For DL, it meant that during the learning process, the possible boundaries of the solution space had to be scanned to have a higher probability of interpolation afterwards and minimize extrapolation processes.

Overall, all models based on an internal or external control or learning loop traditionally

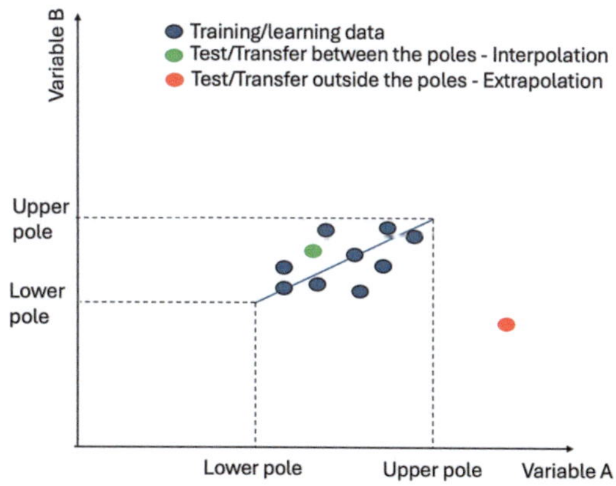

Fig. 2.3 Interpolation–Extrapolation

assume a person- and time-independent ideal. In the best case, the target value is adapted to age, body size, or learning level. Nonetheless, this is only an intermediate step toward individuality, and therefore, it is even more problematic to transfer it to individual treatment in physiotherapy. Errors must be avoided and minimized. Fluctuations are considered detrimental. How the learner minimizes the difference between the actual and target values, however, is largely up to the learner. The actual learning process is therefore most similar to the trial-and-error learning model (Ashby 1947, 1960), sometimes called discovery learning, which is interchangeably used with exploratory learning, which was fostered by reform pedagogy to allow the learners to find solutions on their own.

2.3.1.7 The Contextual Interference Model

Another model for motor learning within the framework of first-order cybernetics, in which the information coming from outside is the same for everyone, is the model of contextual interference (CI). The model of CI learning, or interleaved practice, which was developed at roughly the same time as the VP model, has its roots in the field of language acquisition research (Battig 1966). It is originally characterized by the fact that the repetition of a single sequence of letters to be learned (text) is interrupted by additional learning of other sequences of letters (con-text), thereby supporting learning. This led, after the eponymous context, to the second eponymous phenomenon of interference (Battig 1979). During acquisition, although there were disadvantages (interference) compared to blocked (CI-1: IV1, IV1, IV1, IV2, IV2, IV2, IV3, IV3 … within a single invariant or CI-2: I, I, I, K, K, K, L, L, L, ... with different invariants) learning immediately after the practice phase in random order (IV1, IV2, IV3, IV2, IV3, IV1, IV3, IV2, IV1… or I, K, L, L, K, I, K, L, I, … cf. Fig. 2.1), there were advantages (Fig. 2.4) in later memory tests. A transfer to fine motor movements (Shea and Morgan 1979), e.g., pressing key sequences or knocking over wooden blocks in a certain order, led to similar results (Brady 2004; Magill and Hall 1990).

With this transfer, it was no longer just the stabilization of a single learning object that was examined but the parallel stabilization of several movements, including those that were originally only intended as a context. In contrast to later approaches, it is essential here that, in accordance with the classic information-theoretic model by Shannon and Weaver, no deviations from the target movements are permitted, and incorrect executions must be repeated (Schöllhorn 2016; Shea and Zimny 1983). Advantages of the randomized exercise sequence on the results of the retention test could be shown for movements with sDGF, but the phenomenon of interference immediately after acquisition is rarely observed (Ammar et al. 2023). Systematic effects on the transfer of both CI phenomena to gross motor results have not yet been shown (Ammar et al. 2024). Isolated effects during sports movements (Goode and Magill 1986) are mostly associated with the use of specific working memories related to a focus on sequences with dominant visual–spatial content, as defined by Baddeley (2018), Baddeley and Hitch (1974).

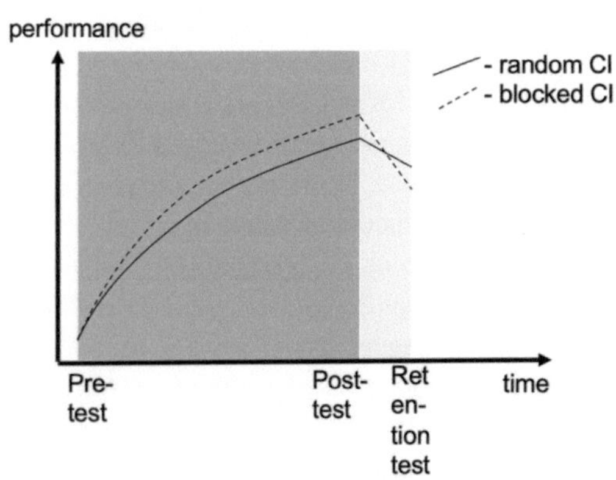

Fig. 2.4 Schematic performance development during the acquisition and retention phase with blocked and random sequences during acquisition

Three psychophysiological models have been proposed to explain the advantages of CI learning after the learning phase, during the retention tests. The elaboration model (Shea and Zimny 1983) assumes a more extensive exploration of the solution space due to the additional movements. The reconstruction model (Lee and Magill 1983) assumes that the positive effects on the learning phase stem from the constant redesigning of the movement plan to be learned. This model is often associated with the forgetting model (Lee and Magill 1985), which, however, contains the additional aspect that the movement plans must always be designed from changed initial conditions due to forgetting and, theoretically, only switched to the reconstruction model if forgetting is complete (Schöllhorn et al. 2022). However, the extent to which the overloading of working memory is a prerequisite for the three proposed models has not yet been clarified or addressed. Indirect evidence of both effects of CI from the neurophysiological side has so far only been provided by a few magnetic resonance imaging (MRI) studies (Lin et al. 2018), as the measurement methodology only allows small motor movements with sDGF.

The cause of the interference phenomenon immediately after the practice phase in the posttests is assumed to be an overload of the cognitive working memory when practicing in random order. The problem here is that the CI phenomenon occurs less frequently in children, for whom a smaller working memory can be assumed, and therefore, at least the first effect should be more pronounced (Apidogo et al. 2023). In addition, the effect is even reversed in DL, in which significantly more different movements are performed, including erroneous ones, during the practice process, which should lead to even more overloading of the working memory that should go along with an even larger decrease in performance after the acquisition phase. However, if one considers the fact that even repetitions cause larger fluctuations at the beginning of the learning process in children and beginners in accordance with the DL model, it becomes problematic to identify differences relative to variable CI training.

Another issue is likely due to an undifferentiated reliance on the prevailing model of working memory at the time, which was proposed by Baddeley and Hitch in 1974 (Baddeley and Hitch 1974). The original model for working memory is based exclusively on experiments on sequential, visual–spatial content. Studies by Goodale and Milner (1992) provided the first indications of a limited area of application for the working memory model. Baddeley himself recently confirmed (Baddeley 2018) that his model has not yet been tested for the processing and storage of sensory information in the areas of proprioception, kinesthetics, and tactile perception. A review of parallel processing of both areas is also still pending (Apidogo et al. 2023).

For physiotherapists, this information is particularly relevant, as much of our work involves proprioception, kinesthetic awareness, and tactile feedback. Relying solely on models of working memory developed from visual–spatial tasks might overlook key aspects of motor learning and rehabilitation. The gaps identified in the working memory model suggest that a deeper understanding of how the brain processes bodily sensations and movements in parallel could lead to more effective therapeutic interventions. Thus, it is important to remain open to new research that explores these specific cognitive processes, as it may have a direct impact on improving patient outcomes.

Although the concept of context is a central element of the structure of the exercise sequence, there have been few studies on this topic to date. Studies with up to six tasks practiced in parallel (Ollis et al. 2005) indicate no influence of the number of exercises on the CI effect. It would be of great interest to increase the number of exercises above the "magic number" of 7, as the chunking effects (Miller 1956) that might then occur could shed further light on the mechanisms of CI learning.

A possible influence of the similarity of the movement sequences to be learned is suspected (Wood and Ging 1991). When the exercise sequences had less visually determined, figurative similarity with each other, the CI effects were greater. The problem of the subordination of motor skills to the visual objective, as investigated in the Gestalt psychological work on the motor outline of visual shapes (Kern 1933), is not addressed (Apidogo et al. 2021). Walking and forming a word in the sand or snow or writing it with the hand or mouth only has visual correspondence in the result but very little motor correspondence. Neurophysiologically, the two activities are also assigned to different areas of the brain that can act widely independently of each other in different contexts.

The attempt to combine the variability of practice (VP) model with the CI model follows in a similar direction, based on phenomenological similarity. Here, the practice of different GMPs in randomized order, called high CI, led to clearer effects than the blocked variation within a GMP, which corresonds to classical VP, called low CI (de Croock et al. 1998). Interestingly, like the schema theoretical model, this could so far only be systematically observed for movements with sDGF. The fact that this may be reversed for movements with large number of degrees of freedom (lDGF) indicates an optimal amount of variation (Apidogo et al. 2023; Apidogo et al. 2021). In movements with lDGF (e.g., volleyball, handball, and basketball), randomized practice of more similar exercises, which correspond to variations within a single GMP, shows greater effects compared to repetitive practice than randomized practice of dissimilar exercises, which correspond to different GMPs (Apidogo et al. 2023).

The model of CI learning can be assigned to first-order cybernetics, as the characteristics of the learner are neglected and learning is assumed to take place independently of the learner's specificities through numerous repetitions, interrupted by other exercises, but nevertheless through repetition of an externally prescribed ideal. Feedback is given in the event of incorrect execution and must be repeated correctly to achieve the same number of correct repetitions (Shea and Zimny 1983). A more recent approach, in which there is a successively increasing frequency of alternation between a given number of exercises, e.g., from blocked to serial to randomized exercise sequences (Porter and Magill 2010), tries to exploit the principle of optimal learning by means of an optimal subjective information rate, as proposed in cybernetic pedagogy and second-order cybernetics, which will be explained in the subsequent chapter (von Cube 1965; Weltner 1970).

While in the methodical series of exercise (MSE) approach (Gaulhofer and Streicher 1924), the optimal subjective information rate is primarily regulated by a successive increase in the amount of subjective information to be processed in parallel, the progressive switching frequency in the increasing CI (iCI) approach modulates the amount of information to be processed successively. In contrast to MSE, where it is about the acquisition of new movements, the starting level is adapted individually, and the progress to the next level of difficulty is made dependent on the individual mastery of the lower-level exercise, in the iCI approach, all the movements need to be mastered from the beginning, and after a certain number of cycles, all learners progress to the next level. In addition, the problem of task similarity and the simultaneous close connection to subjective information are not considered in the iCI model.

From the perspective of cybernetic pedagogy, with the increasing disorder in the sequence in iCI, the subjective information rate should be kept at a corresponding level. Since the variance of the individual movements also increases with the alternation between two movements, the increasing disorder also changes the *noise,* as required by DL. A study comparing the execution variance of the first and the second tennis serves shows exactly this (Janssen et al. 2010). When the serves were executed in a blocked manner, the respective execution variance of both serves was significantly smaller than when the serves were executed in an alternating order.

The motor learning models provided by sport psychologists by the end of the last century either focused on the variation of movement metrics (variability of practice model) or neglected the relative similarity of movement topology (contextual interference model), although, with the recommendation of different GMPs for more effective CI learning, different topologies were used to stabilize single movements. Bernstein's famous quote about "*repetition without repetition*" was restricted to movement metrics because the possibility of quantifying movement topologies was misjudged, and all studies were conducted only on single movement topologies (Bernstein 1935, 1967). Furthermore, all these models were inadmissibly generalized to all types of movements because the specific model purposes were ignored (Schöllhorn et al. 2022) and the underpinning statistics were misinterpreted (Acree 2021; Ammar et al. 2023; Gigerenzer 2004, 2018; Schöllhorn et al. 2022). The individuality of movements served primarily as an excuse for unidentifiable groups and explain unexpected deviations from the average.

Whereas sport psychologists with a strong focus on visual perception research - and much of sports practice, particularly in the United Kingdom, influenced by the political climate under Margret Thatcher (1979 - 1990), when an estimated 5000 playing fields were sold -continued to follow the cognition-driven, teacher-centered model until the early 2000s (Simon 1999), sports pedagogy in mainland Europe had increasingly adopted the learner-centered model since the 1960s. Nation-specific and cultural differences can be traced back to the varying length and strength of military and political influences (Bowen 1919; Chapman et al. 2024; Virchow 2006). Despite some liberation from oppressive, dogmatic pedagogical methods since the 1970s in coach education (Chapman et al. 2020), until the twenty-first century, most coaches in the United Kingdom (Chapman et al. 2024) and many physical education teachers in the United States had a military background (Gordon and Newby 2019). Against this background and with limited access to non-English literature, to some extent, it is understandable that the democratic educational methods are being developed anew under a different name by sport psychologists from these countries.

From the perspective of traditional training control in therapy and sports practice, fluctuations were interpreted in both areas as errors and, when passing a certain threshold, indicated by classic error measures such as standard deviation or variance. Errors were interpreted as detrimental, which had to be avoided and minimized through corrections. In the case of fluctuations, they were referred to as functional variability, without specifying them in more detail, mainly to encode the fact that they were measured, but we do not know exactly what they were for. Giving a problem a name does not solve it. To distance oneself from the prescriptive instructions, the motor learning process was redefined as a "search strategy" (Newell et al. 1989) that had to be found by science. A problem here was the associated assumption of a concrete target movement that was to be found. First, the search had to be tailored to the individual learner, but no specifications for the criteria for finding it were provided. Second, nothing was said about what to do once the solution was found, and third, the temporal changes of the individual "solutions" were neglected as well.

Researchers in sports pedagogy and physical education conducted research in parallel to sport psychology but mainly separated from high-performance sports because of the different aims connected to the target groups, with few exceptions (e.g., (Newell and Rovegno 2021)). Sports psychology research was dominated by skill stabilization in performance sports and was strongly influenced by the legacy of research on optimizing assembly line work during the Cold War between the East and the West. In contrast, sports pedagogy focused primarily on the multifaceted aspects and the application of versatile methods from reform pedagogy of skill acquisition, with strong emphasis on learner-centered teaching, such as problem-based and discovery learning or the laissez-faire style of teaching (Brodtmann 1984; Mosston 1966). For a more extended discussion of the issues on physical education and sport pedagogy, see (Hardman and Green 2011; Kirk 2010; Kirk and Tinning 1990).

Until the turn of the millennium, in the field of sports psychology, only the models of repetition and contrast learning and exercise variability and contextual interference learning were being discussed (internationally), with practice recommendations in extracurricular exercise and sports research. Their model restrictions were largely ignored, and applications were recommended for all movements.

A model that could actually also be assigned to the field of psychological approaches and from which the idea of external focus (Wulf et al. 2000) was derived is the model of common coding (Prinz 1990) and its further development, the model of event coding (Hommel et al. 2001). Since both are very close to the theory of mirror neurons (di Pellegrino et al. 1992; Rizzolatti et al. 1996) and relate only to a single condition of a movement execution and not to the timing and content of the exercise sequence, they are discussed in Sect. 2.2 (neurophysiological principles).

Overall, apart from the fact that the models were only developed for movements with sDGF, the models of movement learning based on first-order cybernetics were characterized by the fact that they increase the variation of the metrics in the learning process but only to stabilize already mastered skills and not to acquire new skills or refine them, and it is assumed that the increased information is the same for all learners (Schöllhorn et al. 2022). While the variations in the VP model related exclusively to the movement metrics of a single movement topology (in movements with sDGF), the CI model suggested variations between different movement topologies but only to learn them exactly through repetition, with distracting interruptions.

2.3.2 Applications of Second-Order Cybernetics in Motor Learning Research

Von Foerster's (1974) introduction of second-order cybernetics not only established a connection to semiotics (Atkin 2008; Peirce 1991)—the study of the relationship between a sign and its meaning—and pragmatics, which examines the relationship between a sign and its interpreter, but also incorporated a subjective dimension into cybernetics. While Anglo-Saxon sport psychology research used the model of the cybernetic control loop (Miller et al. 1960) primarily to map motor control and steering processes onto learning processes from the perspective of an external observer in the sense of first-order cybernetics, cybernetic pedagogy in the Franco-German-speaking world focused more on the subjective aspects of the learner than on those of the internal observer (Jumarie 1978; Jumarie 1990; Ungerer 1971; von Cube 1965).

In contrast to the previously discussed learning models offered from sports psychology, a distinction was introduced in cybernetic pedagogy in the sense of second-order cybernetics between the given learning material and the prior knowledge of the learner in the form of *objective* and *subjective* information for modeling, teaching, and learning processes (von Cube 1965). This distinction was introduced with a delay in the theory of telecommunications as relative information (Jumarie 1990) and is now experiencing a renaissance in the context of educational cybernetics in connection with the latest technological developments around multimedia usage and e-sports (Bilek and Simanova 2012; Cope and Kalantzis 2022). While objective information corresponds to Shannon's definition (probability of occurrence of characters of an alphabet), that is to be distinguished from subjective information that is assigned to syntax, semantics, and pragmatics (Bischof 1995), or as Shannon and Weaver put it: "*Information is not to be confused with meaning*" (Shannon and Weaver 1949).

Transferred to a cognitive linguistic example of movement research, the term "motor equivalence" with its 14 letters would contain a certain amount of objective information. Subjectively, however, the information would be comparatively smaller for an educated movement researcher who knows that the term serves to describe the phenomenon of task-equivalent configurations of an effector (Lashley 1933). Applied to the motor domain, balancing on a beam, for example, objectively contains the same information for everyone. Subjectively, however, this task will contain different information for children and beginners in this area than for an Olympic champion in balance-beam gymnastics. Subjective information can therefore be understood as what is new for the individual learner. The proportion of known information on the part of the learner is understood as redundancy and, thus, learning as a gain in redundancy (von Cube 1965).

Against this background, the subjective information, the relatively new information, constantly decreases during repetition learning, whereas the objective information always remains the same. If a (complex) movement is newly learned, objective and subjective information are the same at the beginning of the learning process. With each repetition, the learner gradually becomes familiar with more and more parts of the movement, and the subjective information becomes less and less, whereas the objective information is still the same. The redundancy for the patient or learner, therefore, increases with each repetition, and less and less new information can be used for learning. When the movement is completely mastered, the redundancy is at a maximum, and the subjective information is minimized. Several studies point to an individually subjective amount of information for optimal learning rates (Miller et al. 1954; Weltner 1970).

While in the cognitive area, the alphabets (character sets) for letters (e.g., a–z) and numbers (e.g., 0–9) had already been created and were used to determine objective and subjective information (von Cube 1965), the situation with whole-body movements was, and is, somewhat more complex due to the lack of an alphabet. Isolated and highly simplified approaches proposed decisions for changes in the direction of individual movement sequences and segments as the basis for an alphabet for determining information in the context of movement (Ungerer 1971; Weltner and Ungerer 1973).

For application in the context of programmed learning as a derivative of cybernetic pedagogy (Farrell 1970; Neuman and Singer 1968), it was necessary to take prior knowledge into account. Without explicitly determining the subjective information, the prior knowledge or learning level in sports was determined by the mastery of exercises with varying degrees of difficulty, and the initial level was derived from this. The mastery of a learning step was mainly judged by its stability (or variance). Essentially, first, the methodical exercise and, later, the game series were transferred to programmed lessons (Daugs 1979; Fetz 1987; Hubert-White 1966; Kunze 1970; Neuman and Singer 1968; Ungerer 1971) with programmed instructions in physical therapy (McDaniel 1968) and physical education (Evaul 1964; Penman 1968; Vargas and Vargas 1991). A longer learning path was divided into subgoals, each of which was to be achieved by appropriate copying and repetition. The characteristic of each program-oriented learning series was the consideration of individual deficits at each learning step and self-pacing. Different error patterns still present after each repetitive exercise block were identified and forwarded accordingly to different sequences of movement tasks. What has recently been increasingly realized individually with smartphones and video feedback was already largely implemented with preprinted station cards at the time. One basic assumption, in line with the prevailing teaching approach at the time, was that all learners should ultimately arrive at a uniform solution and that the error patterns should be successively reduced along the various paths, also with video support (Dietrich 1969). Programmed learning should therefore always lead to the same goal in different but constrained paths. In line with the traditional teacher-oriented physical education, this approach was developed for the acquisition of unskilled movements or forms of games at schools. The learning steps were usually geared toward the slowest and weakest learners, and the pedagogical intention was for everyone to reach the specified target. Once the target technique or major game tactics had been achieved, there was only a choice of increasing the volume and intensity for further improvement, in line with the prevailing philosophy of training science, which was more strongly influenced by the military (Chapman et al. 2024).

More recent studies in physiotherapy, particularly in home-based (tele-)rehabilitation, have reintroduced this approach in a less individualized format. They generally find similar clinical effects between conventional and digital approaches, but reduced financial expenditure for the programmed digital intervention (Bennell et al. 2019; Cui et al. 2023; Fatoye et al. 2020; Lambert et al. 2017; Snoswell et al. 2020).

2.3.2.1 Models from Sport Pedagogy and Physical Education

Before we begin to classify sports pedagogy, we must first make a historical distinction between the education of adults (andragogy), primarily in connection with the military, and the education of children (pedagogy) at schools. While andragogy was primarily characterized by obedience education with many repetitions and punishments, the education of children at school was originally associated with musing, leisure, fun, and discussion. The application of the former to children at school is often confused with the latter. This has its origins, among other things, in the Age of Enlightenment, when children were regarded as small adults, and the primary aim of education was to turn children into intellectuals with adults' minds as quickly as possible. The application of andragogy methods, also known as black pedagogy (Rutschky 1977), is best classified as first-order cybernetics due to its similarity to behaviorism, in which the characteristics of the learner do not play a role.

Interestingly, in parallel to the period of implementing political doctrines, the reform pedagogy arose in the eighteenth century (Rousseau 1762) and shifted the focus from teacher-centered to learner-centered education. With the shift toward the learner, the original understanding of pedagogy experienced a renaissance and very soon made its way into physical education and sports training (Basedow 1774; Pestalozzi 1781–1787). By emphasizing the active role of the learner in building knowledge, adapting to feedback, and encouraging self-regulation, the second-order cybernetics was practically anticipated. In the fields of sports pedagogy and physical education in schools, various learner-centered models were known. Among these modes were the methodical series of exercise (Gaulhofer and Streicher 1924) and methodical game series (Mahlo 1965), which were both influenced by reform pedagogical thoughts on learner-centered teaching. Also, the model of teaching games for understanding (Bunker and Thorpe 1982) that combined the methodical game series with cognitive and psychologically guided discussion, the model of problem-based learning with its root in labor schools (Brodtmann 1984; Dewey 1903; Kerschensteiner 1912), and the model of open physical education (Brodtmann and Frankfurter Arbeitsgruppe 1982) were known. Interestingly, the spectrum of movement variants seen in these fields was mainly associated with different movement topologies that were only treated qualitatively and simply applied in practice. All these approaches originated from the practice of creative teaching in school and were more oriented toward the outcome of the learning process. Depending on the culture, physical education in schools was used to achieve different holistic goals. While the German "*Leibeserziehung*" had always included the holistic education of "body," "mind," and "soul" in German-speaking countries from the beginning of reform pedagogy, in many countries, the focus was much more constrained to the body part (e.g., "physical education"). An open question that was always topical in all these approaches was the question of when to take the next learning step and how big it should be.

2.3.2.2 Motor Learning: The Art of Relaxation

Deciding when to move on to the next exercise in the learning step sequence was generally determined based on the frequency of correctly executed movements and movement consistency. Therefore, the former can be defined by exceeding a higher threshold value of the latter. In the absence of quantitative measurement methods, both criteria were dependent on the visual sensitivity and threshold setting of the therapists, teachers, or trainers. While qualitative thresholds were always subject to subjective criteria, the phenomenon of movement consistency provides an approach for quantitatively determining and supporting the decision-making process, especially with the new pattern recognition methods combined with artificial intelligence methods.

From a biomechanical perspective, the constancy of movement in complex mechanical systems requires extensive damping elements to prevent its destruction through a reciprocal buildup of different forces (Zucca and Firrone 2014). The stiffer a system is, the more force transmission takes place. If you drop a wooden stick (high stiffness) lengthwise onto the ground, it will bounce up again. This will not happen if you drop a piece of rope (low stiffness) in the same way. Better long jumpers generally show greater muscle stiffness in the moment of takeoff than jumpers who are not as good. Nonetheless, if the directions of the forces are not coordinated through appropriate tension and relaxation of the necessary muscles, this leads to correspondingly large and undesirable movement amplitudes, which reduce the consistency of movement. Movement coordination can therefore also be understood as the art of targeted relaxation.

When babies see an attractive toy for the first time, the whole body reacts relatively uncoordinated, and the object of interest is not grasped in the expected way. In adults, on the other hand, all but the minimum necessary muscles are relaxed, and the object of desire is grasped with high precision (Thelen et al. 1993). A distinction must be made between the constancy of movement execution and the constancy of a possible movement goal (Beckmann et al. 2010), whereby an improvement in goal constancy can be accompanied by an increase in movement variance (Cowin et al. 2022). However, in this context, the joint-specific effects and different distinction thresholds were not considered (see Chap. 3). It should be noted that spatially, goal-oriented movements are only a subset of all movements. Numerous movements are oriented toward criteria such as speed maximization, energy or jerk minimization, or artistic expression (Flash and Hogan 1985; Nelson 1983; Viviani and Flash 1995).

2.3.2.3 Constancy of Movement: A Side Effect of Variable Learning Progress

The ability to repeat a movement with minor deviations has been considered an indicator of learning progress since the first records of learning processes. Unfortunately, this was also frequently regarded as the cause of success in most cases for a long time (Lee et al. 1991; Snoddy 1926). It was out of focus to consider the increasing constancy of a movement as a possible side effect of the deviations experienced. The first quantitative indications of a dependence of the learning level on movement consistency in sports in the long term were provided by the studies on Gestalt psychology (Voigt 1933), in which adults showed significantly less variation than children in an experiment on target long jumping. More recent studies on various sports provide evidence in the same direction (Bartlett et al. 2007; Marineau et al. 2024; Schorer et al. 2007; Wagner et al. 2012). Parallel to motor skills research, movement constancy was a fundamental component of medium- and long-term performance development in training practice. In contrast to physiotherapy, where it is more often about acquiring new patterns after injuries or surgery, in sports, it is more about refinement. Nonetheless, from a systemic point of view, it is only a different timescale with phases, where existing movement patterns are destabilized first (classical approaches would talk about being broken up), then the new elements are included, and at the end, the new elements are automated or stabilized again. In sports, this timescale can last several years, whereas in physiotherapy, the timescale is limited to the prescribed regimen. While in sports, normally attention is paid to movement constancy during an ongoing competition period, the time between competition periods is used to incorporate new elements into the movement technique, physical strength, or the team's tactical behavior. This period is usually associated with a loss of constancy of behavior. The athlete's behavior becomes unstable to regain more constancy of movements in the following competition period. In physiotherapy, e.g., a patient with chronic back pain may have adopted a stiff, guarded posture to avoid pain. The therapist begins by guiding and explaining to the patient how this posture is contributing to muscle imbalances and further discomfort. By demonstrating the benefits of improved mobility and showing the patient alternative, healthier movement patterns, the therapist "unfreezes" the patient's rigid reliance on their current habits. Once the patient is open to changing the movement habits, the therapist introduces core strengthening exercises, postural correction techniques, and stretches aimed at restoring balance and mobility. The patients are guided through this process, slowly integrating these new movements into their daily life, replacing the old, ineffective patterns. Lewin suggested a similar process in his model for changing social behavior, derived from the area of locomotion: unfreeze, change, and freeze again (Burnes 2020; Lewin 1947). Here, unfreezing can be seen as a destabilization of the system before the changing process is started to achieve a different stable state.

2.3.2.4 A Key Role in the Learning Process: Subjective Information Rate on Two Timescales

From a first-order cybernetic perspective, not only the objective information of the movement (I) is important in the context of a motor learning process, but also how quickly (dt) the information (I) must be processed during execution (timescale 1), i.e., the information rate ($R = dI/dt$). In contrast, in second order cybernetics where learning is about gaining redundancy, the focus is on subjective information (sI) that relates to new information for the individual learner dependent on the prior knowledge (Schöllhorn et al 2022). Regarding subjective information, in contrast to pure prior knowledge, a further subjective component is added here, namely the individual speed of retrieving known information during the movement sequence (timescale 2). When this subjective information, sI, is retrieved quickly (dt is small), the subjective information rate, $sR=dsI/dt$, is correspondingly increasing, as familiar information is accessed quickly, and vice versa. This has corresponding consequences for memory models in the context of movements and argues against a disjunctive separation of short-term and long-term memory in connection with movement control. A proposal to differentiate working memory into declarative and procedural working memory has been proposed recently (Oberauer 2009).

Of practical interest is the fact that the subjective information rate can be changed by the speed of a single movement execution ($dsI/dt_{movement}$) and by the number of stimuli presented ($dsI/dt_{var.mov}$), which could also be varied with the same speed of movement. The subjective information rate can also be varied with the amount of subjective information (sI), e.g., by the number of parallel or sequential movements and by the number of movement consequences. As movement speed increases, the required rate of sensory processing increases. If the speed remains the same, this subjective information rate can be increased by more parallel stimuli, visual, acoustic, and proprioceptive. This varies for the motor action, which is dependent not only on the **muscular forces** but also on the **gravitational** and **inertial** forces. In consequence, passively guided and actively performed movements in different directions provide a rich source of variable training for the central nervous system (CNS).

On a longer timescale that relates to learning step design in the context of methodical exercise or game series, the subjective information rate ($dsI/dt_{sequence}$) can also be controlled by the size of the learning step to the next, more advanced, or simply different exercise. This step is dependent on the similarity of the movements and the time between executing them. If the learner (patient or athlete) is overwhelmed by a step that is too large or with too short a break in between, i.e., the subjective information rate becomes too big, the learner usually responds by reducing the subjective information by stiffening subareas to adapt the subjective information rate to the available processing capacity. Stiffening subareas by fixing the corresponding joints is, in turn, accompanied by a reduction in damping behavior during complex movements, which leads to correspondingly larger amplitudes at the end of the movement chain. This is reflected in a decrease in the consistency or smoothness of the movement and can often be observed in sports or therapy practice in neuromuscular fatigue processes. If patients or athletes become mentally tired, e.g., toward the end of a therapy session or a game, gait, sprinting, and running movements are often observed with increasing unsteadiness in the upper body movements, which indicates a decrease in the ability to adapt flexibly or a lack of compensation for a wide range of forces in the trunk area (Möhler et al. 2021; van Dieën et al. 2012). However, the response could also be the opposite because it depends on the experience of the learner. When the patient is used to relaxed states, this provides less subjective information and will be preferred. The neglect of an individual patient's or learner's history and the connected amount of subjective information rate may explain ambiguous findings related to the model of freezing and unfreezing degrees of freedom (Guimaraes et al. 2020).

In contrast to repetition learning, with variable learning, the objective information is often changed correspondingly, and thus, the subjective information rate is kept at a higher level in the long term, thereby increasing the chance of learning. The coordination of the variation of the objective and subjective information or the objective and subjective information rate with an individually optimal level can be interpreted as the adjustment of two signals. This can be displayed as a resonance curve, in which the extent of variation that occurs in the exercise sequences associated with the learning models is plotted against the learning rate in the form of, for example, increasing or decreasing movement consistency. If we consider the known motor learning approaches, such as exercise sequences with different temporal and content-related variations (Schöllhorn 2005; Schöllhorn et al. 2006, Schöllhorn et al. 2009), and their effect on the learner's movement constancy in the movement to be learned, this should lead to different responses with an optimum for a certain range of variation of an exercise sequence, according to the different subjective information rate. If there is too much variation in a short period, the rate of subjective information becomes too high, while too little variation results in a rate that is too low for optimal learning. In summary, the optimum noise not only depends on the individual and situation but also on the complexity of exercise (sequential-parallel, metrics-topology, left-right, upper-lower body, etc.), the speed of movement execution (slow-medium-fast, etc.), and the time structure of the exercise variations (linear, stepwise, saw tooth, square wave, random, etc) including break durations between.

Future research should determine whether classical measures of movement consistency and practice variability are more suitable for this purpose than complexity-based metrics (Hausdorff et al. 1996; Stergiou 2004; Strogatz 1994). Various entropy measures (e.g., sample, distribution, and permutation entropy) to describe the disorder in a time series, which can be used to describe an exercise sequence, are suitable due to their proximity to Shannon's original definition of information. Originally proposed by Boltzmann to describe disorder in gas molecules, entropy is now closely associated with information (Shannon and Weaver 1949). In Shannon and Weaver's information theory, the entropy as a measure for disorder is used as a measure of the expected amount of objective information required to describe the state of the variable, considering the distribution of probabilities across all possible states. In difference, second order cybernetics relates more to Wiener's interpretation of information where information increases with growing order, namely the negentropy. Learning then corresponds to gaining internal order.

Analogously, the exercise variation can also be presented in relation to achieved performance, learning progress, performance increases, or learning rates, which are often chosen as a measure of learning success. Regardless of the representation, both variables can be understood as stochastic functions that need to be coordinated within the framework of a therapy or learning process. In the DL model, this was described as stochastic resonance (Beckmann and Schöllhorn 2006; McDonnell et al. 2008; Schöllhorn et al. 2006). As it became apparent early on that the individual optimum for exercise variation depends on numerous individual factors, such as emotions, fatigue, and music (Horst et al. 2016, 2017a; Jäger et al. 2003; Janssen 2017; Janssen et al., 2008, 2011), it was assumed that there is a corresponding temporal adjustment of the variety of exercises, as described in studies with adaptive stochastic resonance (Krauss et al. 2017; Mitaim and Kosko 1998). In addition to individuality, the individual situation must also be considered here. The above-mentioned machine learning (ML)-supported analysis methods based on process-oriented data provide promising tools for this purpose. By considering the aspects of subjective Information rate as well, the optimum noise not only may depend on the individual and situation but also on the complexity of exercise (sequential-parallel, metrics-topology, left-right, upper-lower body, etc.), the speed of movement execution (slow-medium-fast, etc.), and the time structure of the exercise variations (linear, stepwise, saw tooth, square wave, random, etc) including break durations between the exercises and between the sets. Whether all these variants can be described by different colors of noises needs to be shown in future research.

2.3.2.5 Motor Learning by Amplifying Errors

One approach that first became internationally known with the publication of Milanese (Milanese et al. 2016; Milanese et al. 2008) and could be considered close to DL is the approach of Movement learning through the Amplification of Errors (MAE). This approach, originally developed in the 70 s and 80 s of the last century by Bragagnolo (1928–2018), formerly a professor at the University of Verona, largely corresponds to contrast learning, the second form of learning mentioned by Plato, and serves not to explain to the athlete what is correct but to allow them, similar to DL, to directly feel the consequences of the error so that they can correct it themselves. Due to the continuous adaptation of interventions to the individual's errors, this approach could be classified as a second-order cybernetic approach. However, the prerequisite for this would be that the errors can also lead in an unexpected direction as a target movement. If it remains pure contrast learning, it would rather be classified as first-order cybernetics. In contrast to DL, however, the approach is still based on the dichotomy of right and wrong and is highly dependent on the experience and visual perception of the coach, as feedback and practice focus only on the largest errors identified by the coach. However, it remains unclear what must happen once the errors have been eliminated and when they are no longer errors. Independent of how to continue, by executing the contrast, the noise level is increased too, not only by scanning the probable border of the boundary conditions but also by coming back to the "correct movement," similar to the CI approach. By switching between "wrong" and "right" movements, the noise of the wrong version and the noise of the right version are increased and would train the underlying neural network for more stability.

The MAE approach claims to combine motor learning with the Far Eastern philosophy of being in the moment to make movement learning more effective by bypassing consciousness (Scemma 2020). The exact connection between reinforcing mistakes and staying in the moment is not explained in detail but rather formulated as an inspiration. Both DL and MAE have their origins in the training practice of high-performance sports, where these topics have been connected for long, especially in Far Eastern martial arts. Meanwhile, DL offers a bridge between the fluctuations and Far Eastern mental states. This will be discussed in Chap. 3.

2.4 Systems Theory and Movement Science

Systems theory, with its origins in biology, the science of living systems, is the transdisciplinary study of systems. From early on, the general system theory (GST) was developed to overcome the overspecializations of modern times, unraveling the commonalities of different sciences. Originally conceived analogous to cybernetics and information theory, as a bracket for all sciences and as a meta-language, more recently, highly specialized systems theories have increasingly developed again, mostly in ignorance of their roots, and thus, actually contradict the original idea of a holistic view in system thinking.

Systems theory is an approach originally published in German by the Austrian biologist and philosopher Bertalanffy in the 1930s and derived from ancient Greek (*systema*—"*whole composed of several parts*"), in which the fundamental principles of systems are used to describe and explain complex phenomena. Systems are understood as "*complexes of elements in interaction to which certain system laws can be applied*" (von Bertalanffy 1968). A system divides the world into two parts: Inside the system is everything that is enclosed, and outside is everything that is not enclosed (Tranquillo 2019). Going beyond the theory of single systems in biology, physics, or society, systems theory is a science that deals with the comparative study of systems across disciplines.

This very general formulation implicitly refers to analogies at different levels of observation, according to which each subsystem can, in turn, consist of further subsystems. In systems theory, a distinction must be made between two mental operations for this process: abstraction and interpretation (Bischof 1995). Abstraction should ensure that (a) the quality of the system variables is not considered and (b) the determination of the system processes remains at least partially open. Interpretation as a downstream thought process consists of (a) assigning foreign qualities to the variables as meaning and (b) understanding the processes as intended by the system (Bischof 1995). Both operations are essential for a transfer between different science disciplines, e.g., the behavior of heated liquids to the behavior of cyclic finger movements and, from these, to learning processes.

Bertalanffy placed particular emphasis, as a system characteristic, on strong (Rapoport 1966) and nonlinear (Simon 1962) interactions, which often elude a linear cause–effect relationship through circularity due to nonlinear feedback. This, for example, is the case in therapies when dealing with patients and the patient or athlete can no longer move due to pain, but the symptoms get worse and worse without movement. Concrete examples are tendinopathies or fear avoidance. For example, Achilles tendinitis is another example where nonlinear interactions occur. Overloading the tendon can cause inflammation and pain, but under-loading (through rest) can lead to tendon weakening, reducing the tissue's ability to handle stress. This creates a loop where both overuse and disuse lead to further injury. Another example of nonlinear feedback can be observed in the fear avoidance model. Some patients with musculoskeletal injuries develop a fear of movement (kinesiophobia) due to the belief that it will worsen their pain or injury. This fear leads to avoidance behavior, causing muscular atrophy, joint deconditioning, and even psychological distress, all of which contribute to increased pain and functional limitations.

With the GST, cross-disciplinary similarities and relationships were integrated within science, whose "prototype of their description is a set of coupled nonlinear differential equations," which, with few exceptions, are not uniquely solvable (von Bertalanffy 1951a, 1968). Interestingly, Bertalanffy constantly emphasized the mathematization of the systems models. Verbal models were not preferred and only considered as a start but "... *were better than nothing*" (von Bertalanffy 1968). In contrast to the differential equation for unrestrained exponential growth that is used for describing the behavior of different simple systems, e.g., viruses and algae, or the interest in compound interest calculation, the coupled differential equations for the description of a predator–prey relationship as an example for a more complex system have dynamic solutions, which can be modeled by the Lotka–Voltera equations.

For the description of interdisciplinary similarities, typically analogies and morphisms are used, which are also applied in topology (Vitiello 2014). Analogies are understood as explanations that relate something that is not yet understood to something that is understood, and isomorphisms are used when common characteristics, structures, and organizational forms of indifferent systems coincide (Skyttner 1996), i.e., when there are formally identical laws that govern the functioning of materially different phenomena. Only partial correspondences are referred to as homomorphisms. In case of self-similarity, as an endomorphism and a specific case of isomorphism, structural equality within the same system but on different scales in time or space of observation is described.

More recently, the demand for more holistic considerations, especially in specific parts of sport psychology, is frequently used in the context of emergence. Interestingly, the neologism of holism, as introduced by Smuts (1926), already encompassed the phenomenon of emergence since holism, according to this understanding, is defined precisely by what is new beyond the sum of its parts. Emergent phenomena are said to arise from and be sustained by more fundamental phenomena while, at the same time, exerting a "*top-down*" control, constraint, or other kind of influence on those very sustaining processes. For some critics, this has an air of magic about it, as it seems to suggest a kind of circular causality (Kim 1999). Philosophical debates about emergence are often characterized by ambiguity and a lack of common ground (Taylor 2015). Typically, the concept of emergence is used when no certain kind of scientific explanation is available to an observer (Taylor 2015). In sum, **holism** and **emergence** are terms that are used when the observer switches between levels of observations within systems and, therefore, are rather metaphysical phenomena (Corradini and O'Connor 2010; Drack and Pouvreau 2015; von Bertalanffy 1968).

2.4.1 Open and Closed Systems

With the distinction between closed and open systems, the definition of the system and its boundaries implicitly defines its environment and additionally indicates the necessity of exact definitions of the boundary conditions for scientific studies and models (Hempel 1951; Von Bertalanffy 1950). The environment of a system is not to be confused with the environment in everyday language, as Bertalanffy, as an educated biologist, was precisely concerned with viewing living beings and their environment as two elements of the same system. Open systems were originally characterized only by the exchange of matter between a system and its environment. Mainly, a system's environment was considered to be those variables that were or could not be included in the system's momentary analysis. What at first glance may sound plausible, especially regarding the reproducibility of experiments, turns out to be somewhat more problematic on closer inspection and against the background of parallel and later research.

Based on parallel developments that have taken place in the course of the generalization process of provisional systems theory in the field of self-organization since the 1940s (Ashby 1947; von Foerster 1960), the classification of open and closed systems has since undergone further differentiation. When there is no exchange with a system's environment at all, we are talking about self-sufficient systems. Closed systems allow temperature exchange, and in open systems, besides material exchange, informational exchange must also be differentiated.

In a transfer to therapy and training, these distinctions are particularly important in relation to the forms of interaction between the therapist and the patient or the coach and the athlete. While in the first case, the patient or athlete is left completely to their own possibilities and energy resources, in the second case, unstructured energy is supplied to allow the learner to find their own structure. This is done either by the problem-based learning approach (Brodtmann 1984; Heinrichs 2002), where only the problem is given, but the solution is to be found by the patient/athlete by means of the available boundary conditions, or by one of the DL strategies, where many movement variations (diffuse energy) around the possible solution are offered or requested, without giving exact information about an eventual discrete solution. This, in general, also includes not giving information on being right or wrong, which would include discrete information about the expected solution and, therefore, is guidance and no more self-organization. Here, feedback is to be distinguished from emotional encouragement. The same applies to the supply of materials. If this is supplied in the form of food to generate energy for muscle contraction or thinking, it is still regarded as a self-organizing system. But if the material supplied contains discrete information about a specific movement of an athlete's baseball racket, foot positioning, or restricting a patient's trunk movement by means of a corset, then specific information about specific solutions is provided from outside (therapist or coach) for the externally given order. This corresponds to material aids in methodical series of exercise, guides the system to an intended goal, and therefore, is an externally controlled system (Prokopenko 2013). If material aids are used to restrict movements or feedback is given for errors, then it is no longer a self-organizing system. For learning or therapeutic processes, this is of interest because different effects of self-organized and guided learning in the long term are increasingly discussed. A tendency toward longer-term advantages of self-organized learning seems to be crystallizing (Oftadeh et al. 2021). Movements that have been learned in a self-organized manner, such as walking or bicycle riding, appear to be stable for longer than movements that have been instructed and learned through many repetitions.

In a broader sense, this whole classification in the learning–teaching system, which could be analogously transferred to the field of therapies as well, can be associated with the spectrum from learner-centered to teacher-centered education at the most extreme ends of a scale, with all its gradations in between (Mosston 1966). Similarly, the reciprocal interaction in a therapy process can be described with a scale from exclusively patient-centered to therapist-centered and all its gradations in between. The extent to which certain combinations of personalities influence the process and success of therapy would be of great interest from a systems theory perspective (Childre et al. 2007; McCraty and Childre 2010). Studies in the field of brain research indicate individual reactions in connection with these forms of teaching; i.e., some react with stress in the self-sufficient form and others in the teacher-centered form of interaction (Reeve and Lee 2019). The interaction between people, in general, is increasingly becoming the focus of research interest since Bronfenbrenner's transfer of Lewin's field theory to ecological sociology (Tudge et al. 1996).

2.4.1.1 Person and Environment as Elements of One System

Against this background, the structuring of intervention possibilities according to the organism, environment, and task (Magill 1983; Newell 1986) served as a pedagogically valuable and inspiring framework for coaches, teachers, and therapists, summarizing the interventions used up to that time. However, in later interpretations, it did not significantly advance research into the complex interactions between humans and their everyday environment. Essentially, only the approaches from sports pedagogy were transferred to training in competitive sports, with slightly modified terminology. The suggested model represents a section of Lewin's model (Burnes 2020; Lewin 1935), which depicted the diversity of human behavior as an interaction between the environment and the person under a wide variety of possible personal and sociological conditions. Gibson and Bronfenbrenner, in their ecological approaches, were inspired by the work of Lewin, the first in perception and the second in social interactions (Tudge et al. 1996). More recent lip services to the inseparability of the individual and the environment ("perceiving affordances" - despite inseparability of individual and environment) in primarily environment-related interventions within narrow interpretations of the suggested model, disguised in the form of affordances, may give therapists and coaches a feeling of having the therapy or coaching process under control, but actually, it only follows the original affection for behaviorism that Gibson already had (Lobo et al. 2018). A closer look to the origins shows that affordances are mainly a renaming of application of the resonance principle to perception (e.g. "... perception is governed by the brain so that the whole system of input and output resonates ..." (Gibson 1966) - see also "perceptual resonance" in Schütz-Bach and Prinz 2007). From a pragmatic and scientific point of view, this makes a distinction from behaviorism and its assumption that behavior is a reaction to a stimulus problematic. Ultimately, in terms of practical consequences, it becomes confusing with regard to scientific progress in sciences such as pedagogy, which have been dealing with teaching and learning processes for quite some time, when the same practical recommendations have long been available with different terminologies (Basedow 1774; Dewey 1903; Froebel 1826).

In addition to the category error—where the task functions as a mediator, as a specific form of behavior, between the organism and the environment, rather than being an equal category (Hackfort 2017; Nitsch and Hackfort 2016)—there are several aspects to consider. These aspects complicate the distinction between the human subsystem and the environmental subsystem, making a strict separation problematic. In principle, movements of any physical body on the Earth are influenced by gravitational forces, which are a measure of the attraction between two masses and, therefore, cannot be separated per se. Energy is always consumed to overcome the gravitational force, which is accompanied by temperature and gas exchange and, therefore, always involves an exchange of energy and material with the environment. It is therefore often assumed in movement analyses that changes in these latter parameters occur on longer timescales and can be neglected in momentary biomechanical analyses. Conversely, environmental temperature fluctuations affect muscle activation and flexibility, while metabolic heat from movement raises local ambient temperature and humidity, creating a feedback loop between performer and environment. (Bell and Ferguson 2009; Decostre et al. 2005; Malak et al. 2023; Ranatunga et al. 1987). Recent studies in the field of nerve stimulus conduction even indicate a high dependence on mechanical conditions and the temperature of the neuron (Heimburg 2022a, b), which, in turn, depends on the temperature exchange with the environment.[1]

Furthermore, if we also consider more recent findings in the field of biological and terrestrial/planetary interactions (Alabdulgader et al. 2018; Jaruševičius et al. 2018; McCraty et al. 2017; Danho et al. 2025; Schöllhorn et al. 2022), to which we have not yet been able to assign any known direct sensory system in humans, problems with a precise distinction between person and environment as two separate systems become obvious. These more recent examples merely broaden the spectrum of interactions and essentially confirm the need for a holistic view, as has been pursued since the Gestalt theory (Wertheimer 1925), the systems theory (Von Bertalanffy 1950)

[1]A general requirement of Hempel and Oppenheim since 1948 (Hempel, C. G. 1965). *Aspects of Scientific Explanation and Other Essays in the Philosophy of Science*. The Free Press, Hempel, C. G., & Oppenheim, P. (1948). Studies in the Logic of Explanation. *Philosophy of Science*, *15*(2), 135–175. http://www.jstor.org/stable/185169) within the scheme named after them is, to list all boundary conditions that describe both the initial conditions and the intervention conditions to ensure the reproducibility of experiments in science. This was, and is, also true for sports science. Turning this process around and marketing it as a new approach that is guided by constraints indicates a problematic understanding of scientific theory and serves to confuse rather than enlighten.

and the approaches to a more holistic perception derived from it (Gibson 1979), and the eco-sociological approach (Bronfenbrenner 1983).

Depending on the mental state of a person, corresponding physiological changes can be observed in another person or animal (McCraty 2003). The mental states are reflected in corresponding changes in heart activity, which, in turn, leads to a change in the associated heart magnetic field (McCraty 2022). These appear to be identical up to a distance of 1 m with the heart magnetic fields of other people. In addition, several studies have indicated that heart rate variability is influenced by fluctuations in the Earth's magnetic field, which, in turn, is massively manipulated by the solar wind (Russell 2000). If one compares the magnetic field strengths of these systems, the assumption of large-scale interactions is obvious. The Earth's magnetic field fluctuates in a range of 10^{-6} Tesla; for comparison, MRI or fMRI scanners have a magnetic field strength of 1.5–12 Tesla. The magnetic field strength of the heart is in the range of 10^{-9} Tesla, and that of neurons is in the range of 10^{-15} Tesla. Initial indications of the influence of the Earth's magnetic field on brain activity are provided by a study by Ruhenstroth-Bauer and coworkers (Ruhenstroth-Bauer et al. 1993; Wang et al. 2019). The influence of magnetic fields on neuronal growth is already being used in the field of rehabilitation research (Khan and Cohen 2019; Polak and Shefi 2015).

Based on these recently developed physical measurement methods, the more recent findings impressively confirm numerous statements that were theoretically derived a long time ago based on observable phenomena. Against this background, Lewin's equation of behavior, as a function of the interaction of person and their environment, and his complex topological approach, in which both are regarded as inseparable, interacting subsystems in every behavior, takes on a much broader meaning. For Lewin, perception was controlled by individual needs, and his idea of perception was a more asymmetrical act, in which the environment is relativized to one's own possibilities. This idea was shifted normatively by Gibson (1979) toward a symmetry of the perceiver and the environment with a direct perception. While Gibson's model describes the interdependence of the subsystems of the person and the environment in a symmetrical way, the models of Lewin (1935)), von Foerster (1974), and Stachowiak (1973) shift the asymmetry toward the person with second-order cybernetics and the General Model Method, including its epistemological basis of pragmatism, without neglecting the whole (Stachowiak 1973). Philosophical developments in connection with constructivism and findings from neurophysiology point in the same direction (Quartz and Sejnowski 1997; Westermann et al. 2007). To illustrate this, the metaphor of an elephant is often used, which is studied by scientists from different fields to demonstrate the dominant influence of the perceiver despite the same object being presented.[2]

In light of ongoing debates about affordances—including the "invitation" reading and behaviorist drift (Chemero, 2001; Oliver, 2005; Withagen et al., 2012)—these findings raise a systems-level question: do nonconsciously perceived factors that modulate performance count as affordances, or are they background conditions shaping effectivities? Proposed mechanisms—prenatal neurodevelopment influenced directly by geomagnetic fields or indirectly via magnetically modulated maternal cardiac rhythms—remain speculative and underdetermined without independent measurement/manipulation in ecologically valid tasks and preregistered mediation analyses. Moreover, if affordances are "quicksilvery" (Chemero and Turvey, 2007)—"affordances are dynamic and fleeting"—the concept risks eluding scientific verifiability and sliding into unfalsifiability. The commitment to direct perception is also strained by acoustic orientation an basic spatial vision: perceived distance depends on binocular dispar-

[2]The interdependence of humans and their environment was already an early topic in experimental perception research. Perception (germ. *Wahrnehmen*) was no longer understood merely as a passive influx of stimuli but as an active process that is controlled to the highest degree by the perceiver, which is reflected (at least) in the German root of the word: "*Sich das Wahre nehmen*" (engl. Taking the truth). It is an active process, which inspired Wundt (Wundt, W. M. (1874). *Grundzüge der physiolgischen Psychologie*. Engelmann. , ibid.) to introduce the term "apperception."

ity and vergence-based computations that compare the two retinal images to recover depth—an inferential process rather than unmediated pickup. Unless affordances are operationally distinguished from internal computations and generic state variables (e.g., arousal, temperature, circadian phase), extending the label to every performance-relevant factor obscures the very boundary the theory aims to clarify. Systems theory, with its roots in biology, was conceived and developed for such examples, which are characteristic of living beings.

2.4.2 From Static to Dynamic Systems Theory

While static systems do not change their state within the timescale of interest, dynamic systems are subject to change over time. In dynamic systems theory, the change of the system over time is the focus of interest. Similar to the relativity of stable and unstable, static and dynamic are to be understood relative to the timescale under consideration. Static systems can change but on a much larger timescale compared to dynamic systems. Static systems are, therefore, in a quasi-equilibrium state, while dynamic systems are far from equilibrium. Hereby, the dynamics of time should not be confused with dynamics as a physical force.

The concept of system dynamics originally goes back to Forrester's modeling of business processes in the 1950s (Forrester 1961) and specifically emphasizes the complex temporal developments and dependencies in this area. However, due to his training as an electrical engineer, in these models, similar to the information theory model of Shannon and Weaver, noise was regarded exclusively as a disturbance, and it was recommended to be removed by appropriate filtering. System dynamics, as it is currently applied and discussed in the field of motion research, in which noise is viewed more constructively, goes back to the work of Kugler, Kelso, Turvey, Newell, Haken, and Schöner in the 1980s (Haken et al. 1985; Kugler et al. 1980; Newell 1986; Schöner et al. 1986; Zanone and Kelso 1992). However, despite the constructive interpretation, the fluctuations were considered for long as a more or less passive side effect that are observable during phase transitions. This work focused on dissipative systems, i.e., systems that are involved in energy exchange with their environment. They are based on methods and phenomena of statistical physics, such as phase transitions and critical states.

To illustrate the principles in the context of systems theory thinking (abstraction and transfer of commonalities), examples in the field of system dynamics of the convection flow of fluids and cyclic finger movements are explained in the following sections.

2.4.2.1 Self-Organization in Materials: The Rayleigh–Benard Experiment

One of the most popular experiments to explain the phenomena associated with the self-organization of convection flows is the Rayleigh–Benard (RB) experiment (Bénard 1901; Rayleigh 1916). This involves a thin layer of liquid that is slowly heated from below (You can try the experiment yourself with a clean, smooth pan and a little oil). During heating, the warm, low-volume elements rise to the top, and the heavier, cold ones fall to the bottom. Initially, this happens randomly over the entire surface. As the heat increases, rolls of the liquid with different diameters form to equalize the temperature more effectively.

If a critical temperature is exceeded, we suddenly see that all the liquid rolls, so-called convection cells, have a uniform diameter; one roll diameter has prevailed over the others, and the others have been subordinated or, in the language of synergetics, enslaved (Haken 1983). An order has arisen solely due to the properties of the liquid (in this case, a certain viscosity) and the supply of diffuse energy (closed system with energy exchange with the environment). If the system is cooled down again, it returns to its original state. If it is heated again, it may return to this order, but it can also change to an order in which the convection cells rotate in the opposite direction. The system is guided through the order states by the different diameters of the convection cells, with the temperature as the control parameter.

This can be described with a potential landscape: at low temperature, state points diffuse roughly isotropically, and the accessible phase-space volume grows approximately linearly as the potential broadens. At a critical temperature Tc, the landscape changes qualitatively—bifurcating into two minima—so that two stable states emerge (Fig. 2.5).

In the critical temperature range, many different convection cells with different diameters can be observed. In this transition state, the system becomes unstable before it changes to one of the two stable states with a further increase in temperature. The originally stable state is now unstable, as every small fluctuation leads to one of the other two states (Schöllhorn et al. 2017a, b).

> Attention must be paid here to the specific use of the term potential. Unfortunately, there is often a mixture of applications in three different areas. Colloquially, the term potential in connection with sport and exercise or school development is usually associated with as yet unused opportunities that may be available in the future. In a mathematical context, a potential is a quantity whose gradient (greatest change) is a scalar or vector field (abstract function). In a physical context (lat. *Potentia*, "*power, force, performance*"), on the other hand, it is the ability of a conservative force field to perform work; i.e., in contrast to the mathematical potential, a physical effect must be attributed to the field (observable and measurable). The description of finger movements using a mathematical potential must therefore be interpreted differently from a physical or colloquial potential.

A self-organized structure can also be observed when rice is cooked in a pan. After the water has been absorbed by the rice, evenly distributed holes can be observed in the rice pan. This structure is also self-organized due to the properties of the substance, without anyone telling the liquid particles where they should move.

2.4.2.2 Self-Organization in Human Movement: The Cyclic Finger Experiment of Haken–Kelso–Bunz

In early system-dynamics work related to movement, Bernstein's 'degrees-of-freedom' problem was reinterpreted. The associated question is how the human nervous system coordinates the many degrees of freedom of the locomotor (musculoskeletal) system. This shift placed greater emphasis on motor control, on the assumption that understanding it is a prerequisite for purposeful change (learning and development). To this end, the Coordinative Structures model was introduced qualitatively (Kugler et al. 1980), in which muscles, joints, and body segments that work together to produce coordinated movements are grouped into functional groups. These structures are not assumed to be rigid but rather dynamically formed and reorganized depending on the task. This task-specific adaptation is seen as a theoretical key feature of how humans and animals very generally coordinate their movements under different conditions. They maintain their structure through the constant exchange of energy and matter with the environment. They are dissipative by nature (Prigogine and Nicolis 1971). This idea was adopted from Prigogine's work on the thermodynamics of dissipative systems, where systems far from equilibrium can spontaneously organize themselves. Accordingly, coordinated movements are self-organized from the interaction of several systems and are not preprogrammed. Overall, the work laid the foundation for a system-oriented view of movement control. Effects on the understanding of learning, the acquisition of movements, and motor development were nonspecifically suggested until the end of the 1980s.

With the Haken–Kelso–Bunz (HKB) experiment (Haken et al. 1985), this became quantitative and more specific. Its origins lie in the finger tapping experiments of Yamanishi et al. (1979, 1980) and examine the specific behavior of cyclical finger movements with increasing movement frequency. These were analyzed with methods from stochastic physics, with special consideration of a noise component. If the two index fin-

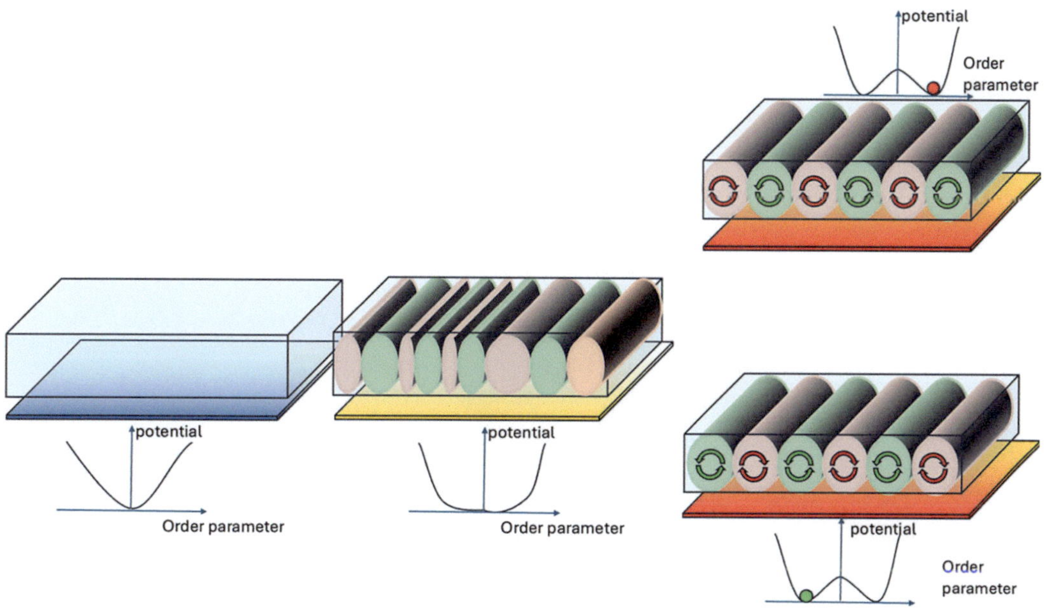

Fig. 2.5 Schema of the Rayleigh–Benard experiment with potential description. Here, the diameter of the convection rolls corresponds to the order parameter and the temperature to the control parameter

gers or both hands (Fig. 2.6) with outstretched fingers are moved in parallel from left to right and the movement frequency is successively increased, the movement pattern changes to an antiparallel one from a critical frequency. As these are cyclical movements, it makes sense to describe them using a sine function ($f(\varphi) = \sin(\varphi)$; φ:angle). If these show a temporal shift, this is also referred to as a phase shift δ ($f(\varphi) = \sin(\varphi+\delta)$). In the first case, this is referred to as antiphase (δ = 180°), as the flexors of one hand and the extensors of the other hand are activated at the same time. In the second case, due to the simultaneous activation of extensors in one direction and flexors in the other direction, one assumes in-phase behavior (δ = 0°). Although the shift from 180° to 0° relative phase is a qualitative change in rhythmic movements that could be considered a change in topology, compared to different topologies in the visual domain, this shift corresponds only to the rotation of a triangle by 180° and not a change in topology or shape, where it would have to be a change from a triangle to a square or a circle. This was one of the problems in transferring the findings of the rhythmic movement studies to ballistic whole-body movements.

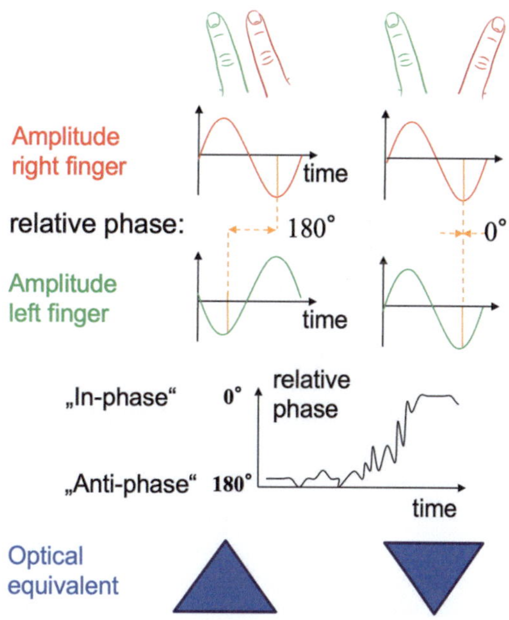

Fig. 2.6 Cyclic finger movement shifting from antiphase to in-phase mode. The phase is related to the activation of left- and right-hand extensors/flexors or ab–/adductors

These phenomena can be represented in a similar way to the convection currents in the Rayleigh–Benard experiment with the help of a

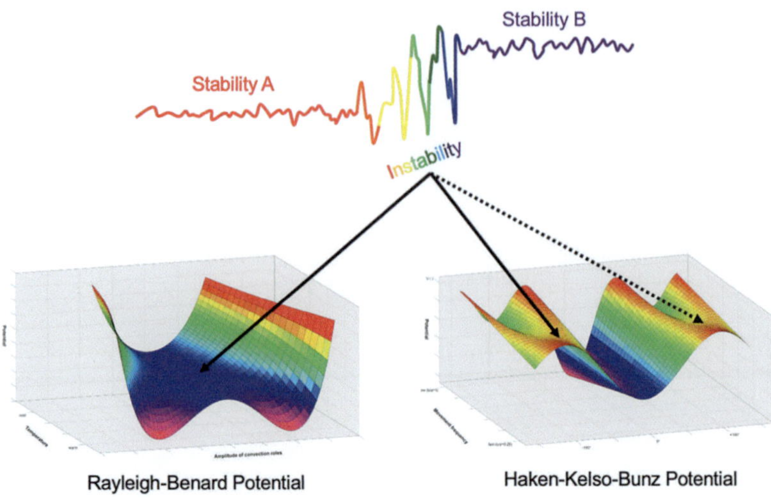

Fig. 2.7 Potential landscape of Rayleigh–Benard (left) and the Haken–Kelso–Bunz finger experiment (right)

mathematical potential. In the following, the relative phases refer to the muscle activity. The geometrical explanation is used here because of a later step when shifting to similarity. The shape of the corresponding finger's Haken–Kelso–Bunz potential (Fig. 2.7) should show two minima, one at 360°/0° and one at 180°, according to the measurements at slow speed, and only one minimum at high speed. As it is irrelevant in the slow range, whether the phase is determined from the left hand to the right, or vice versa, a symmetry of the potential must be formulated at slow speed. Minima occur, therefore, where the finger movements show the least fluctuations, i.e., the highest stability. Mathematically, these requirements for the potential could be mapped using a Fourier series ($V(\varphi) = - a*\cos(\varphi) - b*\cos(2\varphi)$), which was terminated after the second summand, as further summands no longer made any significant contribution. The ratio of the parameters a and b to each other was assigned to the frequency of movement. For $b/a < 0.5$ (corresponding to a higher speed), the potential had one minimum, and for $b/a > 0.5$, the potential had two. The potential model thus depicts the phenomena that occurred during the experiments.

The same phase transition phenomena can be observed with cyclical flexion-extension movements of an arm. If the elbow is initially flexed and the wrist extended and, from here, the elbow is extended and the wrist flexed with increasing frequency, the movement changes with increasing speed into a flexion–flexion and extension–extension pattern (Kelso et al. 1991). When cyclic flexion and extension movements of both elbow and knee joints were tested, all pairs showed stable in-phase and antiphase patterns, with the coupling between both legs or both arms being slightly stronger than that between arms and legs (Jeka et al. 1993; Kelso and Jeka 1992; Schöner et al. 1990). The fact that these phenomena can be strongly influenced by visual perception decoupled from tactile perception was shown in an inspiring experiment in which the movement of the test subjects was altered with the aid of a gearbox so that subjects saw something other than their own movement (Mechsner et al. 2001, 2004). With this arrangement, the test subjects were also able to move other relative phases in a stable manner.

At first glance, one could dismiss these phenomena as more or less conscious switches between two movement programs and attempt to classify the findings in the model of cognitive–psychological programs. On closer examination, however, additional phenomena became apparent, which were difficult to relate with these traditional models but instead showed analogies to stochastic physics and were observed in numerous other dissipative systems. These typical phenomena were:

Stability and Loss of Stability

If the cyclical finger or hand movements are started with in-phase mode and become faster and faster, no change to a different movement pattern can be observed. This is an indication that the in-phase movement is more stable than the antiphase movement, which can only be performed at slower movement frequencies, whereas the in-phase movement can be performed at both slower and faster frequencies.

Learning to play a musical instrument provides an analogy in another area. If a piece of music can be played quickly and slowly, we assume that the movement pattern is more stable than if it can only be played slowly. The same applies to the acquisition of handwriting.

A further indication of the different stability of the two movement modes was provided by the measurement of the continuous deviations of 0°/360° and 180°, for which the measure of variance is often selected. Here, the 0° condition shows a smaller variance than the 180° condition. In addition, a strong increase in variance was observed during the transition from the antiphase mode to the in-phase mode, which was significantly greater than the variances of the in-phase and antiphase patterns. This means that the system loses stability during the transition. A significant increase in variance is a characteristic of instability. Overall, the two areas of greater stability, displayed in the form of valleys in Fig. 2.7, at slow and high movement speeds have a more attractive effect on the system than the neighboring relative phases and are, therefore, designated as attractors of the existing coordination dynamics. Attractors are characterized by a catchment area and can be interpreted as movements that are very stable. If you enter this area with a very similar relative phase, the system tends to move toward this attractor over a longer period of time. However, these attractors only describe momentary states and are transformed through learning.

Fluctuations, Intermittencies, and Increase in Fluctuations

When determining the variances, it was also noticeable that the movements in both cases are subject to constant fluctuations and intermittencies (occasionally larger fluctuations), although these are simple movements compared to everyday and sports movements. This can also be understood as an indication that we are virtually incapable of identical repetitions. The increase in fluctuations in the transition from antiphase to in-phase movement is also an indication that a change from one stability to another stability takes place via instability.

This phenomenon can also be observed in everyday life when relearning, especially in young children when they are learning something new. If a movement technique or habit is changed, a relapse to old patterns mixed with the new movement technique or habit can often be observed at the beginning, before the newly learned skill can be recalled in a stable manner. More recent studies on injury forecast in football also provide indications of an increase in fluctuations before injuries occur (Fonseca et al. 2020). Nonetheless, not all increases in fluctuations led to injuries, indicating that a change of state seems to be accompanied by increased fluctuations. The same can be observed on a larger timescale at a sociological level when political or economic systems change (Hemelrijk 2005; Schmidt 1992; Weik and Lang 2003).

Hysteresis Effect

A hysteresis effect is a phenomenon where a system's current state depends not only on its present input but also on its history. From the Greek hysterēsis ('lagging behind'), hysteretic systems have states that depend on the path of change—i.e., whether the input is increasing or decreasing. Related to the finger experiment, once we are in the in-phase movement and slow down the movement frequency again, there is no change back to the antiphase pattern. The same phenomenon can be observed when we try to walk faster and faster and switch to running at a certain speed; this change usually happens at a different speed than the speed at which we begin running and slows down (Frank et al. 2015; Janssen 2017). Transferred to physiotherapy, the sequence of exercises within a session has an influence on the movement coordination and on the learning process. Walking on a soft mat will prepare the muscle activation of the lower leg muscles in a different way than walking on an uneven solid surface. Similarly, jumping on a trampoline first leads to problems with jumping on solid ground, whereas the other way around is less problematic.

Critical Slowing Down

The phenomenon of critical deceleration is closely associated with an increase in fluctuations. This phenomenon describes a behavior that can be observed in dissipative systems in the critical area of a transition (critical point) from one stable state to another. In this area, processes to return to the original state after disturbances (relaxation time) slow down, and the intentional change between states also slows down (Scholz et al. 1987; Schöner et al. 1986). If, for example, the finger movements are disturbed in this critical frequency range, it takes considerably longer to return to the original state than if the finger movements are disturbed in the more stable in-phase or antiphase modes. The time required for a system to return to its original state after a disturbance is therefore also regarded as a measure of stability. The same applies to the time a system needs to consciously switch between two states. In the case of finger movements, it takes more time to switch from the in-phase mode to the antiphase mode than in the opposite direction. Switching to the more stable movement, because there is less variance, is faster than switching from the stable to the less stable movement.

Analogous phenomena have also been observed in horses during the transitions between walk, trot, and gallop (Schöner et al. 1990), as well as in the production of speech (Kelso et al. 1986a; Tuller and Kelso 1989).

In the terminology of synergetics, which deals with complex open systems and was introduced by Haken (1975, 1983) as the theory of interaction, such system behavior is described by means of control and order parameters. Order parameters determine the dynamics and behavior of the overall system, while the control parameters describe the effect of the environment on the system under consideration and are the variables of the system that can be influenced least directly (Haken and Schiepek 2006). The movement frequency in the finger experiment represents the control parameter that guides the system through the movement landscape without providing specific information about the actual execution of the movement. In the case of Rayleigh–Benard convection, this role is taken over by the temperature. In both cases, the control parameter can be increased and decreased at will. The relative phase represents the order parameter that can be used to classify the movement patterns of the fingers or the convection currents, even during the transition. It is generally up to the creativity of the researcher to choose both order and control parameters for the specific problem (Haken 1991).

The approach was also simulated on discrete goal-directed movements (Schöner and Kelso 1988a, b) with a single effector by replacing the relative phase with the relative timing of the actuators involved as the order parameter. The velocity of the goal-directed movement was chosen as the control parameter. Thus, if a discrete goal-directed movement was repeated and executed increasingly faster, a transition to a movement pattern with altered relative timing was observed in the simulation experiments. The approach was limited to short, goal-directed movements of individual effectors, which could only be distinguished by the relative phase or relative timing.

With relative timing as an order parameter for discrete movements, similar problems arise with respect to the generalization or transfer to sports, as those discussed in the schema theoretical model and the above-mentioned process-oriented signal analysis. For example, it remained unclear to what extent the changes in relative timing in a faster movement are caused by a variety of changes in the relative force components (e.g., muscular, gravitational, and inertial) (Schneider et al. 1989), as part of a learning process, or to which biomechanical characteristic the relative timing should generally refer. Does it refer to the muscular forces or to the overall forces? If it is related to the total forces, the muscular forces must be constantly adjusted, as the gravitational and inertial forces are constantly changing, which makes them problematic as candidates for invariants. As part of a learning experiment in which an object was to be moved around an obstacle as quickly as possible in a vertical direction, passive forces were used as learning progressed (Schneider et al. 1989). With this study, the limitations of the schema theory, whose invariants were exclusively based on muscular force parameters, to movements without gravitational and inertial forces became obvious (Schmidt 2003; Schöllhorn 1998). The passive forces become particularly important for faster movements and movements that are both fast and in a vertical direction. Interestingly, most movement-related studies in psychology are conducted in the horizontal plane on a desk and at a very slow pace compared to sports. The problem becomes many times greater if it is not just an arm movement with two or three segments but a whole-body movement, such as in tennis serves or javelin throws, because, for example, the arm could also be accelerated only by a torso or leg movement, and the same change in the relative timing of the arm movement can therefore be attributed to multiple causes. However, if several subsystems are involved in the acceleration, the number of possible combinations and compensation options for the relative timing increases accordingly, and a clear diagnosis of state changes becomes correspondingly complicated and uncertain. If, in addition, the velocity curves of the subsystems change in such a way that the number of maxima and minima changes, the problem of assigning them accordingly is added (cf. process-oriented curve analysis: see Chap. 1).

2.4.2.3 System Dynamics and Learning a Given Relative Phase

In the next step, Kelso and coworkers studied the process of learning a prescribed relative phase of cyclic finger movements that differed from the in- and antiphase patterns of 0°/360° and 180°; i.e., the participants had to learn a 90° relative phase movement (Zanone and Kelso 1992). In a very traditional way, learners had to try to repeat the new relative phase as often as possible by receiving feedback from a metronome. This process followed the classic paradigm of learning through the knowledge of results (Schöner et al. 1992) to create a new stable movement pattern (attractor) in the internal movement landscape.

An increase in fluctuations was also observed during the learning process but as a side effect of correctly executing the specified relative phase. Most importantly, because the exact target phase was given by the experimenter, there was no self-organization, and this term was also not mentioned in this context in all these studies. Accordingly, it did not lead to any practical consequences until the end of the twentieth century, and a transfer to sports remained limited to reformulations of known phenomena with new terminologies and recommendations to sport scientists (Handford 2002; Handford et al. 1997; Zanone and Kelso 1994; Zanone and Kelso 1997).

A transfer of the later renamed coordination dynamics to the learning of specific relative phases of cyclic finger movements was initiated with predictions about phenomena that were already known from state changes in stochastic physics and dissipative systems (Schöner et al. 1986, 1992) and were an impressive demonstration of systemic abstraction. Those should also be observed during and after the learning of a new relative phase (Schöner et al. 1992; Zanone and Kelso 1992, 1994). To determine the internal dynamics of movement in the form of stable and unstable areas, the relative phases from 0°/360° to 180° were scanned for stability. Relearning a 90° relative phase resulted in a change in the stability of the original coordination dynamics, which was associated with intermittent instabilities such as abrupt changes in performance. The studies provided evidence that the learning process depends on the initial internal coordination dynamics of the learner's cyclic finger movements at the beginning of the learning process (Kostrubiec et al. 2012; Kostrubiec and Zanone 2002; Zanone and Kelso 1994; Zanone and Kelso 1997). If a subject not only had stabilities at 0°/360° and 180° but also at 90°, then learning 45° could lead to the destabilization of the other stabilities. On the other hand, if there were only two stable areas at the beginning, learning 90° could lead to additional stability in this area (Kostrubiec et al. 2012). Similar phenomena are known in sports, where the parallel learning of two similar movements can hinder each other, e.g., in gymnastics, learning the flic flac and back flip or, in athletics, learning discus and shotput rotational technique in parallel. Interestingly, the relative phases to be relearned were always located in areas where the system was less stable. This can be understood as an indication that unstable areas, where the fluctuations are larger, have a higher potential for learning (Schöner and Kelso 1988a, b). Structurally, of even more importance, the acquisition of new unskilled movements differed fundamentally from the studies on the models of variability of practice and contextual interference learning, which exclusively investigated the stabilization of already mastered movements (Schöllhorn et al. 2022).

While in the studies on cyclic finger movements, the similarity of the relative phases to be learned with the existing stability ranges also showed an influence on the learning process in the longer term (Kostrubiec et al. 2012), these were only observed in the short term in analogous studies on two-arm cyclic elbow movements (Fontaine et al. 1997). Recent studies on juggling provide an indication of an even stronger differentiation of the learning process of cyclical two-handed movements, in which the amount of information to be processed simultaneously increases massively due to the involvement of several joints of the arms (e.g., hand, elbow, and shoulder joints) and the information of the visual perceptual component, depending on the rhythm and number of balls (Beek and van Santvoord 1992; Yamamoto et al. 2020). Various responses to the same instructions and the difficulties in finding groups in these experiments with relatively small sample sizes were interpreted in all studies as an indication of a dependence of the learning processes on individual characteristics in the sense of weak individuality. In the end, the speculative assignment of individual stability distributions to individual internal movement dynamics (Kostrubiec and Zanone 2002; Schöner 1989; Zanone and Kelso 1992, 1994) created an analogy to second-order cybernetics in the field of movement research, in which subjective prior knowledge was now mapped in the form of individual distributions of more stable movement zones expressed by less movement variance or, in physics terms, an internal attractor landscape.

For therapy and sports practice, this confirmed the evidence from sports pedagogy of differences at the beginning of learning processes, but in practical terms, the studies on coordination dynamics still limited the actual learning process to the achievement of precisely specified and person-independent goals, which had to be achieved by imitating and repeating the specified goal. In all the learning experiments conducted by the working groups led by Kelso and Zanone (2002), Kostrubiec and Zanone (2002), Zanone and Kelso (1994), Zanone and Kelso (1992), attempts were made to achieve precisely specified relative phases using a metronome, following the knowledge of result learning paradigm. In addition, the initial fluctuations diminished by more than 70% in all participants within the 5 days, as with any model-based learning process associated with the acquisition of a new skill or the formation of a new attractor in the internal landscape dynamics. The logic of deriving the "*... practice under a range of constraints ...*" from this experiment to "*... widen an (existing) attractor ...*" (Davids et al. 2008) is difficult to follow and does not coincidentally fall at a time after having been introduced to the DL approach (Schöllhorn 2000, 2003; Schöllhorn et al. 2006).

From a therapeutic and practical sports perspective, this system dynamics approach corresponds to a compromise between repetitive learning and a methodical series of exercises. In both cases, the initial conditions were designed individually (according to the identified zones of stability), but then an attempt was made to achieve the specified (partial) goal through imitation and repetition. The fluctuations occur incidentally and are not used in a targeted manner.

This knowledge is important and in contrast to therapy and sport in that the movements that result at the end of therapy or training are not as clear and definite as the given relative phase of finger movements, and even more importantly, they have individual and situated characteristics. This means that in therapy and sports, the target is not as constrained as in the relative phase experiments because of individual solution characteristics (Fig. 2.8). By precisely specifying the learning objective, the approach in the system

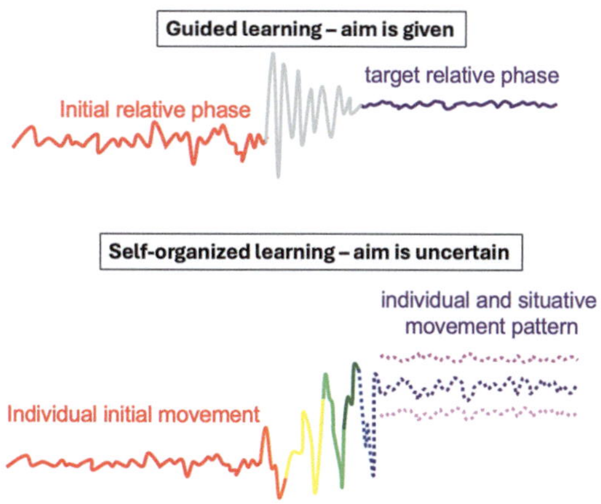

Fig. 2.8 Schematic representation of (top) guided learning based on the knowledge of result (e.g., learning a 90° relative phase (Zanone and Kelso 1992)) when the aim is clearly defined and achieved by constraining the path toward the aim and (bottom) self-organized learning (e.g., learning a running pattern (Schöllhorn et al. 2001a, b)) when the aim is uncertain and is achieved by intentionally increasing the noise

dynamics experiments still corresponded to the prescriptive approach in obedience-oriented teaching and coaching. In contrast, when the aim is uncertain and we can expect individually different solutions, then self-organization by means of increased fluctuations is more plausible.

Interestingly, at the same time, another study pursued an alternative approach more closely related to intervention methods and whole-body movements in its experiments in the early 1990s (van Emmerik et al. 1989; Vereijken et al. 1992a, b). The researchers used a slalom-type ski movement on a ski apparatus to compare discovery learning with approaches based on repetition or systematic variation. One group was asked to practice the movement with an oscillation frequency determined individually based on body size and weight, while other groups practiced with higher, lower, and successively increasing frequencies. Another group, the discovery group, was not given any guidelines. After 4 days of practice, none of the methods used was actually superior to discovery learning, although the training methods did influence the course of learning (Vereijken and Whiting 1990). These experiments provided an impressive example of convergent learning with the guided discovery approach (Mosston 1966), in which the learner can explore the possibilities in relation to a given goal within the given task constraints by means of appropriate restrictions. This must be clearly distinguished from divergent discovery learning, which is inherent in the emergence of something new in the context of self-organization.

One aspect that is often overlooked but has had a major influence on the problems of transferring the system dynamics approach to everyday and sports movements is the use of the **order** and **control parameter** concept of synergetics in connection with learning. Until the beginning of this century, attempts were made in sport psychology to fulfill analogies to the formalities of the system dynamics approach and find equivalents for the terminology rather than take into account the necessary assumptions and the associated limitations of these concepts. Colloquially, the control parameter was associated with the hope of finding simple parameters (e.g., "*key control parameter*" (Handford et al. 1997)), with which, analogous to the diffuse energy in the earlier mentioned two experiments, a learning system could be brought into a new state. The order and control parameter concept of synergetics was previously developed primarily for systems that can adopt different states that are already "present" in the system by changing a specific control parameter. Then, the control parameter can be increased or decreased linearly as desired. In both the Rayleigh–Benard (RB) and the HKB experiment, an increase in the control parameter leads to a phase transition to a different state, in which the system remains even if the control parameter is increased further, before eventually transitioning to a chaotic or completely different state if even more energy is added. In the HKB experiment, however, this transition is dependent on the initial condition. The phase transition cannot be observed if we start with the in-phase mode. Both systems also react differently when the control parameter is reduced again. While in the case of the RB experiment, the system always returns to the initial state, this is not the case in the HKB experiment. Once the fingers or hand movements have switched to in-phase mode, they remain in this mode even if the movement frequency is reduced again. The additional introduction of an intention term is then required for adequate modeling (Schöner et al. 1986). For the modeling of the learning process, terms for memory and the environment were formally added, analogous to the internal dynamics term, but modeling based on the order control parameter concept is still pending. One difficulty here is that the internal dynamics changes permanently after a successful learning process and cannot be reversed in the same way. Using time as a control parameter does not seem to be appropriate in this context because of its asymmetry in living systems. A similar problem arises with the processes of forgetting or aging, i.e., with all events that take place on longer timescales. By formally taking them into account in the equations as a change in the internal dynamics in the form of a weakening of the attractors, the phenomenon can be modeled retrospectively. Although the increased fluctuations that could be observed during a phase transition were recognized as a phenomenon for diagnosis, there was no new practical consequence derived.

2.4.3 Coordination Dynamics and the Transfer to the Practice of Therapy and Sports

2.4.3.1 Initial Problems with the Transfer of System Dynamics to Therapy and Sports: State of the Art in Various Research Areas Before the Introduction of DL

Before the first paper on the DL model was proposed in a high-performance sports journal for practitioners in 1999, as a summary of already applied practice in different sports with different performance levels, including rehabilitation processes in high-performing athletes since 1986, several academic disciplines did research on cognitive and motor learning. Despite specific assumptions for each study (Stachowiak 1973), the erroneous tendency to make false generalizations based on a faulty understanding of the underlying statistics dominated (Acree 2021; Gigerenzer 2004). It was probably no coincidence that Ioannidis' 2005 (Ioannidis 2005) study heralded the beginning of the replication crisis in life sciences (Feest 2019; Gigerenzer 2018; Korbmacher et al. 2023; Tackett et al, 2019). The main approaches that had an influence on the development of the DL model will only be roughly outlined here and are always considered with a view to possible consequences for therapy and sports practice. It would go beyond the scope of this book to describe them in detail. The approaches that were already mentioned in the context of first-order cybernetics will shortly be placed in the temporal context.

2.4.3.2 The Coordination Dynamics Approach: Powerful Theory Without Practical Consequences for Therapy and Training

Due to the limitation of the studies to experiments with cyclic movements (Kelso 1995) and single simulations of discrete movements (Schöner 1990), the system dynamic approach (later called coordination dynamics) was criticized for long in the field of therapy and sports science under the term "*motor-action controversy*" and, mostly, was judged for not being ready to be applicable in these areas (Davids et al. 1999; Meijer and Roth 1988; Schmidt 1988). From 1986 to 2003, various attempts were made to transfer the approach of system dynamics, as investigated by the groups of Kelso and Turvey with cyclical movements, to sports. Although it was considered attractive in some cases, by the turn of the millennium, neither had it been transferred to therapy or sports practice nor had any new practical consequences been derived for therapeutic and sport motor practice.

Primarily known phenomena were reinterpreted and described using the new terminology (Davids et al. 1999; Handford et al. 1997; Kugler et al. 1980; Newell 1986). Alternative methods were proposed for analyzing the data, with the focus on the structure of their variability (Newell and Molenaar 1998; Slifkin and Newell 1999, 2000; Stergiou and Decker 2011).

Recommendations and numerous opinion papers for future research goals were published, which were characterized by the hope of transferring the system dynamics approach into sports practice (Davids et al. 1999, 1994; Handford et al. 1997).[3] As late as 2001, the vague and generalized recommendations like "... practice should be structured to preserve the relationship between such (information-movement-coupling) variables" (Davids et al. 2001) reflect the proximity to methodological practice series and the adherence to familiar traditions. Very general pleas for an integration of system dynamics findings and vague calls for more exploratory learning (Handford et al. 1997), repeating earlier calls (van Emmerik et al. 1989; Vereijken and Whiting 1990; Vereijken et al. 1992b), also show the uncertain state of the research landscape, searching for an exit, especially regarding practical consequences at this time. Accordingly, Rosenbaum warned in 1998 that the system dynamics approach was in danger of degenerating into curve fitting (Rosenbaum 1998).

Following the publication of the DL model (Schöllhorn 1999b, 1999c, 2000, 2003, 2005; Schöllhorn et al. 2009), which focused on the amplification of differences between two successive movement executions, and after proponents of the constraints-led approach (CLA) received publications on and an introduction to DL practice since 2001, Newell's original model was reinterpreted by specifying the differences from the DL model with the three categories of organism, environment, and task.

Until then, fluctuations were only used to describe the known pedagogical approaches with new terminology, albeit with many restrictions and guidance (Handford 2002; Handford et al, 1997). This only covered a small part of DL that was associated with the increase of possibilities for the learner (von Foerster 1997). After having been introduced to DL, the handling of fluctuations and errors in practice changed fundamentally in the context of the CLA approach and only led to practical consequences some years after the introduction of DL, which were already proposed and experimentally tested in studies on DL (e.g. Beckmann and Schöllhorn 2003; Schöllhorn et al. 2001b; Schönherr 2003; Trockel 2003).

Following the research on coordination dynamics in the research groups of Kelso, Haken, Schöner, Turvey, and Thelen, a reinterpretation of system fluctuations (Newell and Corcos 1993; Riley and Turvey 2002; Slifkin and Newell 1999; Thelen and Smith 1994) and the application of

---

[3] Quotes related to the uncertain situation until 2003 on how to transfer system dynamics to sports by CLA proponents: (For ongoing inconsistencies and contradictions within the theoretical foundations of CLA, see Collins et al. 2025)

... the embryonic stage of theoretical development presently ***restricts the scope for serious hypothesis-testing****, increased research effort is needed to evaluate the practical impact of the main tenets of an ecological perspective in the sport and exercise context.*—Handford (1997)

... a major task is to discover the ***control parameters which act to constrain the order parameters*** *of the body as a dynamical system.*—Handford (1997)

To summarize ***... it is still unclear*** *... whether discrete movements are open to dynamic modeling like rhythmical movements.*—Davids (1999)

Quotes related to the restrictive character (in contrast to self-organisation) and stronger focus on the search for key features as control parameters of the constraints-led approach:

...new forms of coordination emerge through changes in ***certain system variables – so-called control parameters –*** *which, when scaled, can trigger transitions in coordination."*—Newell (1986). *One principle that can be generalized across different sports is that* ***practice should be structured*** *to preserve the relationship between such variables.*—Davids (2001)

... environmental and task structure are ***manipulated to channel the search*** *through the workspace ...*—Handford (1997)

Furthermore, system allocation of different "attentional weightings" to each component, ***while maintaining an overall minimization****, may contribute towards an explanation of variable muscle forces and joint kinematics* ***during successful repetition of the same task***—Handford (1997)

The search process involves the ***modification and perfection of movement solutions from trial to trial*** *without identical performance, a type of '****repetition without repetition****'*— Handford (1997)

... to act to tune the action systems directly ***until the desired kinematic outcomes are attained*** *and the set of task constraints is satisfied*—Handford (1997)

...coaches should ***seek to identify the key control parameters***—Handford et al. (1997) ***the preservation of key dynamical relationships*** *between joint segments...*—Handford (2002)

alternative measures, such as sample entropy or approximate entropy, occurred in the early 1990s but primarily for the analysis of movement that provided data series that were long enough for their application, such as those used in walking (Costa et al. 2003) or climbing paths (Cordier et al. 1994) and in balancing tasks (Collins and De Luca 1993; Hausdorff et al. 1996). In connection with motor learning and learning step design, the adaptations were essentially limited to renaming variations as functional variability and interpreting differences in execution as individual variants or various sources of variance (Müller and Sternad 2003), again in a speculative weak individuality because of not having found any group structure. Variations caused by fatigue, emotions, or music were not in focus, mainly because of methodical problems. In sum, no new consequences for practice were associated.

An initial rough proposal for structuring developmental boundary conditions and classical interventions was made by Magill (1983) and Newell (1986) with the three categories of constraints, the individual, environment, and task, similar to Lewin's (1935) behavioral model, where behavior is considered a function of the person and the environment (B = f(P,E)). From a systems theoretic point of view, this model can be assigned to static systems theory, where the individual is considered the system that directly defines its environment, which interacts with the individual via the task. This mainly mirrors the fact that it was known and obvious that therapy or training takes place by manipulating the boundary conditions involved. **Early on, the open questions in motor learning research did not relate to whether boundary conditions need to be varied for optimized learning, but rather to what extent, how often, and which constraints should be changed.** While the first part was linked to the problem of quantifying metrics and topology, the second question was linked to the problem of different timescales for activities and relaxation, and the third was related to the complexity and individuality of the movement technique. At this time, the advantage of using various timescales for the analysis of motor learning processes was raised theoretically by Scholz et al. (1987), but only after 2001 (Newell et al. 2001; Schöllhorn et al. 2009), did it experience increasing attention in the motor learning area.

The first indications of the influence of the parameter of time on learning behavior and performance in sport psychology came from the model of distributed practice with its modified breaks between learning sessions in connection with forgetting (Bjork and Allen 1970; Ebbinghaus 1913) and the model of contextual interference learning with the distinction between blocked, serial, and randomized exercise sequences (Shea and Morgan 1979). While the second model exclusively refers to the timescale of a single intervention and the relative similarity of the exercises, the first model refers to two timescales in accordance with the parallelly studied memory models. One timescale relates to forgetting within an intervention measure from exercise to exercise, whereas the second timescale relates to forgetting between two intervention measures from day to day or longer.

The temporal changes during phase transitions in system dynamics address this aspect by considering both time and order, including the similarity of specific exercises (Schöner 1989). The relative phase as a measure of similarity (Rosen 1988) and its increase in variance during the switch from one stable pattern to another stable pattern for the first time were treated together (Fig. 2.9).

Both aspects, the relative similarity and their dependence on time, were then transferred from cyclic finger movements to ballistic whole-body movements with the time-course-oriented pattern recognition approach (Bauer and Schöllhorn 1997; Schöllhorn 1993a, b, 1995, 1997; Schöllhorn and Bauer 1998a, b, c; Schöllhorn et al. 2001a), and shortly after this, they became central subjects of the DL model with its focus on differences in a double sense: first, on the quantification part related to the similarity of two subsequent movements and, second, regarding the design of exercise processes, with increasing differences between two consecutive movements dependent on stochastic resonance. The consideration of all interventions as various levels of noise allowed to unite several motor learning models under the umbrella of noise in the sense of second-order cybernetics, where the noise of

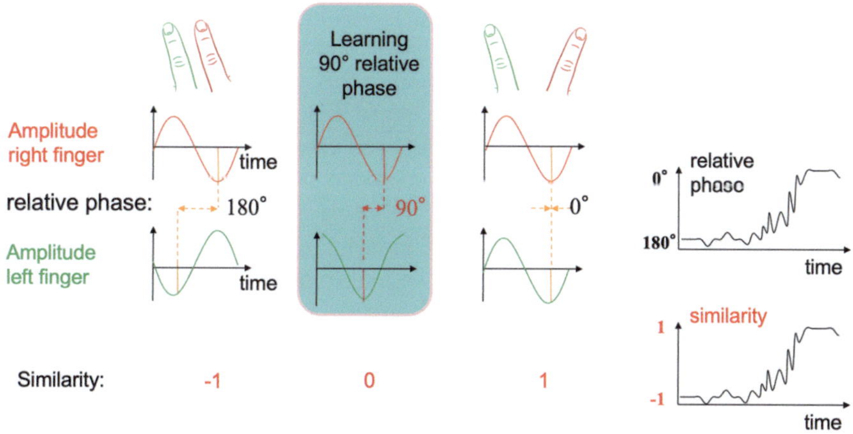

Fig. 2.9 Replacing the relative phase by similarity for describing the cyclic finger movements

the exercises has to be adjusted to the variance of the learner (Beckmann and Schöllhorn 2006; Schöllhorn 2005; Schöllhorn et al. 2006, 2009).

Therefore, three pending problems prevailed by the end of the twentieth century:

- First, on the one hand (classical movement research), to have a restriction of movement variation to metrics (Bernstein 1967; Schmidt 1975) and, on the other hand (coordination dynamics), to deal with fluctuations in qualitative changes in movements that were mainly cyclic (Kelso 1995). Because of this restriction, it was too early to consider this a topological change, as a shift from 0° to 180° relative phase would correspond in the visual field to a rotation of a triangle (or another geometric shape) by 180°, which would still be a triangle, just with a different orientation.
- Second, on the one hand, there was still an orientation toward group trends, while on the other hand, there were increasing signs of strong individuality (Bates 1996; Brisson and Alain 1996; Schöllhorn 1993a, b; Schöllhorn and Bauer 1998a, b, c; Schöllhorn et al. 1999).
- Third, on the one hand, there was the orientation toward movement ideals independent of the individual and situation that were achieved by feedback learning (Adams 1987) and, on the other hand, self-organization during the relative phase transition (Haken et al. 1985).

2.4.4 Opening the Door to New Consequences in Practice

Before looking in detail into the crucial progress that led to crossing the threshold from theoretical description to massive changes in training, therapy, and motor learning, the key phenomena from system dynamics research are summed up. Applying the systems theoretical abstraction of system dynamic principles, the most relevant ones lead to the first DL model and the corresponding practical consequences (Schöllhorn 1999b, c, 2000, 2003).

(a) Fluctuations are an essential component of living systems (Prigogine and Nicolis 1971).
(b) The range of fluctuations provides information about the relative stability of a movement (Schöner et al. 1986).
(c) The fluctuations of the relative phases correspond to specific qualitative changes in the movement patterns (Kelso et al. 1986b).
(d) Fluctuations can increase in the transition from one stable state to another (Kelso et al. 1986b).
(e) The increase in fluctuations leads to instability and a self-organization process (Ashby 1947; von Foerster 1960).
(f) Motor learning studies began the learning process in unstable areas (Kostrubiec et al. 2012; Schöner et al. 1992; Zanone and Kelso 1992).

(g) Motor learning studies set a concrete relative phase without using self-organization (Kostrubiec and Zanone 2002; Zanone and Kelso 1992).

The central phenomena that were interpreted in the DL approach (Schöllhorn 1999b, 2000, 2003) in different and new ways can be clustered into four areas.

A. The exploitations of fluctuations for learning (a, b, and f).
B. The influence of instability during transition (d) based on.
C. More general quantification of qualitative changes (c) using the previously developed pattern recognition approach, based on process-oriented data to quantify movement topology.
D. The identified individuality in high-performance movements (g) by means of self-organization (e).

2.4.4.1 Fluctuations Are Instabilities that Are Deemed to Be the Major Sources of Learning (A)

In principle, identical repetitions do not contain any information. Since a learning process is understood as a permanent change in behavior or attitude, learning must contain, by definition, new information. New information means something distinct from the current state of the learner, which automatically associates the new aspect with the subjective information, i.e., information that depends on the learner's prior knowledge, emotional experiences, or momentary motor abilities. From this information-theoretical perspective, random fluctuations already represent the provision of information, and an amplification of this represents even more information. However, a maximal trend with a constant linear increase of the amount of information is limited by the subjective information-processing capacity, which leads to an optimal trend (Von Cube 1965). In consequence, observed fluctuations and their amplification contain essential information for a learning process.

Strangely enough, the advantage of fluctuations had already been used extensively in physiotherapy since the 1980s in the context of fall prevention and stabilization training of the lower extremities by giving patients variable tasks on different surfaces. If physiotherapy had followed the idea of repeating a prototype model, the patients would have had to stand for a long time on a single leg. Why the logic of variable balance training has not been transferred to other areas earlier remains an open question. From this point of view, the current proposal by CLA proponents to make the training exercises as similar as possible to the target model under the guise of representativeness seems like a relapse into old thought patterns that is even more emphasizes by including the 1935 written quote of Bernstein ("repetition without repetition"). Even without specifying how similar the exercises should be and which of the subsystems must be similar and which ones must not be, such statements again show the earlier normative character of master theories rather than the intention to advance science.

From a traditional perspective, fluctuations would be interpreted as "errors." Here, it is important to remember that the concept of error requires the existence of something that is correct (right–wrong dichotomy) and is always negatively connotated because the supposedly correct target has not been achieved and is typically associated with frustration (Broadbent et al. 2017; Maxwell et al. 2001). The asymmetry between right and wrong had already been the basis of the falsification hypothesis of Popper's philosophy in *The Logic of Scientific Discovery* (Popper 1935), with which he refuted the logical positivism of the Vienna circle, by which Brunswik's model of representativeness (Brunswik 1955) was also strongly influenced (Tolman 1956).

The identification of individual gait patterns in adults (Horst et al. 2016, 2017a; Schöllhorn 1999a; Schöllhorn et al. 2002) as well as the differentiation of individual elite athletes (Bauer and Schöllhorn 1997; Schöllhorn and Bauer 1998a, b, c) fundamentally questioned the existence of a (single) person-independent correct solution in gross motor movements, **which makes the definition of erroneous movements even more problematic.** Traditionally, errors should be avoided from the outset, as changing movements once they have been learned incorrectly is interpreted as a major problem. Consequently, errors and their amplification, as supported by DL, in theory and practice, still represent an inhibition threshold that is difficult to overcome. Unfortunately, this is also supported and conditioned by traditional school pedagogy that is leaning on military-based andragogy and focuses on correct and often singular solutions in conjunction with rewards and punishments (black pedagogy). The fact that this form of error in movements is only in danger of becoming automated and is difficult to change if it has been acquired through repetition is often neglected (see also the chapter on conditioning in behaviorism). It is a different matter if, constantly, different "errors" are made during DL due to fluctuations. Treating mistakes primarily as negative exemplars—'what not to do'—within the constraints-led approach (CLA; Handford et al. 1997), echoes Plato's learning-by-contrast and reintroduces the very right–wrong dichotomy the approach claims to move beyond. In DL, "errors" are interpreted neither as positive nor as negative deviations and are rather amplified actively to make the system unstable for initiating a learning process, thus making it easier to reach a new state in a self-organized manner. Whether the fluctuations are amplified by instructions or by other didactical interventions is related to another (e.g., pedagogical and psychological) level of analysis. In addition, increased noise in the form of various amplified fluctuations is applied continuously to stay adaptive and be able to cope with disturbances that occur anyway. Here, it is important to keep in mind that using noise continuously is not about giving the athlete the experience of what he should not do in the future, as in the original models of CLA or in MAE. **In DL, noise is used continuously on different learning and performance levels (see neuronal bases) dependent on the individual and the situation to make the system more robust against the continuously changing internal and external boundary conditions.**

2.4.4.2 Instability for Initiating Self-Organization Is Actively Induced by Increasing the Noise (B)

Stability is considered the ability of a system to maintain a constant state over time, resist changes, and return to its equilibrium position when disturbed. In classical physiotherapy and training, the aim was to achieve stability by repeating the target exercise as many times as possible. Instability was interpreted as an increase in errors and loss of control that had to be avoided. In consequence, repetitions of ideals, accompanied by numerous corrections, were on the agenda. Since a patient or an athlete can only perceive differences with difficulty during repetitions, as they assume "identical" repetitions, they are dependent on the sensitivity of the therapist's or trainer's perception, who must still identify the small differences (errors) in the repetitions.

A shift of the focus from the actual movements to their fluctuations initiated a rethinking of classical errors (Newell and Corcos 1993). Momentary internal attractor landscapes of movement dynamics were modeled based on the different amounts of fluctuations. The rethinking was supported by the observation of the increase in fluctuations during the transition between two stable states (Haken et al. 1985). An increase in fluctuations could also be observed when using classical learning methods to acquire a new relative phase (Kostrubiec and Zanone 2002; Zanone and Kelso 1992). Thus, only less stable zones in the internal landscape were used for acquiring new relative phases. However, the used learning approach was classically based on a given target relative phase that had to be copied with corresponding augmented feedback learning.

To consider the fluctuations not only as passive consequences in the context of classical interventions in cyclic movements and take advantage of them for the new practical consequences in the DL model, further steps were necessary. In addition to the generalization of the quantification of movement topologies and their fluctuations to gross motor and ballistic everyday and sports movements, these were the alternative interpretations of the three following aspects.

One is related to the physical understanding of stability and instability. In addition to the criteria listed above, stable states are also characterized by the fact that more energy is required to change the state. In contrast, unstable systems are characterized by the fact that little energy is required to change the state of the system. If we consider learning as the change from one stable state to another stable state, this should require less effort if the system is first made unstable.

And this is where the second aspect comes into play. In the cyclic finger experiment, instability meant an increase in variation in topology. If we transfer this to sports or therapy, this corresponds to an increase in the variation of exercises with different topologies and not only the variation of movement metrics.

The third aspect relates to the learning experiments, in which learning processes were always initiated in areas of less stability. Following the systemic abstraction, every fluctuation can therefore be understood as an instability of the system, which can be used to make the system even more unstable, to bring the system into a state in which less energy is required to change the formerly stable state.

In consequence, instead of passively waiting for the destabilization of the system to occur by copying a given role model of given relative phases, as was observed in the experiments of Zanone and coworkers (Kostrubiec and Zanone 2002; Zanone and Kelso 1992), the DL approach was to actively provoke an increase in fluctuations to make the system unstable and deliberately initiate a self-organizing process. This destabilization is achieved in DL by increasing the observable fluctuations (Schöllhorn 2000; Schöllhorn et al. 2006, 2009), which is equivalent to increasing the differences between two successive movements, which gave the DL approach its name.

In addition to the differences between two subsequent movements, differences, in general, were known to be used by the central nervous system in multiple contexts to gain information that supports survival. For example, the difference between the image that we see with the right eye and the image that we see with the left eye provides us with information of the distance, which we do not get from a single image. The problem of one-eyed perception is very common when people with only one eye try to pour tea into a cup. Our auditory system uses the same principle for orientation. If a sound hits the right ear first and then the left ear shortly afterward (due to the speed of sound), our brain calculates the time difference from when the sound source came from the right side for spatial orientation. If the wavelengths of the sound are longer than the distance between our ears, we can no longer localize the source. This is exploited to a certain extent in newer loudspeaker systems by using only one bass speaker since low frequencies (below 100 Hz) fulfill this condition of being difficult to localize. These two neurophysiological examples already stay in conflict with the assumption of direct perception, where no internal processing and no internal representation is assumed (Michaels and Carello 1981). Other phenomena that conflict with these assumptions will be discussed in the chapter on the neurophysiological basis of DL.

How the fluctuations are increased, whether by the learner himself, based on instructions or the problem, or by modifying the environment, at this level of abstraction was of secondary interest. This was mainly considered to be clarified at a different level, as most of these conditions were largely outside the biomechanical point of view, where a vast amount of knowledge related to these topics was offered. These include questions about expectations, evaluation, planning, surprise, intentionality, etc. Similar questions concerned the amount of noise (How extensive may and must the noise be in the different learning phases?) and the noise characteristics (How similar/different should the exercises be? How far apart should the exercises be? Do the exercises or the differences between the exercises have a greater influence on learning?). In this context, the differentiation between inside and outside the learner is primarily a phenomenological approach because, already biomechanically, a gravitational force cannot be distinguished between the two acting objects, and the same counts for interactions of electromagnetic fields produced inside and outside the patient or learner. Above all, however, the individuality and situatedness of the noise were indicated by the findings from the area of pattern recognition (Bauer and Schöllhorn 1997; Schöllhorn and Bauer 1998a, b, c; Schöllhorn et al., 1999, 2001a, 2002).

2.4.4.3 A More General Quantification of the Qualitative Changes Made It Possible to Transfer the System Dynamics to Sports (C)

To build upon earlier theories, we can conceptualize the increase in movement variations as the "variabilization of the learning process." An essential aspect of this new DL approach, however, was that the variation here referred to the topology of the movement, which was excluded from previous models by Schmidt (1975) and Bernstein (1967) for the reasons mentioned above. Both earlier models referred exclusively to the variation of the metrics of a single movement (topology) and served exclusively to stabilize movements that had already been mastered. In the VP model, the movements were even supposed to be automated in advance (Schmidt 1975). The same applies to randomized contextual interference learning, which originally constructed a time related environment (con-text) with additional and precisely prescribed movements to promote cognitive planning processes for a single specific movement topology (text). The parallel practice of several movements with different GMPs also only involves the stabilization of individual topologies, which are practiced through repetition, just with interruptions. The quantification of similarities would be necessary for possible transfers between the practiced GMPs.

In DL (Schöllhorn 1999c), on the other hand, the variations were extended from metrics to movement topology in the application specifically used for the acquisition, stabilization, and performance enhancement of gross motor sports movements (Schöllhorn et al. 2022). This additional extension to the variation of topology provided a bridge between the existing sport pedagogical models, which were primarily

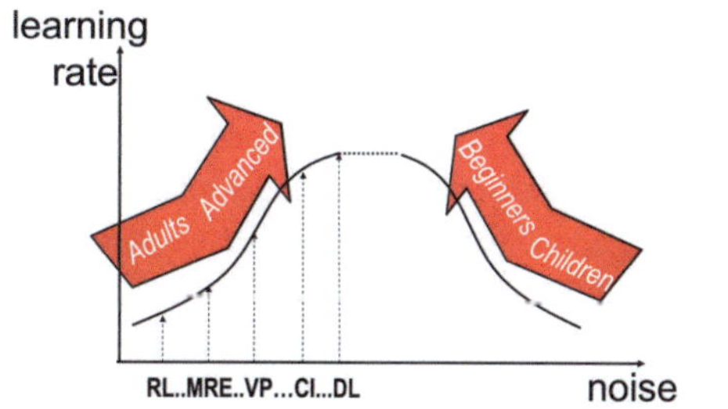

Fig. 2.10 Various motor learning approaches displayed against individual/situation and learning rate. *RL* repetition learning, *MRE* methodical rows of exercise, *VP* variability of practice, *CI* contextual interference, *DL* differential learning

designed for the acquisition of complex techniques using exercises with varying topology, and sport psychological models, which were designed for the stabilization of skilled movements using variable metrics. In consequence, the exercise sequences used in the models could thus be unified under the umbrella of variable levels of noise (Schöllhorn 2005; Schöllhorn et al. 2006). Varying the topology of movements would mean, in the most extreme interpretation, to vary each exercise with a different GMP (in Schmidt's terminology), not completely wild and without limitations but within the boundary conditions of the possible solution space (Fig. 2.10).

In regaining the ability to walk, this would mean not only walking fast and slow or with longer and shorter steps (this would only be a variation of metrics) but also walking in curved lines, with relaxed, stiff, turned or straight feet, only on the heels, or only on the toes or, in a more advanced state, where each step can have one of these characteristics. When learning the finger skills, the variations would not only focus on lighter or heavier and larger or smaller objects but also vary the trunk position and use different fingers, different elbow angles, different head positions, etc.

2.4.4.4 Individuality in High-Performance Movements by Means of Self-Organization (D)

In a parallel step, a fundamental distinction had to be made between everyday and sports movements with regard to the learning experiments on coordination dynamics, in which the relative phase to be learned was specified independently of the person. The individuality of movement patterns found in high-performance sports (Bauer and Schöllhorn 1997; Schöllhorn and Bauer 1998a, b, c) and in walking (Schöllhorn et al. 2002; Schöllhorn et al. 1999) (cf. Chap. 1) were considered the result of learning processes. If the goal is an individually unique movement pattern that is not yet fully known at the beginning of the learning process, it is advisable not to prescribe an initial pattern based on a potentially unsuitable target. Instead, increasing fluctuations can trigger a self-organization process, enabling the patient or learner to discover a solution that aligns with their own boundary conditions. If solutions have already emerged as advantageous, these can be used with all the observed fluctuations.

From a practical point of view, the instability initiated by increased fluctuations has the additional advantage that the system can use and combine the variants that seem most favorable for the new state from the variety of variants offered and can thus find its own new order, even without concrete external information (von Foerster 1960). This phenomenon was described by Foerster as early as 1960 as "*order from noise,*" whereby the noise or random disturbances help a self-organizing system find more stable states in its fitness landscape (Schöllhorn et al. 2009; von Foerster 1960). In contrast to the learning experiments of Zanone's research group (Kostrubiec et al. 2012; Kostrubiec and Zanone 2002; Zanone and Kelso 1992, 1994, 1997), the target movement was not exactly prescribed in the form of a relative phase in connection with sports due to the studies on the recognition of individuality of movements, and thus, self-organization through noise was possible.

Due to the holistic systems approach, the same principles could be applied not only to the overall system but also to subsystems. For example, if there were abnormalities in the hip area when walking, the fluctuations could be concentrated in this area. However, due to the holistic complexity of large motor movements, at least the neighboring joints must always be involved.

The extent to which fluctuations in the movement topology or in the movement metrics can cause destabilization more or less effectively, depending on the learning stage, is a problem that needs to be clarified in future research and has so far been left to the sensitivity and creativity of the therapist or the trainer. A similar question was, and is, the extent of the necessary fluctuations, which is very likely to be linked to the learning stage and still requires some effort in terms of topology.

The central step for the transfer of system dynamics principles first into sports and later into physiotherapy practice was the intentional and targeted increase of noise/fluctuations to destabilize the system, not only in movement metrics but also in the movement topology to initiate a real self-organizing process.

Questions

1. What are the key philosophical and scientific differences between first-order and second-order cybernetics in movement learning?
2. How does differential learning reinterpret the role of variability and error in the learning process?
3. In what ways does DL challenge the repetition- and correction-based assumptions of traditional training models?
4. How do cybernetic principles—such as feedback loops—shape classical motor learning theories like the schema theory?
5. What is the significance of subjective information, and how does it influence learning step design in DL?
6. How does DL relate to natural learning processes observed in infants and children?
7. Why does DL reject the necessity of augmented feedback, and what alternative learning mechanisms does it promote?
8. How does DL integrate concepts like stochastic resonance and noise into the learning process?
9. What are the implications of DL for coaching and therapy practices that prioritize standardized goals and outcomes?
10. How do systems theory and artificial intelligence inform modern, individualized approaches to movement variability and learning?

2.5 Neurophysiological Basis of Differential Learning

Wolfgang I. Schöllhorn
Institute for Sport Science, Johannes Gutenberg-University
Mainz, Germany
e-mail: schoellw@uni-mainz.de

Agnė Slapšinskaitė-Dackevičienė
Department of Sports Medicine, Faculty of Nursing, Medical Academy, Lithuanian University of Health Sciences
Kaunas, Lithuania

Faculty of Public Health, Health Research Institute, Medical Academy, Lithuanian University of Health Sciences
Kaunas, Lithuania
e-mail: agne.slapsinskaite-dackeviciene@lsmu.lt

Abstract This chapter presents the neurophysiological foundations supporting **Differential Learning (DL)**, with a focus on how sensory systems, perception, and brain plasticity contribute to motor learning. It highlights the **active, subjective nature of perception**, emphasizing that movement learning is not simply a response to external stimuli but a dynamic interaction between internal neuronal processes and sensory inputs. The role of **mechano-sensors**, **reafference principles**, and **afferent–efferent pathways** is discussed to show how information flows between the body and the brain. The chapter also explores the **somatosensory and motor cortices**, **mirror neurons**, and **plasticity mechanisms** that shape learning and adaptation. Integrating concepts from **second-order cybernetics**, **constructivism**, and **systems theory**, it argues that each individual's learning is shaped by their unique history and context, supporting the DL approach that embraces variability and nonlinear progression. The reader can expect an in-depth physiological rationale for shifting from repetition-based to individualized learning frameworks in therapy and training.

Keywords Perception – Sense – Mechanosensors – Afferent-efferent pathways – Somatovisceral information – Somatosensory and motor cortices – Plasticity – Mirror neurons – Systems theory

2.6 Introduction

The following chapter provides a coarse overview of the neurophysiological mechanisms of movement and perception as one basis for Differential Learning (DL) in physiotherapy. This chapter is not intended to be exhaustive; rather, it serves more as a reminder presented in a slightly different context. Emphasis is placed on the neurophysiological correlates of the characteristics that provide the basis for the central nervous adaptational processes. Here, the mechano-sensors are assigned a special role, as they enable the connection between the mainly external biomechanics and the internal neuronal coding of the same information. The neurophysiological correlates can also be approximated biomechanically (from the outside) and enable the formation of a connection between biomechanical movements and artificial neural network (ANN) models for modeling and simulating learning processes (Schöllhorn 1998).

In principle, the two subsystems, "*person*" and "*environment,*" within the system "*moving/behaving person*" (moving is understood here in the physical sense as a change in space and time and, thus, includes the environment and the situation) exchange information in a wide variety of ways. For this exchange, the human senses play a special role. The senses enable people to absorb information from their own bodies and the environment and control the state of their organism within it. Thus, contact with the environment is a highly active process and is far from passive. References to the subjectivity of perception can be found early on in the literature. William Shakespeare (1564–1616) summarized this knowledge with "*The eye sees all, but the mind shows us what we want to see,*" and Lessing's (1729–1781) *Nathan the Wise* states: "*The scientist's eye sees only what it wants to see.*" Heinz von Förster (1911–2002) expressed this in more modern terms: "*Objectivity is the delusion of believing that an observation is possible without an observer.*" This process is neither malicious nor conscious. Perception per se depends to a large extent on a person's experiences and his/her history because it shapes his/her entire perceptual and emotional apparatus. This applies to the patient and the athlete, as well as the therapist and the trainer, and can be applied without restriction to all other areas and to the present work.

In modern science, this is already reflected in the suggestion of one of the founders of experimental psychology, Wilhelm Wundt (1832–1920), to better use the term **apperception** for taking the active process of human perception into account. Initially understood only as the active control of attention, this developed into an apperception psychology with a "multimodal concept in which sensory, cognitive, emotional, and motivational partial processes are integrated in the highest synthesis of mental processes" (Wundt 1874). With this approach, Wundt already anticipated aspects of second-order cybernetics and constructivism that clearly indicate an asymmetry in the person–environmental perception process toward the perceiver with his/her active part and being the only one that adapts on the relevant timescale of survival.

A more general approach to the interaction of the two subsystems was provided with Bateson's essays collected in *Steps to an Ecology of Mind* (Bateson 1972) and the cybernetics of cybernetics (second-order cybernetics), which also massively influenced the philosophy of radical constructivism (Glasersfeld 1995). For perception, the stimulus usually acts only as a trigger. With the active control of perception, automatically, the perceiver's (the patient's) history of experiences, including all context variables of the specific perception events, moves into the focus of interest. This has been increasingly and impressively confirmed since the second half of the past century and with the development of high-resolution imaging techniques. The sight of a picture of an apple leads not only to the activation of the visual areas of the brain but also to the activation of numerous other areas that, depending on the experience, are associated with an apple in the broader context of previous experiences, e.g., olfactory areas (Sharma and Estes 2024). The same can be observed when looking at emotional images (Phan et al. 2002, 2003) or when observing conspecifics, depending on the activity (Kemmerer 2021). These central nervous activations are highly dependent on experience. When a beginner observes a movement, different brain areas are activated compared to those engaged by an advanced observer. Advanced users activate areas similar to those involved when performing their own movements (Lacourse et al. 2005).

In terms of system dynamics, this corresponds to considering the internal dynamics that need to be taken into account before starting a learning process (Kostrubiec et al. 2012; Schöner 1989). In consequence, an external stimulus is always connected with a subjective impression and a feeling that is highly dependent on the subject and his/her history.

2.6.1 Dimensions of Senses

The impressions from the apperceived environment can be structured into the following (Schmidt 1985):

1. **Spatiality**
2. **Temporality**
3. **Quality**
4. **Quantity**

This classification is not solely for scientific purposes; it also serves as the first foundation for systematically varying the practice of the intervention, on the one hand, and for enabling the systematic transfer of findings to other senses (quality), on the other.

The first two dimensions are used to categorize our sensations and perceptions in our surroundings, not only spatially (environment) but also temporally (situation). Both factors together contribute to the classification within a given context, analogous to general model theory (Hof

2018; Stachowiak 1973), which consistently considers the timing of model information. In this way, a stimulus can be spatially localized, and the temporal beginning and duration of a stimulus and the same at different times (situations) can be perceived accordingly. The first two dimensions are inherent to all material phenomena and, thus, also closely apply to "objective" sensory physiology.

The third dimension, quality or modality, provides selection criteria among the possible sensations. In the context of the statement, organism refers to a living system, such as a human, animal. The statement highlights that an organism does not perceive its internal environment (e.g., bodily processes like digestion, circulation, or cellular activity) or the external environment as a single, unified experience. Instead, it experiences these through specialized sensory organs (e.g., eyes, ears, skin, etc.), which detect specific stimuli (like light, sound, or touch) and relay information to the organism's nervous system for processing. These organs are each adapted to react to a certain range of environmental influences and transmit corresponding information to the central nervous system (CNS). Sensory impressions are divided into modalities according to their similarity.

Such modalities are, for example, the classic "*five senses*": sight, hearing, touch, taste, and smell. Other modalities relate to the sensations of orientation, temperature, vibration, and pain. The number of modalities cannot be precisely defined (Dudel 1980). The individual modalities can be differentiated according to the type of sensory impression or the quality. The modality of sight is categorized into the qualities of brightness and color, while the modality of hearing is distinguished by frequency (pitch) (Schmidt 1985).

The fourth dimension of sensation refers to the intensity or quantity of a stimulus. A quantity for the sense of sight is, for example, the brightness of a stimulus, and for the sense of hearing, it is the pitch (frequency). Physiologically, the quantity of a sensory impression corresponds to the amplitude of a receptor potential or the frequency of an action potential.

2.6.1.1 The Quality of a Sense

Physicochemically, there are five different types of sensors:

- Sensors that register mechanical deformations (in the skin, muscle, ear, and balance organ).
- Sensors that react to photons (eye).
- Sensors that register changes in temperature (especially in the skin).
- Sensors that react to chemical stimuli (taste and smell sensors).
- Sensors that register physically or chemically induced tissue damage, or the nociceptors.

In addition to brightness, color, and the spatial impression of depth, the movement also represents a quality of visual perception. The eye is the only sensory organ that is self-moving and purposeful, and the motor function of the eyes enables specific information and orientation about the spatial environment. The function of eye movement is to bring visual targets into the central (foveal) field of vision and thus to enable sharp (foveal) vision even during head movements and follow moving objects (Kornhuber 1978). The respective position of the eyes is not determined by position receptors but by efference copies. The reafference principle goes back to von Holst and Mittelstaedt in 1950 (von Holst and Mittelstaedt 1950) and states that the efference copy is branched off in the brain from the motor excitation (efference) that leads to eye movements. This neuronal signal should then be offset against the signal of the self-induced image shift (reafference); i.e., the efference copy and the reafference are simply subtracted from each other (Hassenstein 1977; von Campenhausen 1993). This calculation is used to determine the extent to which the environment or the person moves. The reafference principle was later transferred to general movement control.

In addition to the eye's excellent performance in terms of sharp vision at different distances, the perception of rapid rhythmic movements is limited. If a finger is moved back and forth over an angle of 20–30° at a frequency of 4 Hz, the finger becomes blurred because the gaze cannot follow it. If, on the other hand, the head is moved through the same angle with the same frequency while the finger is held still, it is seen sharply because the vestibular stabilization of the eyes is faster than the visual stabilization (Kornhuber 1978). The same can be observed when reading a text. This is not possible or can be done only with great difficulty if you move the text up and down with your arms. However, if you move your head up and down at the same angular velocity, you can read the text without any problems. Both phenomena give clear indications for different internal processing that can hardly be explained by direct processing in the context of the affordance concept (Michaels and Carello 1981; Ullman 1980). This is similar to spatial vision, in which the difference between the images on both retinas provides the information for the distance, or spatial hearing. You can experience this by closing one eye and trying to hit an object with an index finger by approaching it from the side. The same applies to the time difference between the arrival of the sound at the ears. The time difference between the arrival of the sound at the left and right ears only provides information about the orientation of where the sound is coming from through internal processing. These phenomena can so far best be explained with the help of neuronal circuit models for internal calculation and indicate asymmetry between the perceiving system and the environment. The asymmetry relates primarily to the property of adaptability, which is retained even in more complex perceptual processes in connection with movement. An overview of numerous other studies demonstrating the internal processing and its complexity in multisensory tasks was given by Lackner (1985). Just to get an impression of the complex internal processing, two examples are given. When a person stands upright and the Achilles tendon is vibrationally stimulated, the resulting whole-body sensation of concurrent touch and pressure signals can lead to perceived forward rotation, either from the ankles or around the head (Lackner 1985).

Similar phenomena occur in the pseudo-Coriolis illusion. In this illusion, cross-coupled angular accelerations of the semicircular canals are absent during head movements because the subject is not actually turning. However, aberrant head movements are still perceived (Guedry and Benson 1978).

The vestibular apparatus is located in the inner ear and consists of five organs: two macular organs and three semicircular canal systems; while the two macular organs (macula utriculi and matricula sacculi) respond to translational accelerations, the three semicircular canal systems (horizontal, posterior, and superior) respond to rotational accelerations. Due to the fixed relationship of the vestibular apparatus to the skull, the macular organs provide information about the position of the head in space. The three semicircular canal systems are arranged in such a way that one semicircular canal is "responsible" for each spatial direction. The information processing of the eye and vestibular organ functions relatively smoothly when the head is held upright, if each semicircular canal system is assigned to a spatial direction. However, if the head is tilted forward or to the side during a rotation, additional Coriolis accelerations occur in the vestibular apparatus, significantly complicating spatial orientation. A physical description of the semicircular canals was provided by Mayne (1974). The afferent responses of the semicircular canals to various movements of the head can be described with the aid of a differential equation (Eq. 2.1).

$$F = \theta \frac{d^2\varphi}{dt^2} + \rho \frac{d\varphi}{dt} + D\varphi \qquad (2.1)$$

F is the force underlying the rotation of the head, the first term on the right-hand side indicates the inertial force proportional to the rotational acceleration, the second term indicates the internal friction proportional to the rotational velocity, and the third term indicates the elastic restoring force proportional to the deflection of the cupula. The equation can, therefore, be used to estimate the internal afferences from the "externally" observable head movement.

In addition to conscious spatial orientation, the maculae and semicircular canal systems trigger important vestibulospinal and vestibulo-ocular reflexes. The vestibulospinal reflexes, for example, control the trunk and limb muscles to prevent injury so that the body does not fall during translational acceleration. The vestibulo-ocular reflexes allow the eyeball to make compensatory counter-movements when the head rotates; for movements without visual control and precision, such as discus throwing, additional information for spatial orientation is required in addition to the vestibular and visual reflexes. To clearly describe the position of the head and body in space, the vestibular information about head orientation is supplemented by central nervous signals about the position of the body in space. The central nervous information comes primarily from somato-sensors in the neck muscles and joints, which also transmit the position of the head in relation to the trunk. The overall information about the posture of the whole body is supplemented by somatosensory information from sensors in other joints and muscles (Zenner 1993).

The afferent nerve fibers are generally subdivided according to the speed of their adaptation behavior (slow, medium-fast, and fast) to stimuli. After prolonged exposure to a stimulus, the receptor potential usually does not remain constant but falls back to the resting potential over time; i.e., the sensor adapts to the stimulus. The speed of adaptation is indicated by a time constant, which specifies the time in which the receptor potential falls by 63% (1/t). The receptor potential for a constant stimulus is also referred to as the tonic or static stimulus response of the receptor. The receptor potential is not simply a function of the stimulus intensity R but a function of the intensity changes per time t, i.e., the differential quotient dR/dt. If the response to a stimulus is speed-dependent, we speak of a phasic or dynamic stimulus response. In the case of a constant stimulus, the response is referred to as a proportional stimulus response in accordance with the nomenclature of technical sensors and in the second case as a differential stimulus response. If a phasic response is present, the tonic response can only be recorded after it has subsided (Handwerker 1993).

Rapidly-adapting (FA) receptors (short time constant) only show a phasic response. Slowly adapting (SA) receptors show both phasic and tonic responses and are also referred to as proportional–differential receptors.

The somatosensory system comprises three areas (Handwerker 1993):

- Sensory system of the body surface (exteroception and skin sensitivity).
- Sensory system of the locomotor system (proprioception).
- Sensory system of the internal organs (interoception).

The first area provides information about the external world and the second about the spatial position of the body parts. Enteroception, the perception of the internal organs (inner world), is assigned to visceral sensitivity and is used exclusively for unconscious, reflexive regulation.

Exteroceptors include the skin's sense of touch. This sensory modality has four qualities: the sensations of pressure, touch, vibration, and tickling. The mechanoreceptors of hairless skin (e.g., on the palm of the hand and the sole of the foot) and hairy skin (e.g., on the arm), listed in (Fig. 2.11), can be differentiated according to their adaptation behavior.

The Ruffini corpuscles (SAII sensor) belong to the slowly adapting mechanoreceptors with a relatively large receptive field. The receptive

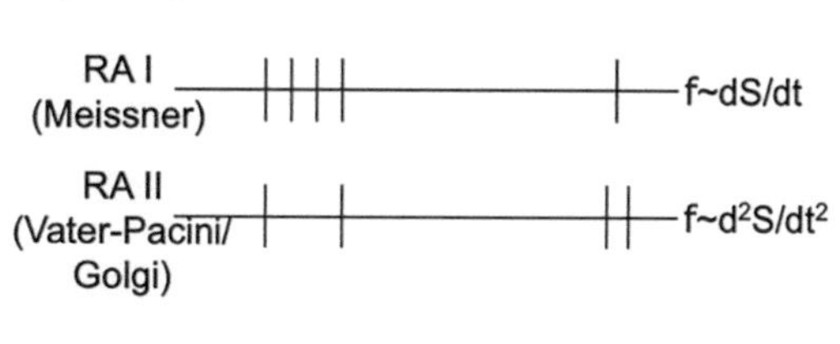

Fig. 2.11 Mechano-sensors (*SAII* slowly adapting II, *SAI* slowly adapting I, *RA* rapidly adapting, and PC: Vater–Pacini corpuscles), their firing patterns (schematic), and their biomechanical analogies. (Adapted from (Johansson and Vallbo 1983))

fields of Merkel cells or tactile discs (SAI sensors), which also adapt slowly, are relatively small and sharply defined; i.e., they can localize a stimulus relatively precisely with a high spatial resolution. Meissner corpuscles belong to the group of rapidly adapting mechanoreceptors with very small receptive fields and, together with the Krause end bulbs, form the so-called velocity detectors. They are capable of constantly perceiving new touches. Vater–Pacini and Golgi–Mazzoni corpuscles are extremely fast adapters and react to changes in the speed of the mechanical stimulus (Zilles and Rehkämper 1993). They perceive accelerations and, as vibration receptors, show a very high temporal resolution of processes and states.

In slow-adapting receptors, the discharge frequency is proportional to the stimulus intensity. Medium-fast-adapting afferents, on the other hand, show a discharge rate that is proportional to the change in mechanical stimulus per time; i.e., they are speed detectors for hair movements or pressure stimuli, and they convey touch sensations. Very-fast-adapting receptors respond adequately to the acceleration of a skin displacement and, together with the hair follicle sensors, are involved in the sensation of vibration. The somatosensory proprioceptors can be divided into three groups:

- The joint receptors.
- The muscle spindles.
- The Golgi tendon organs.

Four types of joint receptors are distinguished:

- The Vater–Pacini corpuscles.
- The Ruffini receptors of the joint capsule.
- The Golgi joint ligament receptors.
- The free nerve endings.

The Vater–Pacini corpuscles are very rapidly adapting vibration receptors (accelerometers) and contribute nothing to the joint position sensation. The Ruffini receptors are located in the joint capsule and are both movement and position receptors. The Golgi joint ligament receptors are purely position receptors. The appropriate stimulus is extension, flexion, or rotation of the joint. Little is known about the numerous free nerve endings of the joints. The last three types belong to the slowly adapting receptors.

Proprioception through mechanoreceptors at the joints certainly plays a role, but it cannot be the sole explanation, as difficulties would then be expected with artificial joints—something that does not occur. The Ruffini corpuscles can be deactivated by local anesthetics in the joint area and in the surrounding tissues without impairing the sense of position. Similar to the eyes, the position is not only determined by position receptors but also by efferent copies (von Campenhausen 1993). The central nervous system receives additional information on position and movement perception via receptors in the muscle and tendon areas.

The muscle spindles consist of two types of specialized muscle fibers in a connective tissue sheath. Because of the connective tissue enclosure, the fibers are called intrafusal muscle fibers, whereas the other muscle fibers are called extrafusal. Since muscle spindles lie parallel to the working musculature, they relax when the muscle shortens, thereby reducing the impulse rate. The corresponding stimulus is the stretching of the intrafusal fibers. Muscle spindles, therefore, take on the function of a length gauge.

Depending on the arrangement of their nuclei, intrafusal muscle fibers are divided into "nuclear bag" fibers (NB fibers) and "nuclear chain" fibers (NC fibers). While the nuclei of NB fibers fill the entire cross section in dense clusters over a short distance, the nuclei of NC fibers are arranged in chains, one behind the other (Schmidt 1972). The two types of intrafusal fibers (NB and NC) are each supplied by two types of efferent γ-fibers (dynamic and static γd and γs) and by two types of afferents (primary Ia and secondary II). Different properties of the bag and chain fibers cause Ia fibers to have more dynamic and II afferents to have more static properties. The same applies to the γd and γs fibers. The γd-motoaxons mainly act on the NB fibers and increase the sensitivity of the spindle for dynamic processes. The γ-axons, on the other hand, increase the static measuring function and, at the same time, reduce the dynamic sensitivity. This rather complicated arrangement of the muscle spindles ensures that the receptor messages from the central nervous system can be influenced separately via the absolute muscle length and the responses to length changes by γs or γd neurons (Ten Bruggencate 1984).

Since muscle spindles are particularly numerous in muscles used for fine motor skills and in neck muscles, it is assumed that they are important for both posture and fine movements. Tendon organs (Golgi organs) lie in series with the extrafusal musculature (Schmidt 1987), usually close to the muscular origin of the tendons, and are thus activated during both muscle stretching and muscle contraction. Passive stretching to the same final tension but at different stretching speeds shows that the pulse frequency of the receptor depends essentially on the strength of the stretch and less on the speed at which the stretch occurs. Even during active contraction of a muscle, the impulse rates of the tendon organs are proportional to the strength of the contraction (Schmidt 1972). Accordingly, tendon organs are tension receptors (Haase et al. 1976), i.e., force sensors (tension = force/area).

Spindle receptors can be excited, on the one hand, by muscle stretching and, on the other, by impulses from the g-fibers. With some receptors, the nervous system can influence the sensitivity of the sensor and thus achieve functionally more favorable adaptation to the stimulus. Such efferent control can also occur without directly influencing the actual sensory cell: Auxiliary structures located in the stimulus transmission pathway to the receptor can be adjusted. Examples of this mechanism include increasing the sensitivity of muscle spindles by motor innervation of the intrafusal muscle fibers (Dudel 1980). Assuming that the muscle spindles and stretch receptors of the tendons provide information about the position of the limbs, the system becomes sensitive and error-prone to external mechanical influences. Vibrating the upper arm flexor at 100 Hz simulated greater stretching of the muscle spindles, creating the illusion that the arm was more extended than it actually was (Goodwin et al. 1972). With the help of the other arm, it was determined that the impression was 30° different from the real angle. The other arm was placed in the same position and showed a deviation of more than 30°. Without vibration, the angular position of both arms was identical.

None of the receptor systems mentioned thus far is capable of providing the necessary information for the corresponding quality on its own (Schmidt 1985). Overall, the proprio- and exteroceptors described serve the mechanical perception of positions (joint and position angles), movements (angular velocities), and forces (accelerations) of individual parts of our body (Handwerker 1993) in the environment (gravitational field of the Earth) and thus supply a large amount of information to the central nervous system.

2.6.1.2 The Quantity of a Sense

In contrast to the measurement of the stimulus intensity or the amplitude or frequency of the stimulus response using physicochemical methods, it is not possible to objectify the intensity of the stimulus response, the triggered sensation, in a physicochemical measurement system. The intensity of sensation is not a physical quantity and, therefore, cannot be measured objectively. This is also shown by the experience that our senses do not provide reliable information about absolute quantities such as weights or orientation. The sensitivity to difference depends on the absolute quantity. According to Weber (1795–1878), the smallest just perceptible deviation dI is a certain fraction of the stimulus I. Weber's law (Eq. 2.2) for the discrimination threshold is

$$dI / I = c \qquad (2.2)$$

The constant c depends on the sensory system and the experimental conditions. When lifting weights, c is 1/50. If the weight is held still without being lifted, the ratio is greater with c = 1/4. This means that the discrimination sensitivity has become smaller in the static situation in comparison to the dynamic condition. Future research will show how closely these thresholds are linked to the extent of fluctuations during movement repetitions. The same applies to sensitivity across multiple joints. These findings have a long tradition in German and European physiological research and can be traced back to the middle of the nineteenth century, long before Gibson's now classic "Observations on active touch" in the English-speaking world (Gibson 1962; Goldscheider 1889; Wagner 2016). When comparing visually the lengths of straight lines, c is 1/60 when viewed alternately, and c is 1/250 when viewed simultaneously (von Campenhausen 1993).

Fechner derived a relationship between the intensity of the sensation E and the stimulus intensity I from Weber's law by integrating eq. 8 over dI and obtaining the Weber–Fechner's law (Eq. 2.3)

$$E = K \log I + C \tag{2.3}$$

The Weber–Fechner law only applies to a limited intensity range and specific senses, however. Since the intensity of sensation could not be measured, Stevens (1906–1973) developed an intrinsic metric by estimating its magnitude. This resulted in Stevens' power function (^{n}Eq. 2.4) with

$$E = k\left(I - I_o\right)^n \tag{2.4}$$

(E = sensation intensity, I = stimulus intensity, Io = threshold stimulus intensity, and k = proportionality factor)

The sensation intensity E is, therefore, proportional to the nth power of the suprathreshold stimulus (I − Io). The threshold stimulus intensity indicates the stimulus intensity required to trigger a perceptible sensation. The modality-specific coefficient n varies between 0.33 and 3.5 in numerical comparison estimates. The increasing slope of the straight line is associated with a decrease in the levels of sensation, i.e., few levels of sensation for pain and many perceptible gray levels for the sense of sight.

Potential functions of the type a^n also characterize the transmission function of sensory neurons. Studies on the sense of taste have shown that the responses of the primary afferents run parallel to the subjective intensity of taste (Ten Bruggencate 1980). This parallelism can be traced to areas of the brain. For example, the mean discharge frequencies of cells in the thalamus during somatosensory activation by joint afferents also show a potential function that is dependent on the joint position (Mountcastle et al. 1963). In the sense of vibration, the amplitude of the stimulus-induced evoked potential is also linked to the external stimulus strength via a power function (Ehrenberger et al. 1966). If these potentials evoked by sensory stimuli are understood as an integration effect of sensory systems, then " ... *there would be an astonishing correspondence between the electro-physiologically detectable cortical information and the contents of consciousness*" (Ten Bruggencate, 1980). The application of Stevens' power function (Eq. 2.4) to multiple stimuli from the same senses at different locations or from different senses is fraught with problems. Here, it is necessary to determine the exponent, if any, of the total population, as two power functions may only be linked linearly if their exponents are identical.

2.6.1.3 The Spatial Dimension of a Sense

Every sensory perception has a spatial component. The ability to localize a stimulus depends on the sensory system. The sense of sight and, to a somewhat lesser extent, the sense of pressure and temperature of the skin can be localized most precisely. Less well-developed are the senses of hearing and smell (Ten Bruggencate 1980). The reason for the localization ability lies in the topographical structure and representation of the peripheral and central parts of the sensory systems. Proprioception can be categorized into different areas depending on the number and type of receptors in the corresponding areas. While the spatial resolution of the sense of touch tends to increase distally to the palm and sole of the foot or in the mouth and lip area, it decreases distally with regard to proprioception (Goldscheider 1889; Hall and McCloskey 1983). This superiority of the proximal joints in terms of proprioceptive accuracy is only present when the position of the joints is specified in angles. However, if one considers the change in position in cm of the distal phalanx (fingertip) associated with the respective angular change of a joint, there is no difference in the sensitivity of the positional sensation of the shoulders, elbows, and metacarpophalangeal joints. The same also applies depending on the flexion speed of the joint (McCloskey 1993). In connection with the dependence of the sensitivity on the conditions (static or dynamic) and on the maximum resolution discussed above, studies on the stability of movements would need to be reconsidered.

2.6.1.4 The Time Dimension of a Sense

One of the main factors influencing sensory intensity is the duration of the stimulus. As the duration of a stimulus increases, the intensity of sensation decreases, showing adaptation to the stimulus process. Adaptation can lead to the extinction of conscious sensation. As early as 1859, Meissner was able to demonstrate rapid adaptation in the sensation of pressure on the skin. When a finger was immersed in a vessel filled with mercury, no pressure was felt at the tip of the finger but only at the surface of the mercury, where there was a change in the constant pressure exerted on the skin. In other words, there is no sensation in the finger due to the pressure as such but only when there is a change in pressure. The experiments were confirmed by Békésy (1970).

Adaptation cannot be traced back to a single process but can be observed on several levels (e.g., spine, brain stem, limbic system, cortex, etc.). In addition to the adaptation of the peripheral receptor, there is a central adaptation that has a much longer time constant and usually outlasts the receptor's adjustment time. The adaptation of the sense of hearing in different central nervous areas was demonstrated by Keidel and Finkenzeller (1984). The longer time constant also applies to de-adaptation; i.e., the subjective sensitivity to the stimulus returns at all levels with a similar time course to that observed for adaptation (Birbaumer 1990). Obviously, frequent stimulus repetition also loses its central effect, both in the short and the long term. Another aspect of the temporal dimension relates to the inertia of the senses. Since the maximum or decay of the intensity of sensation occurs with a time delay, both at the beginning and at the end of a stimulus, this results in a temporal inertia of sensory performance. In the sense of sight, rhythmic stimuli at a frequency of 12–20 Hz merge into a uniform image. The corresponding individual flicker fusion frequency varies but does not appear to depend on eye fatigue (Singh and Wulf 2022). In the sense of touch, frequencies of up to 200 Hz can be perceived (Ten Bruggencate 1980). At this level, too, there is a high degree of individual and situational dependency in perception performance.

2.6.2 Transmission and Central Nervous Processing of Somato-Visceral Information

In what follows, the method of gaining knowledge in the sense of an abbreviated representation of an original model (Hof 2018; Schöllhorn et al. 2022; Stachowiak 1973) should always be considered. The information obtained is, therefore, always simplified under particular conditions. Thereby, the findings on neuronal structures and functions are based on anatomical and cell biological studies, as well as on phenomena that were observed when certain areas failed due to injuries, diseases, or medical operations or with the help of imaging procedures (EEG, MRI, CT, etc.), which were always carried out under specific conditions.

In the processing of messages from the receptors in the central nervous system, two physiological levels are distinguished (Zimmermann 1980):

(a) The level of the afferent systems.
(b) The level of the integrative and efferent systems.

The level of the afferent or sensory system includes various ascending pathways that can be traced via several stations in the spinal cord, brain stem, thalamus, and cerebral cortex. The second level of central nervous processing, the integrative and efferent side, includes four areas that partly overlap anatomically. These include the associative, limbic, motor, and vegetative systems. The essential functions of these systems include the integration of messages from several sensory systems and of stored information (memory) (Zimmermann, 1980).

2.6.2.1 The Level of the Afferent Systems

The afferent system of sensorimotor function essentially receives its information from three sensory systems: the sense of sight (eye), the sense of balance (vestibular organ), and the sense of position (proprioception). A dominant role of the visual system is primarily derived from studies on balance and target movements (Adams 1987). In a large number of movements, however, the visual system is either inferior to other sensory systems or not involved at all because the movement takes place outside the field of vision or is too fast for the visual information to have a modulating effect. For example, Kamen and Morris (1988) were able to demonstrate the superiority of the proprioceptive system in reaction tasks and Rockmann-Rüger (1991) in the reproduction of a skillful movement (60% of the maximum squat jump performance).

Only a part of the afferents of the somatovisceral receptors reaches the conscious mind, i.e., the cerebral cortex. By far the greater part runs in control circuits that are not conscious. They are part of reflexes, which, among other things, counteract the force of gravity as holding reflexes and thus also serve the voluntary motor function. A reflex is a stereotypical and involuntary (automatic) motor reaction to a certain stimulus, which is, however, modulated by certain mental processes (Herbert and Kissler 2010; Stam et al. 1989). A similar asymmetry of the individual and the environment in the perceptual process can be observed in the visual domain, where stimulus rivalry is a common means of investigating visual consciousness. When a constant physical stimulus evokes several different perceptual interpretations (percepts) that alternate over time, such as in optical illusions, the "reflexes" correspond to the percepts rather than the physical stimulus (Naber et al. 2011).

From such neuropsychological findings, models, such as "*direct perception*" and "*without representation*" (Michaels and Carello 1981), in conjunction with the affordances introduced by Gibson, tend to emerge more from a naïve holism (Afriat 2004). This perspective is based on the analysis of perceptual processes while neglecting the underlying neurophysiological findings. A subsequent reinterpretation of previous neurophysiological findings using new terminology (de Wit et al. 2017) does little to change this. In terms of practical consequences, all criticisms of the representation-oriented approaches mainly relied on an outdated black box model of former psychology and did not go beyond implications that had not already been derived from the criticized models (Chemero 2001; Proctor and Miles 2014).

Depending on the structure involved, two types of somato-motor reflexes can be distinguished: (a) spinal cord reflexes and (b) reflexes that are mediated by the brain (Mörike et al. 1991). Depending on the number of synapses involved, a distinction is made between monosynaptic intrinsic reflexes and polysynaptic extrinsic reflexes. The reflexes exert a significant influence on posture, although they are subject to the modulating influence of supraspinal levels (Henatsch 1976).

An essential prerequisite for the correct execution and learning of a movement is that higher sensory and motor centers are informed about the segmental excitation input and the processing of excitation in the spinal cord. The information from the vestibular organ, the skin, and the musculoskeletal system runs centrally in five groups of pathways (Klinke 1985; Silbernagl 1979).

1. The afferent nerve fibers of the vestibular organ (vestibular nerve) project into the brain stem (vestibular nuclei of the medulla oblongata). From the vestibular nuclei, there are connections:
   (a) To the spinal cord (vestibulospinal tract), via which, in particular, motor neurons of the extensors are influenced.

(b) Directly to the motor neurons of the cervical medulla (corresponds to a).
(c) To the eye muscle nuclei (in the brain stem), via which the vestibular-induced eye movements occur.
(d) To the cerebellum (vestibulocerebellum), whose efferents pathways synergistically influence the spinal motor system to maintain balance (Duus 1990).
(e) To the vestibular nuclei of the other side, with the help of which the inputs of both sides are processed.
(f) To the formatio reticularis (in the brain stem), via which the Tr. vestibulospinalis and also the motor neurons are influenced.
(g) Via the thalamus to the posterior central convolutions of the cortex, which serve the conscious processing of vestibular inputs.
(h) To the hypothalamus; these fibers are associated with kinetosis (Klinke 1985).

2. Sensory fibers from the head region (n. trigeminus) also lead to the thalamus.
3. Two pathways lead to the cerebellum (tractus spinocerebellaris anterior and posterior). The fibers of these pathways are among the fastest conductors of all (Duus 1990). Via polysynaptic efferents, the cerebellum influences the muscle tone and the synergistic interaction of agonists and antagonists during walking, standing, and any other movement. In this way, a higher functional circuit is established via the lower control circuits of the spinal cord, which influences motor function but still remains below the threshold of consciousness (Duus 1990).
4. Afferents reach the "conscious" somatosensory cerebral cortex via the posterior pathways in the spinal cord. Since the afferents in these pathways are anatomically and neurophysiologically organized from only one peripheral sensory area at a time and are correspondingly somatotopically related to the sensory cerebral cortex, the entire system is also referred to as the specific system. This lemniscal system forms the basis for all sensory-physiological abilities that require a conscious differentiation of the spatial details of a stimulus. The afferents of the specific somatosensory system run via the posterior cord tracts of the spinal cord through the brain stem (medulla oblongata and bridge) and midbrain (thalamus) to the so-called body feeling sphere in the area of the posterior central convolutions of the cerebrum to the somatosensory regions SI and SII (S = somatosensory).
5. The frontal pathways pass through the brain stem (formatio reticularis) to the thalamus and are transmitted from there to all areas of the cerebral cortex. This system lacks the uniqueness of the afferent influx; i.e., it is excited convergently from all sensory surfaces and is, therefore, referred to as a nonspecific system. In addition to the somato-visceral influx via the spinal cord, there are sensory influxes from all other sensory systems, and there are connections to practically all areas of the cerebral cortex. There are also connections from the thalamus to the vegetative centers in the brain stem and hypothalamus, to the limbic system, and to the subcortical centers of motor function (Zimmermann 1980).

The distinction between the specific and nonspecific systems refers to a number of functional properties that are different in the two systems (Zimmermann 1980). The subdivision does not mean that they can be activated separately. In everyday or sports movements, the systems are always activated together by a variety of sensory stimuli.

2.6.2.2 The Integrative and Efferent Systems

Processes that are not directly related to the processing of sensory input or the activity of the motor centers are referred to as integrative performances of the central nervous system. In the following sections, the functions of the three main areas of the brain involved (Rosenbaum 1991) are described in more detail with special consideration of the sensorimotor system:

- The cerebellum.
- The basal ganglia.
- The cerebrum (cortex).

2.6.2.3 The Cerebellum

With more than half of the neurons in the human brain, far more cells are localized in the cerebellum than in the cerebrum (Barinaga 1996; Blinkov and Glezer 1968; Huggenberger et al. 2019; Ito 1984). The fact that the cerebellum is nevertheless small compared to the cerebrum is due to (a) the thickness of the cerebellar cortex (< 1 mm), (b) the white matter only carrying input and output fibers and no association fibers, and (c) the subcortical gray matter of the cerebellum (cerebellar nuclei) being smaller than that of the cerebrum. The fact that the white matter of the cerebellar cortex carries no association fibers but only input and output fibers indicates that in this part, mainly local calculations are made, and that the task is not to establish as many relationships as possible within the cortex (as in the cerebrum). The stereotypical structure of the neurons and the fact that they are layered in the same way everywhere suggest that this "mapping" takes place in the same way everywhere (Braitenberg and Schüz 1993). One thing that the cerebral cortex and cerebellar cortex have in common is that most synapses are located on dendritic spines and can be influenced by learning. Due to the plasticity of these synapses, it is, therefore, assumed that learned movement strategies for rapid movements or for holding the body upright are stored in the cerebellum (Braitenberg and Schüz 1993).

Afferents and efferents: The cerebellum receives afferents from all parts of the CNS. All afferents reach the cerebellar cortex via two fiber systems (mossy fibers and climbing fibers) after they have previously delivered collaterals to the cerebellar nuclei (Zilles and Rehkämper 1993). The dual access is associated with the assumed learning process. The afferents via the climbing fibers act as a "tutor" during learning (Braitenberg and Schüz 1993). Due to the projection of the cerebellar cortex (Purkinje cells) onto the cerebellar nuclei and their interconnection with specific areas, the cerebellum can be subdivided into three functional subsystems (Illert 1993). In one system (vestibulo-cerebellum), among other things, the transmission of information from the vestibular organ is controlled, and the coordination of eye and head movements is regulated. The muscles of the trunk and proximal extremities are controlled by efferents via the spinal cord (vestibulospinal tracts) to maintain balance. This direct interconnection of the vestibular organ and eye and head movements allows a text to be read even when the head is constantly moving up and down. However, if the text is moved up and down with the hands, reading is no longer possible. Physically, the same stimulus is presented in both situations, but the neuronal circuitry only allows reading when the head is moving. Again, the phenomena indicate a clear asymmetry in the direction of the perceiving individual, which is difficult to explain using affordances in Gibson's sense.

A second system (spino-cerebellum) controls the execution of sequential movements by means of various information from corresponding areas:

1. Information about the cortical movement program from the motor cortex.
2. Information about the progress of the movement programming (spinal interneuronal system).
3. Information about the execution of the movement from the spinal cord, the somatosensory cortex, and the acoustic, visual, and vestibular cortex. It receives an efference copy of the movement performed, which can be compared with an afference copy. The afference copy is made available via the proprioceptive and vestibular afferents and provides information about the length and tension ratios of the muscles as well as the position of the body and its parts in space. By controlling the trunk muscles and the proximal and distal limb muscles, the posture is adapted to the intended movement.

The third system (cerebro-cerebellum) receives afferents from various parts of the cerebral cortex (motor and sensory cortex, posterior parietal cortex, and visual and limbic representation areas). The integration into a loop that runs via the thalamus to the motor fields of the cerebral cortex and back via the brain stem to the cerebellum (Thompson 1990) suggests that this system is involved in the planning and programming of a movement. Due to its internal structure (interconnection of Purkinje cells and parallel fibers), the cerebellum (cerebellar cortex) is able to register the temporal sequence of motor activity and imprint a spatial and temporal pattern on afferents. The topographical arrangement between parallel fibers, Purkinje cells, and neurons of the cerebellar nuclei forms the anatomical basis for muscular synergies during complex movements.

Depending on the size and location of the damage, a failure of the cerebellum results in disorders in the execution of voluntary movements (Duus 1990). Damage to the cerebellum leads, among other things, to target movements becoming too short or too long, the inability to perform rapidly alternating movements, or balance disorders. Functions of the cerebellum can be partially taken over by other areas of the brain (Duus 1990; Ten Bruggencate 1984; Zilles and Rehkämper 1993). Overall, in addition to the "smoothing" (Braitenberg and Schüz 1993) and timing of continuous movements, the creation of new muscular synergies in the context of motor learning is one of the main functions of the cerebellum (Illert 1993; Thompson 1990; Zilles and Rehkämper 1993).

2.6.2.4 The Basal Ganglia

The basal ganglia are subcortical nuclei that control voluntary actions and have been linked to Parkinson's disease. The dysfunctions of the basal ganglia most frequently lead to hyperkinetic-hypotonic (chorea) and hypokinetic-hypertonic (Parkinson's disease) movement disorders. In the first case, there is an excess of movement with uncontrollable and relatively fast movements. The basal ganglia receive their afferents from the entire cerebral cortex (motor, sensory, limbic, and associative cortices), with the most important efferent system projecting back to the motor and prefrontal cortex via the thalamus (Illert 1993). The basal ganglia are thus part of a loop and have access to the efferents of the cerebral cortex (efferent cortical tract systems).

The predominant model for the function of the basal ganglia consists of the direct and indirect pathways that originate from different populations of striatal medium spiny neurons (MSNs) and project to different output structures (Lanciego et al. 2012). These circuits have opposite effects on movement. The activation of the MSN of the direct pathway promotes movement, while the activation of the MSN of the indirect pathway inhibits it. Recent evidence has shown that this model may not fully explain the simultaneous activation of both pathways during movement. Alternatively, a model is proposed in which intrastriatal connections are crucial and the two pathways are structurally and functionally intertwined (Calabresi et al. 2014). Thus, all MSNs could either facilitate or inhibit movement, depending on which form of synaptic plasticity is expressed at a given time. In Parkinson's disease, changes in dopamine-dependent synaptic plasticity could impair this coordinated activity.

2.6.2.5 The Cerebrum (Cortex)

Similar to the cerebellum, the cerebrum consists of white and gray matter. Three types of fiber connections are found in the white matter of the cerebrum:

1. Association fibers, which connect areas of a hemisphere with each other.
2. Commissural fibers, which primarily connect corresponding sections of the hemispheres.
3. Projection fibers, which enter and exit the cerebrum, i.e., both the afferent and efferent pathways. Regarding afferents, two main types can be distinguished:
   (a) The specific thalamocortical.
   (b) The nonspecific thalamocortical and mesocortical fibers.

The thalamocortical afferents are largely topographical, while the nonspecific systems are more diffusely organized. The gray matter of the cerebral cortex, like all core areas, is a switching point for nervous signals (Creutzfeldt 1983). According to their functional importance for the overall function of the brain, both hemispheres are subdivided into smaller areas that are defined by the origin of their afferent inputs and the destination of their efferent outputs. Although some areas are referred to as sensory and others as motor, there is neither a cortical area in which only input fibers arrive nor an area that only sends output fibers (Braitenberg and Schüz 1993). The corresponding regions are therefore often referred to as "moto-sensory or sensorimotor." Several areas of the cerebral cortex are important for the control of movements. They are involved to varying degrees in the direct processing of sensory information or in the integration of cortical output and are referred to as primary, secondary, and tertiary sensory or motor areas (Fig. 2.12). Higher-order areas (secondary and tertiary) are always localized in the immediate vicinity of the primary areas. The distinction between primary, secondary, and tertiary regions refers to levels of increasing complexity and abstraction of sensory representations and motor commands (Wiesendanger 1990).

Since 90% of the cortex has the same structure with vertical columns and six layers (Creutzfeldt 1983; Saladin 2011), which are arranged in topographical maps of increasing complexity, findings that have been extensively derived from the visual cortex can be transferred to the other sensory cortices. The same has been shown for the plasticity of the entire cortex. The plasticity, first identified in the visual cortex as a function of the stimuli presented (Wiesel and Hubel 1963), could also be shown with a slight delay in the somatosensory and motor cortex (Georgopoulos et al. 1982; Merzenich et al. 1984; Schwartz et al. 1988). Implications of neuronal plasticity, e.g., for neurorehabilitation after stroke (Jenkins and Merzenich 1987), for a basic visual discrimination task (Karni and Sagi 1991) or for children with special speech impairments (Merzenich et al. 1996) were successfully derived at an early stage. It was characteristic here that the specific senses were stimulated with a large number of different stimuli. In the case of the visual discrimination task (Karni and Sagi 1991), there were 1000 stimuli per session.

2.6.2.6 Mirror Neurons

The mirror neurons (di Pellegrino et al. 1992; Rizzolatti et al. 1996) fire when an activity is visually observed, activating brain areas similar to those engaged when performing the action. However, their activity is also influenced by various factors, which can be categorized into five groups: the observed action, the actor, the observer, the relationship between the actor and the observer, and the context (Kemmerer 2021). So far, 22 factors have been identified, six of which relate to the action, two to the actor, nine to the observer, four to the relationship between the actor and the observer, and one to the context (Kemmerer 2021). The numerical relationship of the factors alone again indicates the asymmetry of the perception process.

2.6.2.7 Common- and Event-Coding Model

Although these models are classically assigned to psychology, they are dealt with here in the section on basic neurophysiology because of their proximity to the theory of mirror neurons. The common coding model (Prinz 1990, 1997) and its further development into the model of event coding (Hommel et al. 2001) assume that when perceiving an action, a person activates the same representations of motor plans that would also be activated if they were actually performing or even just planning the action. The common coding model assumes that perception and action share common representations. In addition to the Simon effect (Simon and Rudell 1967), several studies now provide confirmatory evidence for the common coding theory (Dayan et al. 2007; Etzel et al. 2008). In psychology, the Simon effect refers to the observation that reactions to stimuli occur more quickly if the stimulus and reaction are in the same place, even if the position of the stimulus is irrelevant to the execution of the task. The model of event coding (Hommel et al. 2001) emphasizes the expected or intended effects of actions. These are represented by the characteristics of their expected sensory consequences (including perceived affect, effort, and motivation), which are integrated with the motor patterns that have elicited these consequences in the past (Hommel and Wiers 2017). From this model, the idea of external focus in motor learning was derived (Wulf 2008; Wulf et al. 2000, 2010). Instead of focusing on body movements or muscle activity, an external focus of attention is directed toward the effect of one's action on the environment. However, despite repeated claims of alleged positive effects, a recent meta-analysis of studies from the past 20 years found little to no systematic effect (McKay et al. 2024). In addition, the model follows the classic idea that external focus would be the more favorable variant for

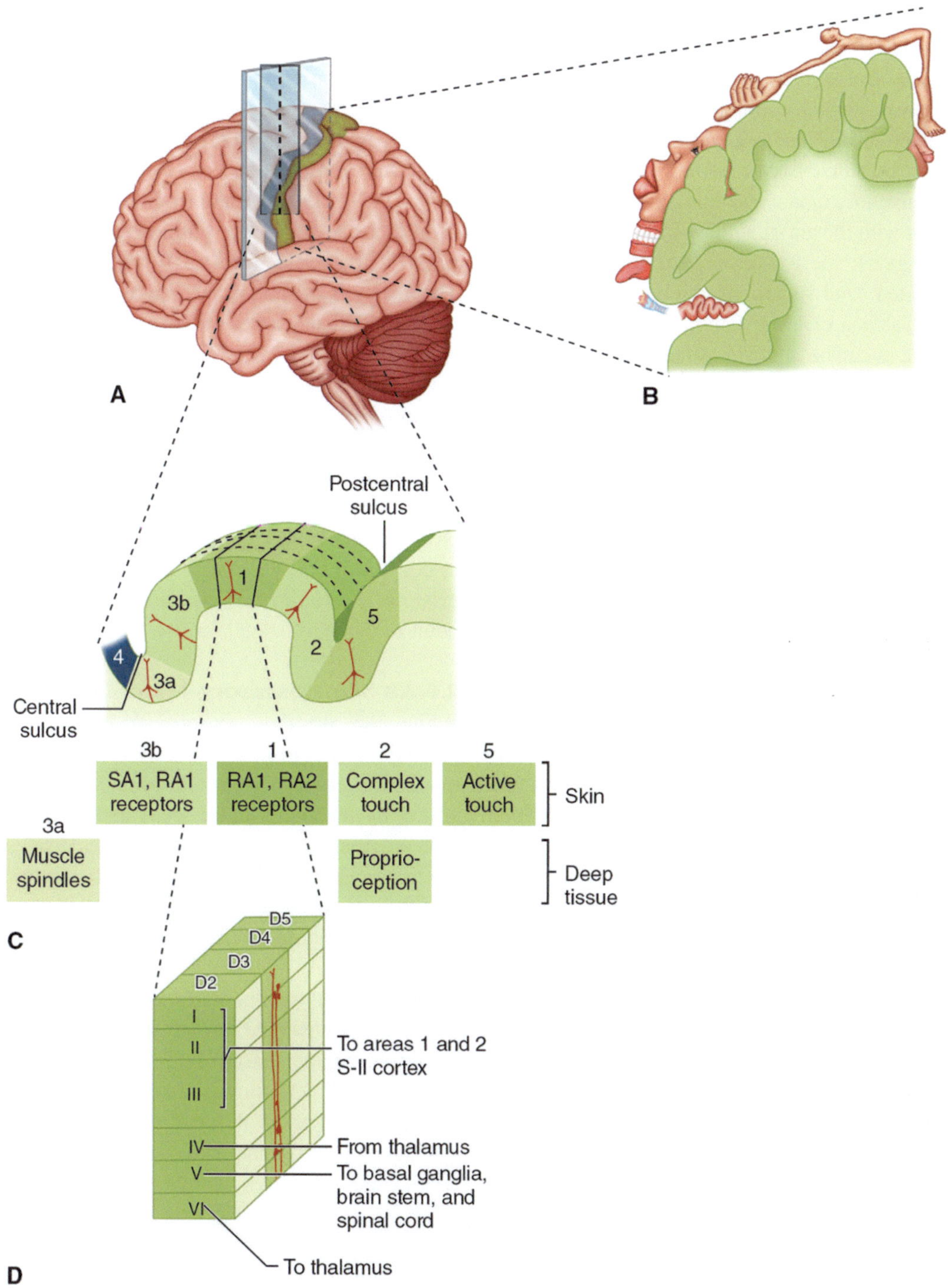

Fig. 2.12 Cortex marked somatosensory and motor–sensory areas and their more detailed anatomical structure

all learners and has not yet been examined with respect to individual specifics or situational conditions. Instead of throwing the baby out with the bathwater and discarding the model altogether, it should motivate us to look at the more precise boundary conditions under which it works or under which it does not work, e.g., looking for person- and context-dependent responses.

All these models and findings agree on the problem of classically separating perception and action. But in addition, they point to the asymmetry of the perception process in relation to the individual and his/her environment, which can be depicted on the part of the individual with the aid of a memory model and in relation to the environment with the aid of a representation model.

Against the background of these cognition-oriented and neurophysiological models, an equivalence or even dominance of the environment, as can be found in connection with isolated interpretations of affordances as invitations (Withagen et al. 2012), is more than problematic. Rather, this type of interpretation resembles an approximation of the outdated model of behaviorism, which assumed that the individual was shaped exclusively by stimuli from the environment. Although this metaphor may give therapists and trainers the illusion of external control over the learning process, the simultaneous use of contradictory models—such as internal dynamics and the affirmation of individual perceptual conditions—not only superficially acknowledges current research trends but also creates confusion and hinders scientific progress due to its contradictory nature. When integrating several models, their mutual contradictions should, therefore, be clarified in advance. The numerous and sometimes contradictory definitions of affordances since Gibson (1979) have so far done little to clarify the situation (Proctor and Miles 2014). If affordances are also characterized as "quicksilvery" (Chemero and Turvey 2007), prone to rapid appearance and disappearance (Shaw et al. 2019), even the ground for scientific verifiability in the sense of replicability is abandoned.

Furthermore, from a pragmatic point of view, the practical consequences derived from the affordance concept in the form of diverse invitations through environmental stimuli do not provide any insights that go beyond an enriched environment, as already suggested by the reform pedagogue Froebel in 1826 when introducing kindergartens for the healthy development of children (Froebel 1826). The same has been extensively confirmed at the neurological level in connection with research on the plasticity of the brain in old age (Altman and Das 1964; Dinse 2004; Faverjon et al. 2002; Garthe et al. 2016; Kempermann et al. 1997). Similarly, training science was recommending a wide range of exercises from early on for a successful sports career (Hirtz 1977; Mechling and Roth 1992). This has been repeated in a more political context in the physical literacy concept of Whitehead (2001). The matching of sports exercises to the skill level of the individual learner was also already the subject of the methodical rows of exercises, as introduced by Gaulhofer and Streicher in 1924 (Gaulhofer and Streicher 1924) and then transferred to the methodical game series by Mahlo (1965). Instead of renaming old findings and ideas, it would be more fruitful for scientific progress and the development of creative practice to derive principles and new consequences from existing knowledge and use them as a starting point for new investigations.

2.6.2.8 Somatosensory–Motor Cortex

While the primary sensory areas primarily receive information about individual sensory modalities, more complex information is integrated in the higher-order areas and compared with previously stored memories (Duus 1990). In the primary somatosensory region (SI), the body surface is mapped several times as a "*homunculus*," differentiated according to the location of the peripheral receptors (somatotopic), in modality-specific columns (areas 3a, 3b, 1, and 2). Area 3a shows the muscle spindles and area 3b the mechanoreceptors of the skin (RA: rapidly adapting and SA: slowly adapting receptors). Mechanoreceptors of deep sensitivity (joint capsule, tendons, and muscles) project to area 2, and area 1 mainly receives afferents from the rapidly adapting receptors. The somatotopy of the smaller secondary sensory area (SII) is coarser than in the primary sensory area, and the receptive fields show much greater overlap. The most striking difference, however, is that in (SII), a representation of both halves of the body is found and not only of the contralateral side as in (SI). In the transition area between (SI) and (SII), vestibular and joint afferents are also mixed

(Creutzfeldt 1983). Moreover, neurons in the somatosensory cortex (SI) react to both active and passive limb movements.

Phasic activations occur during movements and tonic activations during static holding positions. The movement-related activations are not only caused by afferent excitations but occur at least in some of the neurons 50–100 ms before the start of a movement. In particular, the activity of the cells in areas 3a and 2 correlates with electro-myo-graphy (EMG) activity and force (Creutzfeldt 1983). In the case of the secondary somatosensory region (SII), the functional properties of its neurons depend only to a limited extent on the association fiber inputs from the primary region (SI). In the tertiary somatosensory region (area 5), often referred to as the association area due to its long latency, no somatotopic organization of the afferents has been found so far.

Two-thirds of the neurons in area 5 are activated by passive joint movements on the contralateral side of the body. Most respond to a single joint, some to multiple contralateral joints, and a few to joints on both sides. Of the neurons, 10% are excited by skin stimuli, whereby the receptive fields are large. Individual cells can only be excited by muscle pressure or other deep sensory stimuli. More complex stimuli, such as stretching the hand in a certain direction, are particularly effective. Since the neurons of area 5 (analogous to SII) remain excitable even after the ablation of the primary somatosensory areas, it must be a matter of thalamocortical projections and not activation via cortical association fibers (Creutzfeldt 1983). A stronger electrical stimulation can even trigger a flexion synergy of the contralateral arm and the contra- or ipsilateral leg in area 5 with a corresponding latency, as well as a secondary rotation of the head, eyes, and trunk to the opposite side (Foerster 1936).

2.6.2.9 Sensorimotor Cortex

Both the hierarchical (regions of increasing complexity) and the parallel (heterarchical) organization (direct influence of the different areas on the execution of a movement) can also be found in the motor regions. The motor areas are located immediately before (rostral) the somatosensory areas and can be coarsely subdivided into three regions: primary motor cortex (area 4), premotor cortex (area 6aa), and supplementary motor cortex (area 6ab) (also referred to as secondary motor cortex). All three motor areas are organized similarly to the somatosensory areas, with increasingly coarser somatotopies. Recent studies also indicate a modality-specific multiple representation in area 4, at least in the distal sections of the extremities. One muscle zone receives an afferent input from the skin, and another zone receives afferents from deep receptors (muscles and joints) (Creutzfeldt 1983).

Irritations in the primary motor cortex are predominantly limited to individual joints of the opposite half of the body and lead to short movements in a specific direction. Reactions to both antagonistic movements of a joint or neighboring areas are observed less frequently. When stimulating the areas, the allocation of the motor areas depends on the duration (Graziano 2006). Short stimulations of the premotor cortex triggered coordinated muscle contractions across multiple joints (both contralateral and ipsilateral), forming the basis of the classical motor homunculus. In contrast, stimulations of the supplementary motor cortex induced bilateral contractions, primarily affecting the trunk and proximal limb muscles, leading to prolonged postural changes in the limbs. A longer stimulation of a certain area in the motor cortex, e.g., evoked a characteristic hand-to-mouth movement, where the hand movement followed a distinctive bell-shaped velocity profile (Graziano et al. 2005) or was associated with defensive movements (Graziano and Cooke 2006). Longer electrical stimuli in the supplementary motor area even led to turning movements of the head and the trunk to the opposite side, a flexion synergy of the opposite arm, and an extension or flexion synergy of the lower limb (Foerster 1936). Foerster also referred to this type of coarse motor stimulus effects as "movement synergies" (Foerster 1936). The movement synergies are not to be regarded as fixed, however, but as part of a hierarchical system, whose parameters are global at the highest level, usually mechanically defined, and oriented toward the goal of the movement (Bullock and Grossberg 1988; Graziano 2006; Macpherson 1991). These global parameters are involved in the definition of local parameters for the solution of a motor problem at a lower level.

Blood flow (Roland 1981; Roland et al. 1980) and EEG studies (Deecke et al, 1969) confirm the hierarchical relationships of the three motor regions during movement initiation. During simple movement tasks, the blood flow in the contralateral hand area of both the primary motor and primary sensory cortex increased without major changes in the higher areas. When the movements became more complex and involved all fingers of one hand, blood flow also increased significantly in the supplementary motor area. An increase in blood flow in this area was also observed when the subjects merely imagined a movement sequence without performing it. Using electroencephalography with better temporal resolution, Deecke and coworkers (Deecke et al. 1969) were able to show a temporal sequence of activities in the motor areas. Approximately 800–1000 ms before the start of the movement, the Bereitschaftspotential (readiness potential (BP)) can be observed over the supplementary motor and parietal cortex, approx. 90 ms before the premotor activation begins and, immediately afterward, the motor potential in area 4. This motor potential begins between 50 and 100 ms before the actual movement. The readiness potential is a phenomenon that occurs shortly before voluntary movements in the supplementary motor cortex and is interpreted as an expression of activation and preparation processes. The BP suggests that exercises, such as mental training, can stimulate the activation of the motor cortex and can thereby support neuroplastic processes, even when no movement follows (Kline et al. 2020; Lotze et al. 1999).

The study, in which a successive decrease in activation variability in the premotor cortex was observed from the perception of a stimulus to the execution of the movement, points in the same direction (Churchland et al. 2006). When the stimulus and the "go" signal were presented simultaneously, there was a significant increase in reaction time compared to the delayed presentation of the "go" signal. The decrease in activation variability in both cases argues in favor of the stimulus-dependent preparation of the motor action. Although these processes take place in the millisecond range, they are difficult to reconcile with the assumption of direct perception, where "no elaboration" and "no internal representation" are needed (Michaels and Carello 1981).

In addition to the connections to the primary motor cortex, all three areas (area 5, 6aa, and 6ab) also have their own efferents to the brain stem. The existence of two systems, the indirect (hierarchical) and direct (parallel) projections to the motor neurons, has been shown in lesion studies (Creutzfeldt 1983; Wiesendanger 1990). Symptoms of primary motor cortex damage indicate that, aside from the fine control of contralateral distal limbs—particularly the fingers—all functions can be compensated by higher brain regions. Lesions of the pre- and supplementary motor cortices, on the other hand, lead to more complex movement disorders and impair the ability to develop appropriate action strategies (Ghez et al. 1991, 1995). The neurons involved in a movement are not just "start neurons" but are also active during a holding movement.

The higher-order motor areas receive information from the tertiary somatosensory region (area 5, the somatosensory association field), which coordinates somatic and visual sensations and links partial aspects of these sensory perceptions with movements (Kelly 1991). Similar to the assumption that earlier impressions are stored in the adjacent association areas of the somatosensory cortex, it is also assumed for the pre- and supplementary motor cortex that previously learned motor activities are stored here in interaction with the cerebellum and basal ganglia (Duus 1990). Intention and conception of a movement sequence are thus attributed to the premotor (area 6aa), supplementary motor (area 6ab), and posterior parietal cortex (area 5). The actual activation process originates from the primary motor cortex (area 4). The brain stem and spinal cord are the levels at which the common motor end pathway leading to the musculature is reached. The basal ganglia and cerebellum have a modulating and controlling effect on the motor system (Zilles and Rehkämper 1993).

More detailed studies of the primary motor cortex indicate the existence of parallel representations of kinematic and dynamic movement characteristics in the motor and parietal cortex (i.e., different mechanical aspects of a movement are assigned to corresponding neuron populations). Of particular importance here is that the direction of movement, for example, is determined by a whole group of neurons (neuronal network) and not by individual cells (Evarts 1968, 1981; Georgopoulos 1990, 1991). Depending on the direction of movement of a joint (flexion or extension), different groups of neurons are active in the primary motor cortex. The corresponding discharge frequencies of the neuron populations control the force required to execute a movement. In addition to the neurons responsible for force, neurons that react to changes in force (dF/dt) have also been identified in the primary motor cortex. They are supported by neurons in the rubrospinal system and are probably involved in the control of movement speed (Ghez et al. 1991).

Since the neuronal activity is characteristically observed before the contraction of the corresponding muscles, the involvement of the primary motor cortex in the initiation and triggering of movement is also assumed (Ghez et al. 1991). Most neurons (90%) of the primary motor cortex discharge only until the target of a movement is reached or until shortly (30–50 ms) before the movement target is reached, if no resistance is encountered. The increase in neuronal activity is generally proportional to the amplitude and speed of the postural change (i.e., the ballistic movement). To a lesser extent (1/4–1/3), the increase in activity is proportional to the force applied. When moving against resistance, the activation frequency is increased, especially during the tonic phase. Large and small corticospinal neurons show different reactions depending on the type of movement. While the large neurons are predominantly involved in ballistic movements, the small neurons control the finer force exerted during a movement. Different activation patterns exist for the same amount of force and the same movement:

- At the beginning of the movement, predominantly phasic activation.
- Exclusively tonic until the holding phase; physic and ramp like with increasing activity.

Only the activation of all cortical neurons involved in a simple-structured movement correlates under isometric, auxotonic, and isotonic conditions with the motoneuron activity in the muscles involved in the execution of the movement (Creutzfeldt 1983).

2.6.2.10 General Organization of the Cerebrum

In addition to the complexity-dependent, somatotopic, and modality-specific (vertical) organizational criteria on the surface of the cortex, 90% of the cerebral cortex is also structured horizontally in six layers. The six layers generally reflect the structure of the connections within the cortex and between the cortex and other areas of the brain. Fibers with specific target areas originate predominantly or exclusively from cells of a specific layer, and the primary motor and sensory regions differ cyto-architectonically, especially in the fourth layer. In contrast to the motor cortex, the nerve cell density in the fourth layer of the somatosensory cortex is very high. This layer primarily receives afferents from the periphery via the thalamus.

The layers should not be thought of as superimposed and separated cell layers, "*...but as a single-layered network whose elements are arranged on top of each other due to their developmental history, but which can participate in the same activities as cells above and below them* via *dendrites and, on the other hand, inform about their own activity* via *their intracortical axon branches and recurrent collaterals*" (Creutzfeldt 1983). Intracortical connections, which propagate within the cortex without first entering the white matter, give the cortex the property of a network in which the reaction of individual elements is also determined by the activity state of its neighbors and not only by the activity of afferents from the thalamus or via association pathways. Regarding the intracortical connections, no separate volumes or columns can be delineated in the cortex. It is, therefore, also referred to as a "modular structure of the cortex with overlapping structures" (Creutzfeldt 1983). One module is overlaid by another. These modular cortical components cross both the boundaries between the representational fields and the topographical boundaries determined by cortical afferents (Creutzfeldt 1983).

However, the connections of the cortical nerve cells are not only limited to immediate neighbors but also lead to distant nerve cells. The cells belonging to a neuronal network recognize each other through temporally correlated signals; i.e., the affiliation of the cells is expressed by the temporal structure of the neuronal responses (Hebb 1949; Singer 1989; von der Malsburg 1981). In principle, the internal organization of the motor cortex is comparable to that of the visual cortex, probably the best-studied sensory system of the cerebrum (Creutzfeldt 1983). Because most of the cortex is structured horizontally and vertically in the same way, the mechanisms found in the visual cortex can be transferred to all other somatosensory and motor areas. The first foundations for the plasticity of the visual cortex were laid by Hubel and Wiesel's experiments on the visual cortex of newborn cats (Hubel and Wiesel 1962, 1964; Wiesel and Hubel 1963). A practical consequence of the findings on the development and structure of the visual cortex led to the covering or clouding of the better eye in infants with amblyopia (one eye sees significantly worse than the other), not only to train the worse eye but also to slow down the neuronal development of the better eye and thus enable spatial vision. Something similar happens in forced use therapy (Willis et al. 2002).

2.6.3 Self-Organization and Plasticity of the Cortex

The structures of the network-like modules are not strictly genetically predetermined. Even after the developmental modifications of the neuronal architecture have been completed, which in humans lasts until the end of puberty, adaptive mechanisms remain effective and continue to enable changes in the functional properties of connections. These mechanisms form a basis for the learning and adaptive capacity of the mature brain (Singer 1991a, b).

The different forms of experience-dependent changes in neuronal networks are based on common mechanisms. The early structural development of the central nervous system, developmental learning processes such as imprinting and compensatory adaptation phenomena after brain lesions, and synaptic plasticity in the mature system are therefore based on the same principle, the principle of contingency matching and selective stabilization of coherent active neuronal connections (Singer 1989). There are different types of plasticity, which vary with brain region and age. Even the spinal cord displays plasticity, although on a different timescale (Windhorst 1988). The analogy of the similarities between developmental learning processes and learning in adults can be traced back to molecular mechanisms (Singer 1991a, b). At the molecular level, the nerve growth factor (NGF) plays an essential role in the selective stabilization and new formation of synaptic connections (Jessell 1991). At the cellular level, plasticity is attributed to the spines of pyramidal cells in the cerebral cortex, which make up 85% of the cells (15% are stellate cells) (Braitenberg and Schüz 1993).

Recently, there has been increasing research on the influence of the growth factors, nerve growth factor (NGF) and brain-derived neurotrophic factor (BDNF), on the development, function, and plasticity of the nervous system (Barde et al. 1982; Levi-Montalcini and Hamburger 1951; Xiao 2023). Recent analyses indicate a dependence of exercise intensity on BDNF concentration, with resistance training leading to higher levels than high-intensity training, which outperformed aerobic training (Zhou et al. 2022). However, the current evidence primarily focuses on the general effects of exercise and cognitive training on BDNF, rather than explicitly examining the impact of task complexity or coordination.

The selection algorithms for connections of neurons are similar to the modification rules postulated by Hebb (1949) to explain associative learning in neuronal networks. According to these rules, the change in the efficiency of synaptic connections between nerve cells is a function of the coherence of the mediated activities; i.e., connections are strengthened if there is a high probability that the activities in the afferent pathways and in the downstream element are temporally correlated. Genetically, therefore, only the basic connections with excess and strongly overlapping connections are predetermined. From the redundant systems, those nerve connections that show coherent, temporally correlated activity patterns are then selectively stabilized according to functional criteria. In addition to selective stabilization, coherent signals can also lead to the formation of new neuronal connections, some of which run through the entire brain (Roth 1991; von der Malsburg 1987, 1988). The later modular networks, therefore, only form in an epigenetic and self-organizing manner because of the interaction with the environment during brain development (Roth 1991; Singer 1991a, b). Consequently, the brain is not a self-contained, autarch system but a system that uses environmental influences for self-organization based on one's own memories.

The actual model for the consolidation and creation of connections is based on the criterion of the similarity or temporal correlation of the mediated activities. The signals can originate both within the brain and from corresponding peripheral receptors. This selection principle is essentially responsible for the optimization of neuronal circuits and "*...plays a major role in the entire nervous system*" (Singer 1991a, b). If the activities of two afferent pairs, A and B, are not temporally correlated, they engage in competitive interaction. In this process, one afferent group is strengthened at the expense of the other, with the afferent that most effectively excites the downstream neuron typically prevailing. If two afferent subsystems, A and B, are frequently activated together, they will eventually be selectively connected to a common effector, C. As a result of this consolidated connection, the same reaction is triggered by C after the end of the "learning phase" when A and B are activated separately. Thus, a mechanism exists that can evaluate the temporal correlation of activity patterns and form neuronal representations of the corresponding statistical bindings via structural changes (Singer 1988).

The selection process, which is ultimately responsible for the experience-dependent optimization of brain architecture, is influenced by globally organized control systems that integrate activities from different brain areas and distribute the result of this interaction globally back to the brain areas via widely ramified projections. These control systems include selective attention, the motivational state, and the behavioral relevance of the respective activation conditions (Knudsen 2018). An example of the experience-dependent expression of functional properties is the development of the feature selectivity of neurons in the visual cortex. Under normal conditions, the nerve cells of the visual cortex develop highly selectively to contours of a very specific orientation. The orientations are represented with approximately the same frequency, with a slight preference for vertical and horizontal edges (Gonzalez et al. 1993, 2003). However, if a restriction occurs during early development, e.g., through cylindrical lenses, this results in the destruction of the orientation bands. The majority of neurons only react to specific orientations (Hubel and Wiesel 1962). Experiments with neuronal computer networks show analogous results on orientation dependence (Li et al. 2022).

A feature-specific organization of the neurons in the visual cortex exists not only related to the orientation of the perceived structures but also to color (Engel et al. 1997), form (Shen et al. 1999), and movement (Georgopoulos et al. 1982). In the acoustic cortex, a feature-specific organization according to frequencies and other acoustic features can also be observed (Bitterman et al. 2008; Schreiner et al. 2000). Further literature references on the organization and development of neural networks can be found in the works of Grossberg (1980) and Ritter (Ritter et al. 1992). The findings derived primarily from studies on the visual system have numerous counterparts in the sensorimotor area. In the course of ontogenesis, reflexes regress (Creutzfeldt 1983), and the temporary immobilization of fingers leads to an enlargement of the somatosensory cortex areas of the fingers used, which can occupy up to ½ of the entire hand representation (Jenkins and Merzenich 1987; Merzenich et al. 1984). The long-term takeover of functions of damaged sensorimotor cortex areas, even in adults (Nudo 2006; Nudo et al. 2001), by neighboring areas also points to activity-dependent, self-organizing, and plastic mechanisms.

2.6.4 The Power Law of Neural Adaptation

The power law of (neural) adaptation describes how the response of neurons to a sustained stimulus decreases over time in a predictable manner, which can often be approximated by a mathematical power-law relationship (Anderson 2001; Ehrenberger et al. 1966; Stevens 1970). Power-law adaptation has been observed across various neural systems, including sensory neurons (e.g., visual (Gutnisky and Dragoi 2008; Tring et al. 2023), auditory (Drew and Abbott 2006), or mechanoreceptor (Catton and Petoe 1966; French and Torkkeli 2008; Wong 2020) systems) and motor neurons. In the law of power adaptation, two aspects can be differentiated. The first is related to neural adaptation and the second to the mathematical model of this behavior. When a neuron is exposed to a constant or repeated stimulus, its firing rate or activity tends to decrease over time despite the stimulus remaining the same. This process is considered to be conducive to the nervous system reacting sensitively to changing stimuli and not to constant background values. The drop in the response can be modeled (simplified) mathematically using a power function. The response curves fall faster or slower depending on the neural adaptation behavior (Fig. 2.13). Here, a close connection to the scaling of time becomes already evident.

Either way, the most significant adaptations occur during the first three repetitions, which is why, from the outset, up to three repetitions have been recommended in DL. The power law implies that the rate of adaptation does not follow a simple exponential decay but instead follows a slower, scale-free decay (Fig. 2.14; Eq. 2.5)). Mathematically, this is expressed as:

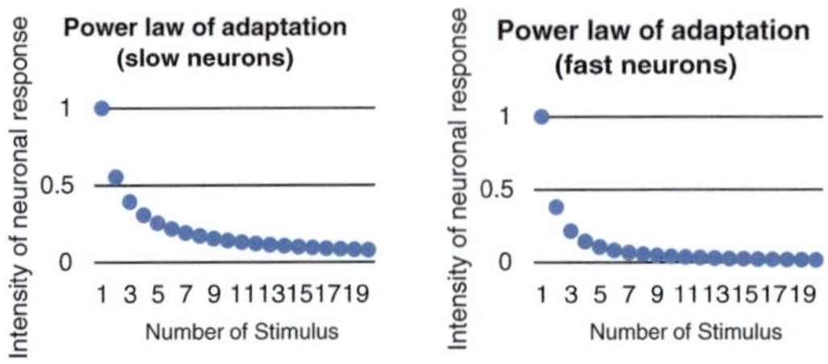

Fig. 2.13 Schematic time courses of slow- (**a**) and fast- (**b**) adapting neurons modeled by means of a power function

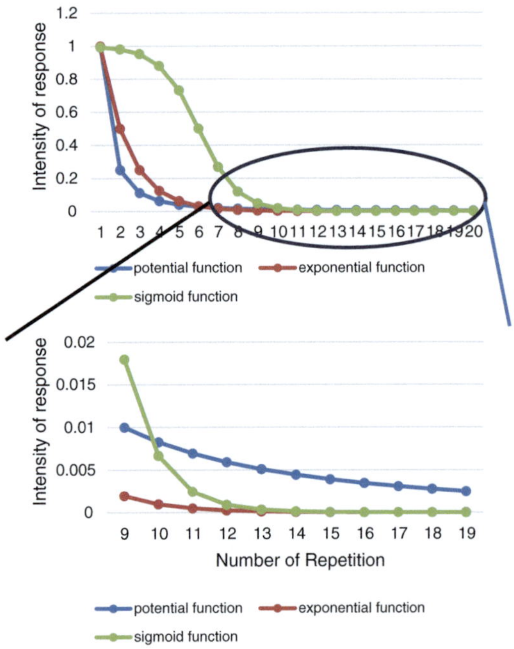

Fig. 2.14 Mathematical models (potential, exponential, and sigmoid) of learning

$$R(t) \propto ct^{-\alpha} \tag{2.5}$$

where R(t) is the neuron's response at time t; α is the power-law exponent, which determines the rate of decay; and t is the time elapsed since the onset of the stimulus c: a constant.

A characteristic of the power law of adaptation is the scale invariance. If the behavior of different subsystems that act on different timescales can be modeled with the same mathematical equation (e.g., 1/f noise), then self-similarity is assumed (Flandrin 1994), a phenomenon for which wavelet analysis is frequently used. On a neuronal level, mostly, the power law appears to be superior to the exponential law (Drew and Abbott 2006). The response decreases more slowly than exponential decay, allowing the system to adapt over a wide range of timescales. This is crucial for neurons to encode dynamic environments that operate on different temporal scales. In addition, the power law predicts that adaptation effects persist for longer durations compared to other decay models, such as exponential or sigmoid functions. By prioritizing changes rather than absolute levels of stimuli, power-law adaptation ensures the efficient use of neuronal resources. It also enables neurons to remain sensitive to new or changing inputs over extended periods, which is critical in natural environments where stimuli vary unpredictably. The exact mechanisms that give rise to power-law adaptation vary by system but generally involve synaptic processes, ion channel dynamics, and network effects.

A direct transfer of the power law of adaptation to the complex learning process of a person is not straightforward due to the different timescales of the neuronal adaptations. In simple terms, it is a matter of adding several adaptation curves in such a way that the envelope, in turn, results in a power-law function too. If we additionally consider, for example, forgetting or fatigue effects, the problem becomes not only more complicated but also much more complex because of their nonlinear interactions. Interestingly, however, populations of neurons and human learning processes can be modeled with the same mathematical functions (Grill-Spector et al, 2006; Tring et al. 2023) (Fig. 2.13). Independent of the type of neuron or type of function chosen as the model, the biggest adaptations occur during the first three stimulations. For this reason, only up to three repetitions were recommended for the DL.

The model of the power law of neuronal adaptation has also been used extensively to describe learning processes (Cattell 1885; Newell 1981; Snoddy 1926; Thurstone 1919). The "power law of practice" model can be considered a derivative of it and models progressively smaller advances with increasing practice (Newell 1981). However, following the general model method (Schöllhorn et al. 2022; Stachowiak 1973), the time (e.g., historical situation) of this modeling must be considered. At that time, the dominant learning method was repetition learning, the phenomenon of which is reflected in the model.

From a second-order cybernetic perspective (see Chap. 1), the neuronal response corresponds to the amount of information that is provided for learning. If we theoretically assume that, during repetition learning, the movement is entirely new to the learner the first time it is performed (where objective and subjective information are equal), then with each repetition, the learner becomes increasingly familiar with it. As a result, the learner's subjective information—and consequently, the amount of new information required for individual learning—gradually decreases. With each repetition, therefore, the redundancy (that equals the known) increases, and thus, the learning rate decreases. If we also consider the individuality of learning rates (learning speed) as subjective information/time, the number of repetitions that are needed for an optimal learning rate can serve to determine the threshold (if the stimuli have the same time interval). If the subjective information rate drops below this individual threshold, i.e., too many repetitions are carried out, this would slow down the learner's progress, and the learning curve becomes flatter. In terms of movements, this becomes apparent when a learner's repetitions become too constant and no longer show sufficient variation. This could also explain why children and beginners, with their increased variation even during initial repetitions, still learn by repetition. If we consider redundancy as something familiar and no longer absolutely necessary for learning, it can be systemically associated with a subjective feeling of security and the feeling of having something under control. In this way, this model of learning as a gain in redundancy also provides an approach for considering different needs for security and control. A greater need for control would, therefore, be associated with a higher demand for redundancy, necessitating more repetitions. The typically prescribed number of repetitions, which corresponds to the variety of exercises, could thus be adjusted to individual psychological characteristics, in line with concepts from second-order cybernetics and stochastic resonance. This could apply, for example, in cases of emotional or daily fluctuations.

Alternatively, exponential or sigmoid functions (Fig. 2.14) have also been used for modeling learning processes (Newell et al. 2001). Similar to the problem of timescales at the neuronal level, the modeling of learning processes depends on the timescale considered in each case. Learning in a single session, also referred to as acquisition in motor learning, seems to follow different principles than learning over several sessions, several days with sleep in between, or several weeks and years, which is only then understood as actual learning in the sense of a change in behavior over time (Schmidt and Bjork 1992).

Regardless of the mathematical model, all learning processes show a decreasing response to repetitive stimuli that goes along with a reduction in learning progress with increasing time. Nonetheless, there seem to be specific learning approaches that keep the subjective information on a higher level during the acquisition process to achieve higher learning rates.

On a more detailed level, one of the challenges of future research will be the study of interactions of the systems, depending on the different timescales. Muscles, ligaments, cartilage, and bones are adapting, each on different timescales ranging from weeks up to a year (Buckwalter 1995; Frank 2004). Similarly, in the neurophysiological area, short-, middle-, and long-term adaptations mirror the various timescales (Cramer et al. 2011; Hedrick et al. 2022; Holtmaat and Svoboda 2009; Kandel et al. 1991). However, the timescales in the brain differ from those related to spinal adaptations (Wolpaw 2010). Still other timescales come from the level of metabolism (Hargreaves and Spriet 2020; Hawley et al. 2014). The extent to which these timescale models may exhibit self-similarity will be a particular issue. For a long time, these systems were fathomed separately. More recent studies point to extensive mutual interactions between the systems. An increasing number of studies support the idea of cross talk between muscles and organs by numerous myokines (Severinsen and Pedersen 2020). Bones produce hormones (e.g., osteocalcin) that have an extensive effect on hormonal processes during psychological stress (Berger and Karsenty 2022). Whole-body exercises with highly coordinative demands, together with a higher weight load, e.g., Olympic weight lifting (Ammar et al. 2024), are associated with different neurological responses than structurally similar exercises, in conjunction with greater endurance load, e.g., cross-country skiing or differential rope skipping (Büchel et al. 2023; John and Schöllhorn 2018; John et al. 2022). Going one step further, this is linked to questions such as the extent to which learning is domain-specific; i.e., are the models only applicable to motor learning, or are they also transferable to cognitive learning, or vice versa? Or are the learning models that have so far been primarily oriented toward phenomena much closer to the neuronal networks in the brain and their plasticity; i.e., with a high cognitive component, are specific learning processes with little transfer more likely to be observed due to the close coupling to the cerebrum, or with a high emotional component and its coupling to the limbic system, are general learning processes with a higher transfer effect more likely to be observed? Similarly, when areas of the cortex are involved that are used in multiple contexts, then the probability of a positive transfer increases. This seems to happen in the transfer of team tactics in games with similar structures (Smeeton et al. 2004) by applying the feeling for rhythm when playing different musical instruments (Levitin et al. 2018) or by sharing mechanisms in speech and music (Fiveash et al. 2021).

2.6.5 Models of Neural Nets

The first attempts to mathematically model neuronal processes go back to McCulloch and Pitts (1943). Shortly afterward, the psychologist

Donald Hebb (1904–1985) proposed the oldest and simplest learning rule, which enables learning in an association of neurons with shared synapses (Hebb 1949). It became known as "*what fires together wires together*" and means that the more often neuron A is active at the same time as neuron B, the more preferentially the two neurons will react to each other. Hebb is, therefore, regarded as the founder of the first model of synaptic plasticity. Interestingly, the model only represents repetition learning, as it was the most used method in animal studies at the time and the easiest to study. However, to conclude from this that repetition is a necessary prerequisite for learning would be a logical fallacy, as other forms of learning were not investigated. Learning through insight or spontaneous learning, as can be observed when learning logical tasks or how to ride a bicycle and other forms of learning, is not represented.

The first calculating machine based on the models of McCulloch, Pitts, and Hebb was designed by American psychologist Rosenblatt (1928–1971) with the perceptron, which had three layers where neurons were assigned different functions: an input layer (sensor unit), a hidden layer (association unit), and an output layer (response unit) (Rosenblatt 1958). Although Rosenblatt had already proposed backpropagation error correction and other researchers were working on it in the 1970s, the breakthrough came with the publication of Rumelhart (1942–2011) and colleagues (Rumelhart et al. 1986). This work led to the widespread use of the gradient descent algorithm for adjusting parameters in multilayer perceptrons (MLPs) with multiple hidden layers. The gradient descent method is a method to find the minimum of a cost function, which optimizes the model. It uses the gradient of the cost function to determine the direction of steepest descent and updates the parameters of the model accordingly. This optimization method is a generalization of the Newton method, which involves descending in the direction of the negative derivative of a single variable, whereas in the gradient method, all variables are considered simultaneously.

As with any model, MLPs that are based on the backpropagation algorithm have various limitations, particularly regarding the backward transferability of their properties to living neurons. First and foremost, an MLP is based on a supervised learning process in which the teacher/trainer of the MLP must specify the target(s) and correct solutions so that the MLPs can adjust the weights accordingly, based on the actual setpoint deviations, analogous to a control-loop model. On the one hand, this involves a very slow learning process that also requires large amounts of data, and on the other hand, once these trained ANNs are trained on new data, the previously learned data structures are forgotten.

Specific attention must be devoted to the problem of finding an absolute minimum. With the gradient descent method on which the backpropagation algorithm is based, it is not possible (or only possible by chance) to find an absolute minimum; i.e., there is a risk of ending up with a local minimum (Fukuoka et al. 1998; Gori and Tesi 1992; Sontag and Sussmann 1989).

We face similar phenomena in therapy or training, where patients or athletes sometimes find a stable solution, but this does not correspond to their individual possibilities, which would be even more economical or effective in the long term. However, the therapist or coach runs the risk of interpreting this into absolute minimums. This problem is also an outstanding question in science as to how this can be recognized. A patient recovering from an anterior cruciate ligament (ACL) injury might adopt a compensatory movement pattern that helps them avoid pain in the short term. However, this pattern may not be the most efficient or beneficial in the long run, potentially leading to other issues, such as muscle imbalances or joint stress. In sports, this problem always becomes apparent when new movement techniques are developed for the same problem, e.g., in the high jump, the straddle being long regarded as the optimal technique until Dick Fosbury showed a more effective alternative or the more recent changes in ski-jumping technique from parallel skis to the V-style.

With the simulated annealing (SAN) approach (Kirkpatrick et al. 1983), similar to the order-from-noise suggestion of von Foerster (1911–2002) in 1960, a proposal was made to minimize the problem of getting stuck in a local minimum. The SAN process begins with an initial solution and then iteratively improves the current solution by randomly perturbing it and accepting the perturbation with some probability. The concept of annealing is derived from metallurgy, where metals are heated and slowly cooled again to rearrange the molecular structure and thus change the physical and chemical properties of the metal. The heating corresponds to adding perturbations in a learning process.

Following Gelfand and Tsetlin (1962), Newell proposed, in addition to the strategies of blind and nonlocal search, the gradient descent method or local search for finding an optimal coordination pattern. Unfortunately, an experimental test of Newell's theoretical proposal is still pending. Levy flights and simulated annealing are algorithmic realizations of the first two search strategies (Palyulin et al. 2014; Pavlyukevich 2007). Although ANNs and theoretical modeling of movement learning use roughly the same mathematical strategy to find a minimum, they differ in detail. In Newell's case, all movements are executed only once, one after the other, and are supposed to lead linearly to a single optimal coordination pattern. A constant comparison of the new movements with the movements stored in an undefined memory regarding the steepest gradient descent ultimately leads to a single optimal coordination pattern for the learner.

When training MLPs, on the other hand, all data is available from the beginning of the training process, e.g., derived from all biomechanically measured movements. The training process runs through several epochs (cycles), in which all weights (synapses) of the MLPs are optimized according to the data. To ensure that the MLPs are used as stably as possible after the training process, the training data should have two key characteristics. First, the training data for the ANN should contain a certain amount of noise, as the use cases are very likely to deviate from the training data, and second, the training data for the ANN should cover such a large area that the use cases will lie within the range of an interpolation (Barnard and Wessels 1992; Haykin 1994; Hertz et al. 1991). This meant that the neuronal networks were not only trained for individual special cases but for a large number of cases that could be expected in future applications.

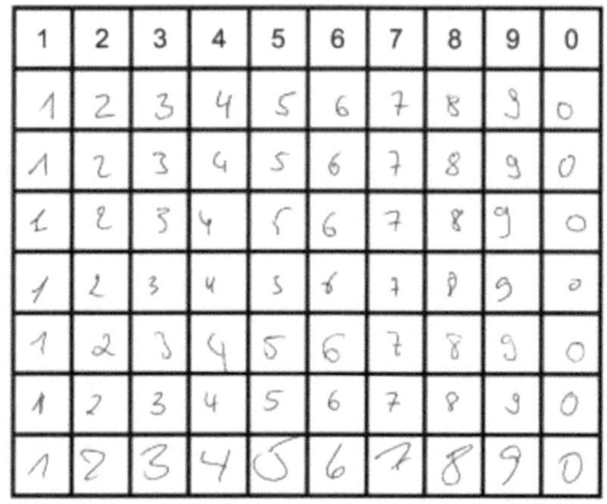

Fig. 2.15 Numbers written with various handwritings for the training of ANNs

One of the first applications of ANNs was in the context of the recognition of numbers in bank transfer forms. For this, the ANNs were trained with numbers from various handwritings, as shown in Fig. 2.15.

Similar phenomena were observed in motor learning studies on transfer after variable practice. Catalano and Kleiner provided evidence of the disadvantages of extrapolation in a visuomotor timing task (Catalano and Kleiner 1984). The further the test speed was outside the trained range (extrapolation), the poorer the performance in the transfer test. Studies with small autonomously moving robots impressively confirmed this successful strategy. If they were trained in a constantly changing environment, they were subsequently able to move into various other environments. If they were only trained for a fixed environment, they subsequently became stuck in a changed environment (Miglino et al. 1995).

In summary, Newell's (1986) proposal still followed the idea of a single concrete optimum, which contradicts the later findings with regard to ideal technique and repeatability (see Chap. 1). It also remained unclear how to proceed once this optimum had been reached. Although a destabilization of this assumption began shortly afterward with the greater tolerance of movement variations (Newell and Corcos 1993), the contradictions to the proposed search process remained unresolved. In contrast, the minimum of the cost function in the MLP model does not represent a point but a valley or an area that also tolerates future deviations. For this, the training data had to have a corresponding variance (or noise) that allowed interpolation between the training data. If this insight is applied systemically to natural neural systems, such as patients, athletes, dogs, or horses, it corresponds to an expansion of the training space. This involves exploring the boundaries of the solution space, on the one hand, and increasing variability during the training process, on the other. Both are achieved in the Differential Learning model by amplifying the noise.

Another type of ANN was provided by Kohonen (1982) with the self-organizing maps (SOMs). They learn without a teacher (self-organizing) and maintain the relative spatial relationships of input data (topology preservation). Similar to the topology preservation in the cortex (e.g., somatosensory homunculus), the input data points are mapped to nearby locations in the SOM grid. They are often used for pattern recognition by projecting high-dimensional data into a lower-dimensional space and learn inherent structures without labeled data. Sometimes, they are also referred to as a nonlinear alternative to a linear factor analysis.

The similarity of the properties also provides an indication of the ability to identify the principal axes of inertia of the inertia tensor of an arbitrarily shaped body. By wielding rods with unknown lengths and shapes, several studies of Turvey and colleagues could show that the subjects were able to identify the principal moment of inertia (Turvey 1996). Neurophysiologically, two mechanisms are used here during wielding. First, sensitivity is improved by movement (see chapter on static and dynamic sensitivity), and second, information about all moments of inertia of the rods in the hand is transmitted through the mechanoreceptors in the skin and muscles to the central neuronal network. From this information, the structure of the neuronal nets allows us to determine the principal axes of inertia that correspond to an eigen-decomposition similar to a principal component analysis. This allows the patient and every healthy person to move with minimal shear forces in the joints. A series of experiments on dynamic touch provided evidence for this ability (Turvey 1996). However, this ability is dependent on the structure and processes of the underlying neuronal net structure of the perceiving person and is hardly to be explained through direct perception in the context of the affordance concept (Michaels and Carello 1981).

Analogous to statistical analysis methods, the ANNs that are supervised (e.g., MLPs or support vector machines) correspond to hypothesis-confirming procedures, whereas the self-organizing ones correspond more to hypothesis-generating or exploratory procedures.

The first recognition tasks in context with movements based on supervised MLPs could confirm the classifications of normal and pathological gait (Holzreiter and Köhle 1993) or level uphill and downhill running (Aminian et al. 1993). A self-organizing map was also applied for classifying walking at various speeds and inclinations on the basis of single trials of several subjects (Aminian et al. 1995). The first pattern recognitions based on self-organizing maps that relied on several trials of the subjects lead to generating the hypothesis of individual and situated movement patterns in discus throw (Bauer and Schöllhorn 1997), javelin throw (Schöllhorn and Bauer 1998b), and running (Schöllhorn and Baue 1997, 1998a). Both the individuality and the situatedness of movement patterns have since been extensively confirmed by means of other supervised learning ANNs (Horst et al. 2016, 2017; Janssen et al. 2008) and have formed a fundamental pillar of DL.

2.6.6 Transferring the Findings into Therapy and Learning Practice

In summary, four main aspects of neurophysiology and related areas had an influence on the derivation of practical consequences for

Differential Learning. Numerous consequences have since been confirmed in other studies (Schöllhorn 1997, 1999a, b, c; 2000; Schöllhorn and Bauer 1998b).

(a) Plasticity of the central nervous system. Extensive findings on the plasticity of the visual system could be transferred systemically to the somatosensory and motor systems.
(b) Complex neuronal circuits with their phenomenal correspondences as well as their behavior in case of failure and their rehabilitation.
(c) The power law of neuronal adaptation.
(d) Training of artificial neural networks.
 - The power law of adaptation suggests that the most significant improvements in motor performance occur within the first few repetitions. This means that the initial phase of motor learning is crucial for the establishment of basic neural patterns. DL tries to create many "initial phase situations" for motor learning by constantly offering new situations and usually no more than three repetitions.
 - Neural plasticity shows that the brain and spine remain adaptable throughout the learning process, although on different timescales. Even after initial gains, continued practice can lead to further refinement and optimization of motor skills.
 - The intricate networks in brain architecture suggest that multiple neural systems work together in motor learning. This complexity enables the development of such sophisticated motor skills that integrate different sensory inputs and motor outputs (Birklbauer 2019).
 - Given the rapid initial adaptations and ongoing plasticity, incorporating variability/noise into motor exercises may help activate different neural pathways and promote more robust skill acquisition.
 - The combination of power-law adaptation and continuous plasticity suggests that while initial progress is rapid, continuous improvement is possible only over longer periods of time.
 - The complex neural connections suggest that learning in one motor domain may have transfer effects on related skills, as the adaptations may involve shared neural circuits (Dayan et al. 2007; Dayan and Cohen 2011).
 - In conjunction with the findings on the individuality and situatedness of movements, the interplay between rapid initial adaptation and ongoing plasticity suggests that individuals may have unique learning curves that are influenced by factors such as previous experience and individual neural architecture.
 - The power law of adaptation and neural plasticity highlight the need for adequate rest periods between training sessions to allow for neural consolidation and the optimization of learned skills.

Structurally, two approaches were successfully used in the training of ANNs to optimize the solutions. Both approaches improved the performance of ANNs and brought them closer to modeling the performance of natural neural nets in specific areas. Both correspond to an amplification of the noise on different scales, which can be assigned to different phases in movement learning, depending on the amount of noise. While during the phases of acquisition and refinement, the amount of noise needs to be bigger (simulated annealing) to find a spatially more distant and possibly more global minimum, for the phase of stabilization, less noise (noisy data) is demanded for finding multiple solutions in the area of a local minimum valley.

If we also take into account the findings on neighborhood preservation (Bauer and Pawelzik 1992) and plasticity (Hubel and Wiesel 1964), in which neighboring neurons have similar functions and, in the absence of input, use it to expand the existing input or, in the event of failure, their function is partially taken over by neighboring neurons, then this has further practical consequences.

It always seems advantageous to activate areas near the impairment through the corresponding peripheral regions. When extended to more complex neural networks and their diverse interconnections, the activation of networks linked to forgotten or lost abilities can help in recalling or regaining them. Babies build up these kinds of networks when they put everything in their mouths. This immediately connects the areas of shape with the areas of texture, taste, smell, fingers, eyes, listening, etc. Similar networks are built up by taking the toe into the mouth or touching other body parts with the opposite side. Touching the foot with the hands builds up a different network compared to touching the foot with the other foot or with the tongue. If language is lost in a stroke, then the patient could be helped to regain it, for example, by singing songs that they had previously sung themselves. Let us assume that during the original acquisition of the song, not only areas assigned to the lyrics and/or the rhythm and the sound of the music were activated centrally but also a whole network that is associated with the situational conditions, such as the spatial environment (for church music in church and for children's songs in kindergarten), the people present (siblings and friends), the emotions, or even the smell (what was mainly cooked or baked at home), and then all these conditions and their corresponding variations could be conducive to regeneration or rehabilitation (Aderinto et al. 2023; Hara 2015). The same applies to the acquisition of reading, where learning could be made more stable and effective by varying the font and its size and the colors of the letters and the background.

All variables for description could be used to produce different levels of noise for providing various stimuli to the neural system to stay adaptive. With little noise, for example, only one letter can be red and all others black; with a lot of noise, all letters can be colored with varying font sizes and different fonts. Contradictory meanings of words and colors (the word red is written in blue colors) can be used not only in the Stroop test (Stroop 1935) but also in a modified form for training and rehabilitating the affected areas. An analogy in the sensorimotor area would be to offer big, light objects in contrast with small and heavy objects, and vice versa.

If we consider each joint as a letter, the approach can be transferred systemically. Changing the size of the letter corresponds to a movement with bigger amplitude, and shifting the position of the letter can be associated with starting a movement from different angles. Similar to the example in Fig. 2.15, handwriting could be trained by writing number/letter variations or, similar to the first steps in learning to write, by drawing large and small circles, vertical and horizontal lines that curve to the left or right, etc. You could do the same by coordinating finger–thumb movements with wrist movements or combining elbow and shoulder movements with different grips with different pens on different papers, different surfaces, etc. (Marquardt et al. 2016; Vehof et al. 2009).

In contrast to reading, most of the human movements involve several joints in parallel. In this case, the metaphor of a score for an orchestral piece is close at hand, in which each joint can be compared to the playing of notes on a musical instrument. This means that all the variations used in music for learning an instrument, e.g., variation of tempi (Largo, Allegretto, Allegro, etc.), volume (pianissimo, forte, etc.), the form of articulation (staccato and legato), and dotting or duration of the notes (quarter, eighth, sixteenth, etc.), can be used as suggestions for the variations of different joints. We should not forget that not every orchestra has a conductor, and it is still an open question as to who the conductor in the orchestra of our movements is or whether we have several conductors depending on the situation, which would be advantageous for evolution if one conductor drops out.

Independent of culture, a large number of children's games are designed for this type of learning, with similar effects on learning in older ages due to the plasticity of the central nervous system into old age.

Conversely, this also points to the advantages of multisensory learning. If an odor is applied during learning, what has been learned is consolidated when the learner is given the same odor again during subsequent sleep (Pin-Barre and Laurin 2015; Shanahan and Gottfried 2014).

This becomes even more obvious if we also consider the structural arrangement and wiring of the brain. Thus, the differences in the range of transferring tasks become clearer. If only the geometric phenomenology of the joint angles of a movement or skin stimulation to be learned is considered and the sensors of speed, acceleration, jerk, texture, temperature, etc. are neglected, the transfer of the learning process remains very limited, hindering the patient's overall progress and adaptation. However, if the learning process leads to changes that take place on similar and multiple levels, such as emotional and expectational, due to the complex central nervous connections with different areas, then more far-reaching transfer can be expected. This differentiation also points to a fundamental problem of representativeness as a training strategy that only relates to the similarity of exercise on the phenomenological level and the to-be-learned movement.

Similar to the differentiation of movement description into metrics and topology, the emotional level can be used as an extra dimension in movement learning. Both the metrics and the topologies can be varied independently of each other with different emotions. More specifically, while physiotherapists often focus on a small subset of this information—such as joint angles or specific movement patterns—"the rest" represents the additional, perhaps less obvious, elements that contribute to the overall stability and success of the learning process. These neglected factors can be crucial in stabilizing learning, enhancing memory retention, or even facilitating recovery and rehabilitation, especially in cases where the body or mind requires support beyond just the mechanical aspects of movement.

More abstractly and holistically, mapping all internal and external conditions of the learning situation to a very long vector, motor learning is frequently restricted to a small excerpt of this vector, and "the rest" is mainly neglected. Very often, it is "the rest of the vector" that stabilizes learning and, in extreme cases, contains the source of recovery or supports rehabilitation. If we extend the vector by the time dimension to a variable-time-matrix in which all conditions become a function of time, then, on the one hand, the complexity of holism becomes clear, and on the other hand, it reflects the variety of possible active variations in the rows and columns of the matrix.

Questions

1. What are the key philosophical and scientific differences between first- and second-order cybernetics?
2. How does Differential Learning reinterpret variability and error within the learning process?
3. In what ways does Differential Learning challenge repetition- and correction-based models of traditional motor learning?
4. How is cybernetic feedback traditionally used in motor-learning theories and how does DL reinterpret it?
5. What is the significance of subjective information in the Differential Learning framework?
6. How do the cerebellum, basal ganglia, and cerebral cortex contribute differently to movement control and learning?
   A. All three act only as passive relays for spinal reflexes.
   B. Basal ganglia fine-tune eye movements, while cerebellum plans speech.
   C. Cerebral cortex stores vestibular reflexes and nothing else.
   D. Cerebellum times and smooths synergies, basal ganglia select/inhibit competing action "programs," and cerebral cortex plans and initiates voluntary movements.
   E. Each structure controls exactly one joint of the body.
7. What role do mirror neurons play in understanding movement and action in others?
   A. They discharge only when we perform an action, never when we observe.
   B. They fire both when we execute an action and when we watch someone else do it, providing a neural basis for action understanding and imitation.
   C. They are vestibular cells that stabilize gaze during rotation.
   D. They inhibit cerebellar plasticity during repetitive drills.
   E. They create muscle twitches in the observer's limbs.

8. How does cortical plasticity support learning even after developmental stages are complete?
   A. Adult cortex becomes anatomically fixed and cannot change synapses.
   B. Neurons lose all dendritic spines once puberty ends.
   C. Training reduces BDNF levels, blocking new connections.
   D. Plasticity survives only in the spinal cord, not in the brain.
   E. Experience-dependent synaptic changes—e.g., neuronal growth modulated by BDNF—allow remapping and skill acquisition throughout life.
9. Why is it problematic to treat perception and action as separate processes in movement science?
   A. Neurophysiological evidence (e.g., readiness potentials, common-coding, mirror-neuron activations) shows tightly coupled, bidirectional loops, so splitting them ignores their integrated nature.
   B. Because perception stops once movement begins.
   C. Action pathways are located only in the spinal cord, perception only in the cortex.
   D. Separating them eliminates all neural noise, making learning impossible.
   E. It is not problematic; the two systems never interact.
10. How does the presented neurophysiological model support Differential Learning (DL) over repetition-based training?
   A. It proves that eliminating variability accelerates synaptic growth.
   B. It shows vestibular dominance makes error-reduction essential.
   C. It emphasizes self-organizing plastic circuits driven by variable mechano-sensory input, aligning with DL's noise-rich, non-repetitive practice rather than uniform correction.
   D. It concludes that efference copies cancel all learning signals.
   E. It demonstrates that augmented external feedback is mandatory for change.

References

Acree MC (2021) The myth of statistical inference. Springer. https://books.google.de/books?id=IQo3EAAAQBAJ

Adams JA (1968) Response feedback and learning. Psychol Bull 70(6 Pt.1):486 504. https://doi.org/10.1037/h0026741

Adams JA (1987) Historical review and appraisal of research on the learning, retention, and transfer of human motor skills. Psychol Bull 101(1):41–74. https://doi.org/10.1037/0033-2909.101.1.41

Adams, J. A., Gopher, D., & , G. (1975). The Effects of Visual and Proprioceptive Feedback on Motor Learning. Proceedings of the Human Factors Society Annual Meeting, 19(2), 162–165. https://doi.org/10.1177/154193127501900204

Aderinto N, AbdulBasit MO, Olatunji G, Adejumo T (2023) Exploring the transformative influence of neuroplasticity on stroke rehabilitation: a narrative review of current evidence. Ann Med Surg 85(9) https://journals.lww.com/annals-of-medicine-and-surgery/fulltext/2023/09000/exploring_the_transformative_influence_of.38.aspx

Afriat A (2004) Duhem, Quine and the other dogma. Preprint. https://philsci-archive.pitt.edu/3967/

Alabdulgader A, McCraty R, Atkinson M, Dobyns Y, Vainoras A, Ragulskis M, Stolc V (2018) Long-term study of heart rate variability responses to changes in the solar and geomagnetic environment. Sci Rep 8(1):2663. https://doi.org/10.1038/s41598-018-20932-x

Altman J, Das GD (1964) Autoradiographic examination of the effects of enriched environment on the rate of glial multiplication in the adult rat brain. Nature 204(4964):1161–1163. https://doi.org/10.1038/2041161a0

Aminian K, Robert PH, Jequier E, Schutz Y (1993) Level, downhill and uphill walking identification using neural networks. Electron Lett 29(17):3. https://doi.org/10.1049/el:1993104.

Aminian K, Robert P, Jequier E, Schutz Y (1995) Estimation of speed and incline of walking using neural network. IEEE Trans Instrum Meas 44(3):743–746. https://doi.org/10.1109/19.387322

Ammar A, Trabelsi K, Boujelbane MA, Boukhris O, Glenn JM, Chtourou H, Schöllhorn WI (2023) The myth of contextual interference learning benefit in sports practice: a systematic review and meta-analysis. Educ Res Rev 39:100537. https://doi.org/10.1016/j.edurev.2023.100537

Ammar A, Trabelsi K, Boujelbane MA, Salem A, Boukhris O, Glenn JM, Zmijewski P, Jahrami HA, Chtourou H, Schöllhorn WI (2024) The effects of contextual interference learning on the acquisition and relatively permanent gains in skilled performance: a critical systematic review with multilevel meta-analysis. Educ Psychol Rev 36(2):57. https://doi.org/10.1007/s10648-024-09892-z

Anderson RB (2001) The power law as an emergent property. Mem Cogn 29(7):1061–1068. https://doi.org/10.3758/bf03195767
Anokhin PK (1935) Problem of centre and periphery in the physiology of nervous activity. Gorky:9–70
Apidogo JB, Burdack J, Schöllhorn WI (2021) Repetition without repetition or differential learning of multiple techniques in volleyball? Int J Environ Res Public Health 18(19). https://doi.org/10.3390/ijerph181910499
Apidogo JB, Ammar A, Salem A, Burdack J, Schöllhorn WI (2023) Resonance effects in variable practice for handball, basketball, and volleyball skills: a study on contextual interference and differential learning. Sports (Basel) 12(1). https://doi.org/10.3390/sports12010005
Ashby WR (1947) Principles of the self-organizing dynamic system. J Gen Psychol 37(2):125–128. https://doi.org/10.1080/00221309.1947.9918144
Ashby WR (1960) Design for a brain, 2nd edn. Chapman & Hall
Atkin A (2008) Peirce's theory of signs. In: Atkin A (ed) Stanford encyclopedia of philosophy
Baddeley AD (2018) Exploring working memory: selected works of Alan Baddeley. Routledge/Taylor & Francis
Baddeley AD, Hitch GJ (1974) Working memory. In: Bower GH (ed) Psychology of learning and motivation, vol 8. Academic Press, pp 47–89. https://doi.org/10.1016/S0079-7421(08)60452-1
Bakker FC, Oudejans RRD, Binsch O, Van Der Kamp J (2006) Penalty shooting and gaze behavior: unwanted effects of the wish not to miss. Int J Sport Psychol 37(2–3):265–280
Ballreich R (1969) Weg- und Zeit-Merkmale von Sprintbewegungen (Distance and time characteristics of sprint movements.). Bartels & Wernitz
Ballreich R (1970) Weitsprung-Analyse (Long jump analysis). Bartles & Wernitz
Ballreich R (1972) Zur Optimierung des sportmotorischen Leistungszustands (For the optimization of the sports motor performance condition). In: Rieder H (ed) Bewegung – LeistungVerhalten. Hofmann, pp 15–28
Ballreich R, Baumann W (1983) Biomechanische Leistungsdiagnostik: Ziele, Organisation, Ergebnisse, 1st edn. Bartels & Wernitz
Barde YA, Edgar D, Thoenen H (1982) Purification of a new neurotrophic factor from mammalian brain. EMBO J 1(5):549–553. https://doi.org/10.1002/j.1460-2075.1982.tb01207.x
Barinaga M (1996) The cerebellum: movement coordinator or much more? Science 272(5261):482–483. https://doi.org/10.1126/science.272.5261.482
Barnard E, Wessels LFA (1992) Extrapolation and interpolation in neural network classifiers. IEEE Control Syst Mag 12(5):50–53. https://doi.org/10.1109/37.158898
Bartlett FC (1932) Remembering: a study in experimental and social psychology. Cambridge University Press
Bartlett R, Wheat J, Robins M (2007) Is movement variability important for sports biomechanists? Sports Biomech 6(2):224–243. https://doi.org/10.1080/14763140701322994
Basedow JB (1774) Das in Dessau errichtet Philantropinum. Crusius
Bates BT (1996) Single-subject methodology: an alternative approach. Med Sci Sports Exerc 28(5):631–638. https://doi.org/10.1097/00005768-199605000-00016
Bateson G (1972) Steps to an ecology of mind: collected essays in anthroplogy, psychiatry, evolution and epistemology. University of Chicago Press
Battig WF (1966) Facilitation and interference. In: Bilodeau EA (ed) Acquisition of skill. Academic Press, pp 215–244
Battig WF (1979) Are the important "individual differences" between or within individuals? J Res Pers 13(4):546–558. https://doi.org/10.1016/0092-6566(79)90015-1
Bauer HU, Pawelzik KR (1992) Quantifying the neighborhood preservation of self-organizing feature maps. Trans Neur Netw 3(4):570–579. https://doi.org/10.1109/72.143371
Bauer HU, Schöllhorn WI (1997) Self-organizing maps for the analysis of complex movement patterns. Neural Process Lett 5(3):193–199. https://doi.org/10.1023/a:1009646811510
Beckmann H, Schöllhorn WI (2003) Differencial learning in shot put mechanics, physiology, psychology – first European workshop on movement science, Münster – Germany
Beckmann H, Schöllhorn WI (2006) Differenzielles Lernen im Kugelstoßen. Leistungssport 36(4):44–50
Beckmann H, Winkel C, Schöllhorn WI (2010) Optimal range of variation in hockey technique traiing. Int J Sport Psychol 41, 5–10.
Beek P (2000) Toward a theory of implicit learning in the perceptual-motor domain. Int J Sport Psychol 31(4):547–554
Beek PJ, van Santvoord AA (1992) Learning the cascade juggle: a dynamical systems analysis. J Mot Behav 24(1):85–94. https://doi.org/10.1080/00222895.1992.9941604
Bell MP, Ferguson RA (2009) Interaction between muscle temperature and contraction velocity affects mechanical efficiency during moderate-intensity cycling exercise in young and older women. J Appl Physiol (1985) 107(3):763–769. https://doi.org/10.1152/japplphysiol.91654.2008
Bénard H (1901) Les tourbillons cellulaires dans une nappe liquide. – Méthodes optiques d'observation et d'enregistrement. J Phys Theor Appl 10(1):254–266. https://doi.org/10.1051/jphystap:0190100100025400
Bennell KL, Marshall CJ, Dobson F, Kasza J, Lonsdale C, Hinman RS (2019) Does a web-based exercise programming system improve home exercise adherence for people with musculoskeletal conditions?: a randomized controlled trial. Am J Phys Med Rehabil 98(10):850–858. https://doi.org/10.1097/phm.0000000000001204

Berger JM, Karsenty G (2022) Osteocalcin and the physiology of danger. FEBS Lett 596(5):665–680. https://doi.org/10.1002/1873-3468.14259

Bernstein N (1935) The problem of the interrelation of co-ordination and localization (in Russian). Arch Biol Sci 38:1–35

Bernstein N (1967) The co-ordination and regulation of movements, 1st edn. Pergamon Press

Bilek MCP, Simanova I (2012) Educational cybernetics or didactics approach to "economy" of human thinking. Probl Educ 21st Century 46(6). https://doi.org/10.33225/pec/12.46.22

Binsch O, Oudejans RRD, Bakker FC, Savelsbergh GJP (2010) Ironic effects and final target fixation in a penalty shooting task. Hum Mov Sci 29(2):277–288. https://doi.org/10.1016/j.humov.2009.12.002

Birbaumer NSRF (1990) Biologische Psychologie. Springer

Birklbauer J (2019) Optimal variability for effective motor learning: A theoretical review and empirical work on movement variability. (1st ed.) (Spektrum Bewegungswissenschaft). Meyer & Meyer Verlag.

Bischof N (1995) Struktur und Bedeutung: eine Einführung in die Systemtheorie für Psychologen ; zum Selbststudium und für den Gruppenunterricht. Huber

Bitterman Y, Mukamel R, Malach R, Fried I, Nelken I (2008) Ultra-fine frequency tuning revealed in single neurons of human auditory cortex. Nature 451(7175):197–201. https://doi.org/10.1038/nature06476

Bjork RA (1994) Memory and metamemory considerations in the training of human beings. In: Metcalfe JSA (ed) Metacognition: knowing about knowing. MIT, pp 185–205

Bjork RA, Allen TW (1970) The spacing effect: consolidation or differential encoding. J Verbal Learn Verbal Behav 9(5):567–572. https://doi.org/10.1016/S0022-5371(70)80103-7

Blinkov SM, Glezer II (1968) Das Zentralnervensystem in Zahlen und Tabellen. Fischer

Blume DD (1978) Zu einigen wesentlichen theoretischen Grundpositionen für die Untersuchung der koordinativen Fähigkeiten. Theor Prax Korperkult 27(1):29–36

Bothmichel E, Nehmer G (1967) Untersuchungen über den Krafteinsatz beim Riemenrudern. Theorie und Praxis der Leistungssports 5(5):16–31. https://open--archive.sport-iat.de/tupl/1967_05_Bothmischel_01.pdf

Bowen WP (1919) The influence of the war upon physical education. Am Phys Educ Rev 24(2):90–92. https://doi.org/10.1080/23267224.1919.10650773

Brachman A, Kamieniarz A, Michalska J, Pawłowski M, Słomka KJ, Juras G (2017) Balance training programs in athletes—a systematic review. J Hum Kinet 58:45–64. https://doi.org/10.1515/hukin-2017-0088

Brady F (2004) Contextual interference: a meta-analytic study. Percept Mot Skills 99(1):116–126. https://doi.org/10.2466/pms.99.1.116-126

Braitenberg V, Schüz A (1993) Allgemeine Neuroanatomie. In: Schmidt RF (ed) Neuro- und Sinnesphysiologie. Springer, Berlin/Heidelberg, pp 1–30. https://doi.org/10.1007/978-3-662-08941-5_1

Brisson TA, Alain C (1996) Should common optimal movement patterns be identified as the criterion to be achieved? J Mot Behav 28(3):211–223. https://doi.org/10.1080/00222895.1996.9941746

Broadbent DP, Causer J, Williams AM, Ford PR (2017) The role of error processing in the contextual interference effect during the training of perceptual-cognitive skills. J Exp Psychol Hum Percept Perform 43(7):1329–1342. https://doi.org/10.1037/xhp0000375

Brodtmann D (1984) Unterrichtsmodelle zum problemorientierten Sportunterricht. Rowohlt. Reinbek.

Brodtmann DD, Frankfurter Arbeitsgruppe K (1982) Offener Sportunterricht: analysieren und planen. Rowohlt. Reinbek.

Bronfenbrenner U (1983) The context of development and the development of context. In: Lerner RM (ed) Developmental psychology: historical and philosophical perspectives. L. Erlbaum, pp 147–184

Brunswik E (1939) Probability as a determiner of rat behavior. J Exp Psychol 25(2):175

Brunswik E (1955) Representative design and probabilistic theory in a functional psychology. Psychol Rev 62(3):193–217. https://doi.org/10.1037/h0047470

Büchel D, Torvik P, Lehmann T, Sandbakk Ø, Baumeister J (2023) The mode of endurance exercise influences changes in EEG resting-state graphs among high-level cross-country skiers. Med Sci Sports Exerc 55(6):1003–1013. https://doi.org/10.1249/mss.0000000000003122

Buckwalter JA (1995) Activity vs. rest in the treatment of bone, soft tissue and joint injuries. Iowa Orthop J 15:29–42

Buekers MJA, Magill RA, Hall KG (1992) The effect of erroneous knowledge of results on skill acquisition when augmented information is redundant. Q J Exp Psychol 44(1):105–117. https://doi.org/10.1080/14640749208401285

Bullock D, Grossberg S (1988) Neural dynamics of planned arm movements: emergent invariants and speed-accuracy properties during trajectory formation. Psychol Rev 95(1):49–90. https://doi.org/10.1037/0033-295x.95.1.49

Bunker D, Thorpe R (1982) A model for the teaching of games in secondary schools. Bull Phys Educ 18, 5–8

Burdack J, Giesselbach S, Simak ML, Ndiaye ML, Marquardt C, Schöllhorn WI (2023) Identifying underlying individuality across running, walking, and handwriting patterns with conditional cycle-consistent generative adversarial networks. Front Bioeng Biotechnol 11:1204115. https://doi.org/10.3389/fbioe.2023.1204115

Burnes B (2020) The origins of Lewin's three-step model of change. J Appl Behav Sci 56(1):32–59. https://doi.org/10.1177/0021886319892685

Calabresi P, Picconi B, Tozzi A, Ghiglieri V, Di Filippo M (2014) Direct and indirect pathways of basal ganglia: a critical reappraisal. Nat Neurosci 17(8):1022–1030. https://doi.org/10.1038/nn.3743

Catalano JF, Kleiner BM (1984) Distant transfer in coincident timing as a function of variability of practice. Percept Mot Skills 58:851–856

Cattell JMK (1885) Über die Zeit der Erkennung und Bezeichnung von Schriftzeichen, Bildern und Farben. Philsosophische Studien 2:15

Catton WT, Petoe N (1966) A visco-elastic theory of mechanoreceptor adaptation. J Physiol 187(1):35–49. https://doi.org/10.1113/jphysiol.1966.sp008074

Chapman R, Richardson D, Cope E, Cronin C (2020) Learning from the past; a Freirean analysis of FA coach education since 1967. Sport Educ Soc 25(6):681–697. https://doi.org/10.1080/13573322.2019.1654989

Chapman R, Cope E, Richardson D, Littlewood M, Cronin C (2024) How did we get here; a historical and social exploration of the construction of English FA coach education. Sport Educ Soc 29(9):1133–1152. https://doi.org/10.1080/13573322.2023.2256754

Chemero A (2001) What we perceive when we perceive affordances: commentary on Michaels (2000) "information, perception, and action". Ecol Psychol 13(2):111–116. https://doi.org/10.1207/S15326969ECO1302_3

Chemero A, Turvey MT (2007) Complexity, hypersets, and the ecological perspective on perception-action. Biol Theory 2(1):23–36. https://doi.org/10.1162/biot.2007.2.1.23

Childre DL, McCraty R, Atkinson MA, Joffe D (2007) Physiological coherence in animals. United States of America Patent No.

Choi JW, Nandram B (2021) Large sample problems. Int J Stat Probab 10(2), 81. https://doi.org/10.5539/IJSP.V10N2P81.

Churchland MM, Yu BM, Ryu SI, Santhanam G, Shenoy KV (2006) Neural variability in premotor cortex provides a signature of motor preparation. J Neurosci 26(14):3697–3712. https://doi.org/10.1523/jneurosci.3762-05.2006

Collins JJ, De Luca CJ (1993) Open-loop and closed-loop control of posture: a random-walk analysis of center-of-pressure trajectories. Exp Brain Res 95(2):308–318. https://doi.org/10.1007/bf00229788

Collins D, Carson HJ, Rylander P et al (2025) Ecological dynamics as an accurate and parsimonious contributor to applied practice: A critical appraisal. Sports Med 55:799–810. https://doi.org/10.1007/s40279-024-02161-7

Cope B, Kalantzis M (2022) The cybernetics of learning. Educ Philos Theory 54(14):2352–2388. https://doi.org/10.1080/00131857.2022.2033213

Cordier P, France MM, Pailhous J, Bolon P (1994) Entropy as a global variable of the learning process. Hum Mov Sci 13(6):745–763. https://doi.org/10.1016/0167-9457(94)90016-7

Corradini A, O'Connor T (2010) Emergence in science and philosophy. Routledge

Costa M, Peng CK, Goldberger LA, Hausdorff JM (2003) Multiscale entropy analysis of human gait dynamics. Physica A 330(1):53–60. https://doi.org/10.1016/j.physa.2003.08.022

Cowin J, Nimphius S, Fell J, Culhane P, Schmidt M (2022) A proposed framework to describe movement variability within sporting tasks: a scoping review. Sports Med Open 8(1):85. https://doi.org/10.1186/s40798-022-00473-4

Cramer SC, Sur M, Dobkin BH, O'Brien C, Sanger TD, Trojanowski JQ, Rumsey JM, Hicks R, Cameron J, Chen D, Chen WG, Cohen LG, deCharms C, Duffy CJ, Eden GF, Fetz EE, Filart R, Freund M, Grant SJ et al (2011) Harnessing neuroplasticity for clinical applications. Brain 134(Pt 6):1591–1609. https://doi.org/10.1093/brain/awr039

Creutzfeldt OD (1983) Cortex ceribri. Springer. https://doi.org/10.1007/978-3-642-68962-8

Cui D, Janela D, Costa F, Molinos M, Areias AC, Moulder RG, Scheer JK, Bento V, Cohen SP, Yanamadala V, Correia FD (2023) Randomized-controlled trial assessing a digital care program versus conventional physiotherapy for chronic low back pain. npj Digital Med 6(1):121. https://doi.org/10.1038/s41746-023-00870-3

Danho S, Vega Leonel JM, Alexander Garzon D et al (2025) Exploratory study on the improvement of jump performance through exposure to schumann frequencies. Cureus 17(9):e92038. https://doi.org/10.7759/cureus.92038.

Daugs R (1979) Programmierte Instruktion und Lerntechnolgie im Sportunterricht. Minerva.

Davids K, Handford C, Williams M (1994) The natural physical alternative to cognitive theories of motor behaviour: an invitation for interdisciplinary research in sports science? J Sports Sci 12(6):495–528. https://doi.org/10.1080/02640419408732202

Davids K, Button C, Bennett S (1999) Modeling human motor systems in nonlinear dynamics: intentionality and discrete movement behaviors. Nonlinear Dynamics Psychol Life Sci 3(1):3–30. https://doi.org/10.1023/A:1022429522099

Davids K, Kingsbury D, Bennett S, Handford C (2001) Information–movement coupling: implications for the organization of research and practice during acquisition of self-paced extrinsic timing skills. J Sports Sci 19(2):117–127. https://doi.org/10.1080/026404101300036316

Davids K, Button C, Bennett S (2008) Dynamics of skill acquisition: a constraints-led approach. Hum Kinet

Dayan E, Casile A, Levit-Binnun N, Giese MA, Hendler T, Flash T (2007) Neural representations of kinematic laws of motion: evidence for action-perception coupling. Proc Natl Acad Sci USA 104(51):20582–20587. https://doi.org/10.1073/pnas.0710033104

Dayan E, Cohen LG (2011) Neuroplasticity subserving motorskill learning. Neuron 72(3):443–454. https://doi.org/10.1016/j.neuron.2011.10.008

de Croock MBM, van Merriënboer JJG, Paas FGWC (1998) High versus low contextual interference in

simulation-based training of troubleshooting skills: effects on transfer performance and invested mental effort. Comput Hum Behav 14(2):249–267. https://doi.org/10.1016/S0747-5632(98)00005-3
De Fazio R, Mastronardi VM, De Vittorio M, Visconti P (2023) Wearable sensors and smart devices to monitor rehabilitation parameters and sports performance: an overview. Sensors (Basel) 23(4). https://doi.org/10.3390/s23041856
de Wit MM, de Vries S, van der Kamp J, Withagen R (2017) Affordances and neuroscience: steps towards a successful marriage. Neurosci Biobehav Rev 80:622–629. https://doi.org/10.1016/j.neubiorev.2017.07.008
Decostre V, Bianco P, Lombardi V, Piazzesi G (2005) Effect of temperature on the working stroke of muscle myosin. Proc Natl Acad Sci 102(39):13927–13932. https://doi.org/10.1073/pnas.0506795102
Deecke L, Scheid P, Kornhuber HH (1969) Distribution of readiness potential, pre-motion positivity, and motor potential of the human cerebral cortex preceding voluntary finger movements. Exp Brain Res 7(2):158–168. https://doi.org/10.1007/bf00235441
Dewey J (1903) Democracy and education; The elementary school teacher, IV, 4. The University of Chicago Press
di Pellegrino G, Fadiga L, Fogassi L, Gallese V, Rizzolatti G (1992) Understanding motor events: a neurophysiological study. Exp Brain Res 91(1):176–180. https://doi.org/10.1007/bf00230027
Dietrich K (1969) Moeglichkeiten des Einsatzes audiovisueller Techniken in der Leibeserziehung. In: Recla J (ed) Methodik der Leibesübungen. Graz.
Dinse HR (2004) Sound case for enrichment. Focus on "environmental enrichment improves response strength, threshold, selectivity, and latency of auditory cortex neurons". J Neurophysiol 92(1):36–37. https://doi.org/10.1152/jn.00213.2004
Drack M, Pouvreau D (2015) On the history of Ludwig von Bertalanffy's "general systemology", and on its relationship to cybernetics – part III: convergences and divergences. Int J Gen Syst 44(5):523–571. https://doi.org/10.1080/03081079.2014.1000642
Drew PJ, Abbott LF (2006) Models and properties of power-law adaptation in neural systems. J Neurophysiol 96(2):826–833. https://doi.org/10.1152/jn.00134.2006
Dudel J (1980) Allgemiene Sinnesphysiologie. In: Schmidt RF (ed) Physiologie des Menschen. Springer, pp 191–208
Duus P (1990) Neurologisch-topische Diagnostik. Thieme
Ebbinghaus H (1913) Memory: a contribution to experimental psychology. Ann Neurosci 20(4):155–156. https://doi.org/10.5214/ans.0972.7531.200408
Ehrenberger K, Finkenzeller P, Keidel WD, Plattig KH (1966) Elektrophysiologische Korrelation der Stevensschen Potenzfunktion und objektive Schwellenmessung am Vibrationssinn des Menschen. Pflugers Arch Gesamte Physiol Menschen Tiere 290(2):114–123. https://doi.org/10.1007/BF00363689
Engel S, Zhang X, Wandell B (1997) Colour tuning in human visual cortex measured with functional magnetic resonance imaging. Nature 388(6637):68–71. https://doi.org/10.1038/40398
Estes WK (1950) Toward a statistical theory of learning. Psychol Rev 57(2):94–107. https://doi.org/10.1037/h0058559
Estes WK (1955) Statistical theory of spontaneous recovery and regression. Psychol Rev 62(3):145–154. https://doi.org/10.1037/h0048509
Estes WK, Burke CJ (1953) A theory of stimulus variability in learning. Psychol Rev 60(4):276–286. https://doi.org/10.1037/h0055775
Estes WK, Suppes P, Mathematics SUA, Laboratory S (1959) Foundations of statistical learning theory: the stimulus sampling model. Behavioral Sciences Division, Applied Mathematics and Statistics Laboratory, Stanford University
Etzel JA, Gazzola V, Keysers C (2008) Testing simulation theory with cross-modal multivariate classification of fMRI data. PLoS One 3(11):e3690. https://doi.org/10.1371/journal.pone.0003690
Evarts EV (1968) Relation of pyramidal tract activity to force exerted during voluntary movement. J Neurophysiol 31(1):14–27. https://doi.org/10.1152/jn.1968.31.1.14
Evarts EV (1981) Role of motor cortex in voluntary movements in primates. In: Brooks VB (ed) Handbook of physiology, vol II. American Physiology Association, pp 1083–1120
Evaul TW (1964) The automated tutor. J Health Phys Educ Recreat 35(3):27–82. https://doi.org/10.1080/00221473.1964.10621757
Farfel WS (1977) Bewegungssteuerung im Sport. Sportverlag. Berlin.
Farrell JE (1970) Programed vs. teacher-directed instruction in beginning tennis for women. Research Quarterly. American Association for Health, Physical Education and Recreation, 41(1):51–58. https://doi.org/10.1080/10671188.1970.10614946.
Fatoye F, Gebrye T, Fatoye C, Mbada CE, Olaoye MI, Odole AC, Dada O (2020) The clinical and cost-effectiveness of telerehabilitation for people with non-specific chronic low back pain: randomized controlled trial. JMIR Mhealth Uhealth 8(6):e15375. https://doi.org/10.2196/15375
Faverjon S, Silveira DC, Fu DD, Cha BH, Akman C, Hu Y, Holmes GL (2002) Beneficial effects of enriched environment following status epilepticus in immature rats. Neurology 59(9):1356–1364. https://doi.org/10.1212/01.wnl.0000033588.59005.55
Feest U (2019) Why replication is overrated. Philos Sci 86(5):895–905. https://doi.org/10.1086/705451
Fetz F (1987) Programmierter Sportunterricht unter einfachsten Verhältnissen. In: Schaller HJ (ed) Sport lernen mit Lernprogrammen. Putty, pp 25–45
Fink C, Schöllhorn WI, Jaitner T (1999) A more pragmatic criterion for filtering data. In: The XVII ISB Congress, Calgary.

Fitts PM, Posner MI (1967) Human performance. Brooks/Cole
Fiveash A, Bedoin N, Gordon RL, Tillmann B (2021) Processing rhythm in speech and music: shared mechanisms and implications for developmental speech and language disorders. Neuropsychology 35(8):771–791. https://doi.org/10.1037/neu0000766
Flandrin P (1994) Time-scale analyses and self-similar stochastic processes. In: Byrnes JS, Byrnes JL, Hargreaves KA, Berry K (eds) Wavelets and their applications. Springer, Dordrecht, pp 121–142. https://doi.org/10.1007/978-94-011-1028-0_7
Flash T, Hogan N (1985) The coordination of arm movements: an experimentally confirmed mathematical model. J Neurosci 5(7):1688–1703. https://doi.org/10.1523/jneurosci.05-07-01688.1985
Fleishman EA (1954) Dimensional analysis of psychomotor abilities. J Exp Psychol 48(6):437–454. https://doi.org/10.1037/h0058244
Foerster O (1936) Motorische Felder und Bahnen. In: Blumke OFO (ed) Handbuch der Neurologie, vol 6. Springer, pp 1–357
Fonseca ST, Souza TR, Verhagen E, Van Emmerik REA, Bittencourt NFN, Mendonça LDM, Andrade AGP, Resende RA, Ocarino JM (2020) Sports injury forecasting and complexity: a synergetic approach. Sports Med 50(10):1757–1770. https://doi.org/10.1007/s40279-020-01326-4
Fontaine RJ, Lee TD, Swinnen SP (1997) Learning a new bimanual coordination pattern: reciprocal influences of intrinsic and to-be-learned patterns. Can J Exp Psychol 51(1):1–9. https://doi.org/10.1037/1196-1961.51.1.1
Forrester JW (1961) Industrial dynamics. MIT
Frank CB (2004) Ligament structure, physiology and function. J Musculoskelet Neuronal Interact 4(2):199–201
Frank TD, Profeta VL, Harrison HS (2015) Interplay between order-parameter and system parameter dynamics: considerations on perceptual-cognitive-behavioral mode-mode transitions exhibiting positive and negative hysteresis and on response times. J Biol Phys 41(3):257–292. https://doi.org/10.1007/s10867-015-9378-z
French AS, Torkkeli PH (2008) The power law of sensory adaptation: simulation by a model of excitability in spider mechanoreceptor neurons. Ann Biomed Eng 36(1):153–161. https://doi.org/10.1007/s10439-007-9392-9
Froebel FWA (1826) Die Menschenerziehung, die Erziehungs- Unterrichts- und Lehrkunst, angestrebt in der allgemeinen deutschen Erziehungsanstalt zu Keilhau. (Human education, the art of education, instruction and teaching, pursued in the general German educational institution at Keilhau). Wiebrad
Fukuoka Y, Matsuki H, Minamitani H, Akimasa I (1998) A modified back-propagation method to avoid false local minima. Neural Netw 11(6):1059–1072. https://doi.org/10.1016/S0893-6080(98)00087-2
Garthe A, Roeder I, Kempermann G (2016) Mice in an enriched environment learn more flexibly because of adult hippocampal neurogenesis. Hippocampus 26(2):261–271. https://doi.org/10.1002/hipo.22520
Gaulhofer K, Streicher M (1924) Grundzüge des Österreichischen Schulturnens. Deutscher Verlag für Jugend und Volk
Gel'fand IM, Tsetlin ML (1962) Some methods of control for complex systems. Russ Math Surv 17:95–117
Georgopoulos AP (1990) Neurophysiology of reaching. In: Jeannerod M (ed) Attention and performance XIII. Erlbaum, pp 227–263
Georgopoulos AP (1991) Higher order motor control. Annu Rev Neurosci 14:361–377. https://doi.org/10.1146/annurev.ne.14.030191.002045
Georgopoulos AP, Kalaska JF, Caminiti R, Massey JT. (1982) On the relations between the direction of two-dimensional arm movements and cell discharge in primate motor cortex. J Neurosci 2(11):1527–1537. https://doi.org/10.1523/JNEUROSCI.02-11-01527.1982
Ghez C, Hening W, Gordon J (1991) Organization of voluntary movement. Curr Opin Neurobiol 1(4):664–671. https://doi.org/10.1016/s0959-4388(05)80046-7
Ghez C, Gordon J, Ghilardi MF (1995) Impairments of reaching movements in patients without proprioception. II. Effects of visual information on accuracy. J Neurophysiol 73(1):361–372. https://doi.org/10.1152/jn.1995.73.1.361
Gibson JJ (1962) Observations on active touch. Psychol Rev 69:477–491. https://doi.org/10.1037/h0046962.
Gibson JJ (1979) The ecological approach to visual perception. Lawrence Erlabaum
Gigerenzer G (2004) Mindless statistics. J Socio-Econ 33(5):587–606. https://doi.org/10.1016/j.socec.2004.09.033
Gigerenzer G (2018) Statistical rituals: the replication delusion and how we got there. Adv Methods Pract Psychol Sci 1(2):198–218. https://doi.org/10.1177/2515245918771329
Glasersfeld EV (1995) Radical constructivism: a way of knowing and learning. Falmer Press
Godde B, Berkefeld T, David-Jürgens M, Dinse HR (2002) Age-related changes in primary somatosensory cortex of rats: evidence for parallel degenerative and plastic-adaptive processes. Neurosci Biobehav Rev 26(7):743–752. https://doi.org/10.1016/s0149-7634(02)00061-1
Goldscheider A (1889) Untersuchungen über den Muskelsinn. Archiv Anat Physiol 3:369–502
Gonzalez F, Relova JL, Perez R, Acuña C, Alonso JM (1993) Cell responses to vertical and horizontal retinal disparities in the monkey visual cortex. Neurosci Lett 160(2):167–170. https://doi.org/10.1016/0304-3940(93)90405-a
Gonzalez F, Justo MS, Bermudez MA, Perez R (2003) Sensitivity to horizontal and vertical disparity and orientation preference in areas V1 and V2 of the monkey. Neuroreport 14(6):829–832. https://doi.org/10.1097/00001756-200305060-00010
Goodale MA, Milner AD (1992) Separate visual pathways for perception and action.

Trends Neurosci 15(1):20–25. https://doi.org/10.1016/0166-2236(92)90344-8
Goode S, Magill RA (1986) Contextual interference effects in learning three badminton serves. Res Q Exerc Sport 57(4):308–314. https://doi.org/10.1080/02701367.1986.10608091
Goodwin GM, McCloskey DI, Matthews PB (1972) Proprioceptive illusions induced by muscle vibration: contribution by muscle spindles to perception? Science 175(4028):1382–1384. https://doi.org/10.1126/science.175.4028.1382
Gordon SP, Newby PJ (2019) Transitioning from the military to teaching: two veterans' journeys through the entry year. Educ Forum 83(2):140–159. https://doi.org/10.1080/00131725.2019.1561965
Gori M, Tesi A (1992) On the problem of local minima in backpropagation. IEEE Trans Pattern Anal Mach Intell 14(1):76–86. https://doi.org/10.1109/34.107014
Graziano M (2006) The organization of behavioral repertoire in motor cortex. Annu Rev Neurosci 29:105–134. https://doi.org/10.1146/annurev.neuro.29.051605.112924
Graziano MS, Cooke DF (2006) Parieto-frontal interactions, personal space, and defensive behavior. Neuropsychologia 44(6):845–859. https://doi.org/10.1016/j.neuropsychologia.2005.09.009
Graziano MS, Aflalo TN, Cooke DF (2005) Arm movements evoked by electrical stimulation in the motor cortex of monkeys. J Neurophysiol 94(6):4209–4223. https://doi.org/10.1152/jn.01303.2004
Gregor RJ, Pink MM (1985) Biomechanical analysis of a world record javelin throw: a case study. Int J Sport Biomech 1:73–77. https://doi.org/10.1123/ijsb.1.1.73.
Grill-Spector K, Henson R, Martin A (2006) Repetition and the brain: neural models of stimulus-specific effects. Trends Cogn Sci 10(1):14–23. https://doi.org/10.1016/j.tics.2005.11.006
Grossberg S (1980) How does a brain build a cognitive code? Psychol Rev 87(1):1–51. https://doi.org/10.1007/978-94-009-7758-7_1
Guadagnoli MA, Lee TD (2004) Challenge point: a framework for conceptualizing the effects of various practice conditions in motor learning. J Mot Behav 36(2):212–224. https://doi.org/10.3200/jmbr.36.2.212-224
Guedry FE Jr, Benson AJ (1978) Coriolis cross-coupling effects: disorienting and nauseogenic or not? Aviat Space Environ Med 49(1 Pt 1):29–35
Guimarães AN, Ugrinowitsch H, Dascal JB, Porto AB, Okazaki VHA (2020) Freezing Degrees of Freedom During Motor Learning: A Systematic Review. Motor Control 24(3):457–71. https://doi.org/10.1123/mc.2019-0060.
Gutewort W, Stürmer H, Thorhauer HA, Wittemann G (1973) Die Objektivierung ausgewählter Stützsprünge im Gerätturnen – Die biomechanische Analyse als Beitrag zur komplexen Leistungsdiagnostik. Theorie und Praxis des Leistungssports 11(5)
Gutnisky DA, Dragoi V (2008) Adaptive coding of visual information in neural populations. Nature 452(7184):220–224. https://doi.org/10.1038/nature06563
Haase J, Henatsch HD, Jung R, Strata P, Thoden U (1976) Sensomotorik. Urban & Schwarzenberger
Hackfort D (2017) Commentary on "towards a grand unified theory of sports performance". Hum Mov Sci 56(Part A):166–168. https://doi.org/10.1016/j.humov.2017.05.003
Haken H (1975) Cooperative phenomena in systems far from thermal equilibrium and in nonphysical systems. Rev Mod Phys 47(1):67–121. https://doi.org/10.1103/RevModPhys.47.67
Haken H (1983) Synergetics: an introduction: nonequilibrium phase transitions and self-organization in physics, chemistry, and biology. Springer
Haken HWA (1991) Die Selbststrukturierung der Materie: Synergetik in der unbelebten Welt. Vieweg+Teubner Verlag
Haken H, Schiepek G (2006) Synergetik in der Psychologie: Selbstorganisation verstehen und gestalten. Hogrefe
Haken H, Kelso JA, Bunz H (1985) A theoretical model of phase transitions in human hand movements. Biol Cybern 51(5):347–356. https://doi.org/10.1007/bf00336922
Hall LA, McCloskey DI (1983) Detections of movements imposed on finger, elbow and shoulder joints. J Physiol 335:519–533. https://doi.org/10.1113/jphysiol.1983.sp014548
Handford C (2002) Strategy and practice for acquiring timing in discrete, self-paced interceptive actions. In: Davids K, Savelsbergh GJP, van der Kamp J (eds) Interceptive actions in sport. Tayler & Francis, pp 288–300
Handford C, Davids K, Bennett S, Button C (1997) Skill acquisition in sport: some applications of an evolving practice ecology. J Sports Sci 15(6):621–640. https://doi.org/10.1080/026404197367056
Handwerker HO (1993) Somatosensorik. In: Schmidt RF (ed) Neuro- und Sinnesphysiologie. Springer
Hara Y (2015) Brain plasticity and rehabilitation in stroke patients. J Nippon Med Sch 82(1):4–13. https://doi.org/10.1272/jnms.82.4
Hardman K, Green K (2011) Contemporary issues in physical education: international perspectives. Meyer & Meyer Sport
Hargreaves M, Spriet LL (2020) Skeletal muscle energy metabolism during exercise. Nat Metab 2(9):817–828. https://doi.org/10.1038/s42255-020-0251-4
Harre D (1971) Trainingslehre. Sportverlag
Hassenstein B (1977) Biologische Kybernetik, 5th edn. Quelle & Meyer
Hausdorff JM, Purdon PL, Peng CK, Ladin Z, Wei JY, Goldberger AL (1996) Fractal dynamics of human gait: stability of long-range correlations in stride interval fluctuations. J Appl Physiol

(1985) 80(5):1448–1457. https://doi.org/10.1152/jappl.1996.80.5.1448
Hawley JA, Hargreaves M, Joyner MJ, Zierath JR (2014) Integrative biology of exercise. Cell 159(4):738–749. https://doi.org/10.1016/j.cell.2014.10.029
Haykin SS (1994) Neural networks: a comprehensive foundation. Macmillan
Hebb DO (1949) The organization of behavior; a neuropsychological theory. Wiley
Hedrick NG, Lu Z, Bushong E, Singhi S, Nguyen P, Magaña Y, Jilani S, Lim BK, Ellisman M, Komiyama T (2022) Learning binds new inputs into functional synaptic clusters via spinogenesis. Nat Neurosci 25(6):726–737. https://doi.org/10.1038/s41593-022-01086-6
Heimburg T (2022a) The effect of stretching on nerve excitability. Hum Mov Sci 86:103000. https://doi.org/10.1016/j.humov.2022.103000
Heimburg T (2022b) The thermodynamic soliton theory of the nervous impulse and possible medical implications. Prog Biophys Mol Biol 173:24–35. https://doi.org/10.1016/j.pbiomolbio.2022.05.007
Heinrichs KI (2002) Problem-based learning in entry-level athletic training professional-education programs: a model for developing critical-thinking and decision-making skills. J Athl Train 37(4 Suppl):S189–s198
Hemelrijk C (2005) Self-organisation and evolution of biological and social systems. Cambridge University Press
Hempel CG (1951) General system theory and the unity of science. Hum Biol 23(4):313–322. http://www.jstor.org/stable/41448004
Hempel CG (1965) Aspects of scientific explanation and other essays in the philosophy of science. Free Press
Hempel CG, Oppenheim P (1948) Studies in the logic of explanation. Philos Sci 15(2):135–175. http://www.jstor.org/stable/185169
Henatsch HD (1976) Bauplan der peripheren und zentralen sensomotorischen Kontrollen. In: Haase JH, Henatsch HD, Jung R, Strata P, Thoden U (eds) Sensomotorik. Physiologie des Menschen, vol 14. Urban & Schwarzenberger
Herbert C, Kissler J (2010) Motivational priming and processing interrupt: startle reflex modulation during shallow and deep processing of emotional words. Int J Psychophysiol 76(2):64–71. https://doi.org/10.1016/j.ijpsycho.2010.02.004
Herrmann C, Gerlach E, Seelig H (2015) Development and validation of a test instrument for the assessment of basic motor competencies in primary school. Meas Phys Educ Exerc Sci 19(2):80–90. https://doi.org/10.1080/1091367X.2014.998821
Hertz J, Krogh A, Palmer RG (1991) Introduction to the theory of neural computation. Addison-Wesley/Addison Wesley Longman
Hirtz P (1976) Die koordinative Vervollkommnung als wesentlicher Bestandteil der körperlichen Grundausbildung. Körpererziehung 26(8/9):381–387
Hirtz P (1977) Struktur und Entwicklung koordinativer Leistungsvoraussetzungen bei Schulkindern (Structure and development of coordinative performance prerequisites). Theor Prax Korperkult 26:503–510
Hirtz P (1988) Koordinative Fähigkeiten im Schulsport – vielseitig – variationsreichungewohnt. Volk und Wissen Volkseigener Verlag
Hof BE (2018) The cybernetic "general model theory": unifying science or epistemic change? Perspect Sci 26(1):76–96. https://doi.org/10.1162/POSC_a_00268
Hohberg V, Kreppke J-N, Cody R, Guthold R, Woods C, Brand R, Dunton G, Rothman A, Ketelhut S, Nigg C (2022) What is needed to promote physical activity? Current trends and new perspectives in theory, intervention, and implementation. Curr Issues Sport Sci 7(1). https://doi.org/10.36950/2022ciss005.
Holtmaat A, Svoboda K (2009) Experience-dependent structural synaptic plasticity in the mammalian brain. Nat Rev Neurosci 10(9):647–658. https://doi.org/10.1038/nrn2699
Holzreiter SH, Köhle ME (1993) Assessment of gait patterns using neural networks. J Biomech 26(6):645–651. https://doi.org/10.1016/0021-9290(93)90028-d
Hommel B, Wiers RW (2017) Towards a unitary approach to human action control. Trends Cogn Sci 21(12):940–949. https://doi.org/10.1016/j.tics.2017.09.009
Hommel B, Müsseler J, Aschersleben G, Prinz W (2001) The theory of event coding (TEC): a framework for perception and action planning. Behav Brain Sci 24(5):849–878; discussion 878-937. https://doi.org/10.1017/s0140525x01000103
Horst F, Kramer F, Schäfer B, Eekhoff A, Hegen P, Nigg BM, Schöllhorn WI (2016) Daily changes of individual gait patterns identified by means of support vector machines. Gait Posture 49:309–314. https://doi.org/10.1016/j.gaitpost.2016.07.073
Horst F, Eekhoff A, Newell KM, Schöllhorn WI (2017a) Intra-individual gait patterns across different timescales as revealed by means of a supervised learning model using kernel-based discriminant regression. PLoS One 12(6):e0179738. https://doi.org/10.1371/journal.pone.0179738
Horst F, Mildner M, Schöllhorn WI (2017b) One-year persistence of individual gait patterns identified in a follow-up study – a call for individualised diagnose and therapy. Gait Posture 58:476–480. https://doi.org/10.1016/j.gaitpost.2017.09.003
Horst F, Janssen D, Beckmann H, Schöllhorn WI (2020) Can individual movement characteristics across different throwing disciplines be identified in high-performance decathletes? Front Psychol 11:2262. https://doi.org/10.3389/fpsyg.2020.02262
Hubel DH, Wiesel TN (1962) Receptive fields, binocular interaction and functional architecture in the cat's visual cortex. J Physiol 160(1):106–154. https://doi.org/10.1113/jphysiol.1962.sp006837
Hubel DH, Wiesel TN (1964) Effects of monocular deprivation in kittens. Naunyn Schmiedebergs Arch Exp Pathol Pharmakol 248:492–497. https://doi.org/10.1007/bf00348878

Hubert-White GM (1966) The application of programmed learning to athletics symposium: a journal of education for Southern Africa. https://hdl.handle.net/10539/27434

Huggenberger S, Moser N, Schröder H, Cozzi B, Granato A, Merighi A (2019) Cerebellum (Kleinhirn). In: Huggenberger S, Moser N, Schröder H, Cozzi B, Granato A, Merighi A (eds) Neuroanatomie des Menschen. Springer, Berlin/Heidelberg, pp 73–84. https://doi.org/10.1007/978-3-662-56461-5_8

Illert M (1993) Motorische Systeme. In: Schmidt RF (ed) Neuro- und Sinnespyhsiologie. Springer, pp 113–149

Ioannidis JPA (2005) Why most published research findings are false. PLoS Med 2(8):e124. https://doi.org/10.1371/journal.pmed.0020124

Ito M (1984) The cerebellum and neural control. Raven Press

Jäger JM, Alichmann M, Schöllhorn WI (2003) Erkennung von Ermüdungszuständen anhand von Bodenreaktionskräften. In: Brüggemann GP, Morey-Klapsing G (eds) Biologische Systeme. Czwalina, pp 179–183

Janssen D (2017) Analyse und Klassifikation der Effekte unterschiedlicher Emotionsinduktionsmethoden auf das menschliche Gangmuster sowie den Übergang zwischen Gehen und Laufen, vol. 9. Kovacs

Janssen D, Schöllhorn WI, Lubienetzki J, Fölling K, Kokenge H, Davids K (2008) Recognition of emotions in gait patterns by means of artificial neural nets. J Nonverbal Behav 32(2):79–92. https://doi.org/10.1007/s10919-007-0045-3

Janssen D, Gebkenjans F, Beckmann H, Schöllhorn WI (2010) Analyzing learning approaches by means of complex movement pattern analysis. Int J Sport Psychol 41(S):18-21.

Janssen D, Schöllhorn WI, Newell KM, Jäger JM, Rost F, Vehof K (2011) Diagnosing fatigue in gait patterns by support vector machines and self-organizing maps. Hum Mov Sci 30(5):966–975. https://doi.org/10.1016/j.humov.2010.08.010

Jaruševičius G, Rugelis T, McCraty R, Landauskas M, Berškienė K, Vainoras A (2018) Correlation between changes in local Earth's magnetic field and cases of acute myocardial infarction. Int J Environ Res Public Health 15(3). https://doi.org/10.3390/ijerph15030399

Jeka JJ, Kelso JA, Kiemel T (1993) Pattern switching in human multilimb coordination dynamics. Bull Math Biol 55(4):829–845. https://doi.org/10.1007/bf02460675

Jenkins WM, Merzenich MM (1987) Reorganization of neocortical representations after brain injury: a neurophysiological model of the bases of recovery from stroke. Prog Brain Res 71:249–266. https://doi.org/10.1016/s0079-6123(08)61829-4

Jessell TM (1991) Neuronal survival and synapse formation. In: Kandel ERS, Jessel JH, T.M. (eds) Principles of neural science. Appleton & Lange, pp 929–943

Johansson RS, Vallbo ÅB (1983) Tactile sensory coding in the glabrous skin of the human hand. Trends Neurosci 6:27–32. https://doi.org/10.1016/0166-2236(83)90011-5

John A, Schöllhorn WI (2018) Acute effects of instructed and self-created variable rope skipping on EEG brain activity and heart rate variability. Front Behav Neurosci 12:311. https://doi.org/10.3389/fnbeh.2018.00311

John AT, Barthel A, Wind J, Rizzi N, Schöllhorn WI (2022) Acute effects of various movement noise in differential learning of rope skipping on brain and heart recovery analyzed by means of multiscale fuzzy measure entropy. Front Behav Neurosci 16:816334. https://doi.org/10.3389/fnbeh.2022.816334

Jumarie G (1978) Théorie relativiste de l'information et télécommunication. Perspectives. Annales des Télécommunications 33(1):13–27. https://doi.org/10.1007/BF02999489

Jumarie G (1990) A theory of subjective information. In: Relative information: theories and applications. Springer, Berlin/Heidelberg, pp 100–127. https://doi.org/10.1007/978-3-642-84017-3_5

Kamen G, Morris HH (1988) Differences in sensorimotor processing of visual and proprioceptive stimuli. Res Q Exerc Sport 59(1):29–34. https://doi.org/10.1080/02701367.1988.10605470

Kandel ER, Schwartz JH, Jessell TM (1991) Principles of neural science. Appleton & Lange

Kaplan RM, Chambers DA, Glasgow RE (2014) Big data and large sample size: a cautionary note on the potential for bias. Clin Transl Sci 7(4):342–346. https://doi.org/10.1111/cts.12178

Karni A, Sagi D (1991) Where practice makes perfect in texture discrimination: evidence for primary visual cortex plasticity. Proc Natl Acad Sci USA 88(11):4966–4970. https://doi.org/10.1073/pnas.88.11.4966

Keele SW (1968) Movement control in skilled motor performance. Psychol Bull 70(6, Pt 1):387–403. https://doi.org/10.1037/h0026739

Keidel WD, Finkenzeller P (1984) Artificial auditory stimulation theories. In: Advances in audiology, vol 1. S. Karger

Kelly JPDJ (1991) Hearing. In: Kandel ERS, Jessel JH, TM (eds) Principles of neural science. Appleton & Lange, pp 481–498

Kelso JAS (1995) Dynamic patterns: the self-organization of brain and behavior. MIT

Kelso JA, Jeka JJ (1992) Symmetry breaking dynamics of human multilimb coordination. J Exp Psychol Hum Percept Perform 18(3):645–668. https://doi.org/10.1037/0096-1523.18.3.645

Kelso JA, Zanone PG (2002) Coordination dynamics of learning and transfer across different effector systems. J Exp Psychol Hum Percept Perform 28(4):776–797. https://doi.org/10.1037/0096-1523.28.4.776.

Kelso JAS, Saltzman EL, Tuller B (1986a) The dynamical perspective on speech production: data and theory. J Phon 14(1):29–59. https://doi.org/10.1016/S0095-4470(19)30608-4

Kelso JAS, Scholz JP, Schöner G (1986b) Nonequilibrium phase transitions in coordinated biological motion: critical fluctuations. Phys Lett A 118(6):279–284. https://doi.org/10.1016/0375-9601(86)90359-2

Kelso JA, Buchanan JJ, Wallace SA (1991) Order parameters for the neural organization of single, multijoint limb movement patterns. Exp Brain Res 85(2):432–444. https://doi.org/10.1007/bf00229420

Kemmerer D (2021) What modulates the mirror neuron system during action observation?: Multiple factors involving the action, the actor, the observer, the relationship between actor and observer, and the context. Prog Neurobiol 205:102128. https://doi.org/10.1016/j.pneurobio.2021.102128

Kempermann G, Kuhn HG, Gage FH (1997) More hippocampal neurons in adult mice living in an enriched environment. Nature 386(6624):493–495. https://doi.org/10.1038/386493a0

Kern G (1933) Motorische Umreißung optischer Gestalten. Neue Psychologische Studien 9:65–104

Kerr R, Booth B (1978) Specific and varied practice of motor skill. Percept Mot Skills 46(2):395–401. https://doi.org/10.1177/003151257804600201

Kerschensteiner G (1912) Begriff der Arbeitsschule n der Pädagogik. Teubner

Khan S, Cohen D (2019) Using the magnetoencephalogram to noninvasively measure magnetite in the living human brain. Hum Brain Mapp 40(5):1654–1665. https://doi.org/10.1002/hbm.24477

Kim J (1999) Making sense of emergence. Philos Stud 95(1):3–36. https://doi.org/10.1023/A:1004563122154

King AC, Stokols D, Talen E, Brassington GS, Killingsworth R (2002) Theoretical approaches to the promotion of physical activity: forging a transdisciplinary paradigm. Am J Prev Med 23(2):15–25. https://doi.org/10.1016/S0749-3797(02)00470-1

Kirk D (2010) Physical education futures. Routledge

Kirk D, Tinning R (1990) Physical education, curriculum, and culture: critical issues in the contemporary crisis. Falmer Press

Kirkpatrick S, Gelatt CD Jr, Vecchi MP (1983) Optimization by simulated annealing. Science 220(4598):671–680. https://doi.org/10.1126/science.220.4598.671

Kline A, Pittman D, Ronsky J, Goodyear B (2020) Differentiating the brain's involvement in executed and imagined stepping using fMRI. Behav Brain Res 394:112829. https://doi.org/10.1016/j.bbr.2020.112829

Klinke R (1985) Physiologie des Gleichgewichts. In: Schmidt RF (ed) Grundriss der Sinnesphysiologie. Springer, pp 272–287

Knudsen EI (2018) Neural circuits that mediate selective attention: a comparative perspective. Trends Neurosci 41(11):789–805. https://doi.org/10.1016/j.tins.2018.06.006

Köhler W (1917) Intelligenzprüfungen an Anthropoiden. Kgl. Akad. d. Wiss.

Kohonen T (1982) Self-organized formation of topologically correct feature maps. Biol Cybern 43(1):59–69. https://doi.org/10.1007/BF00337288

Korbmacher M, Azevedo F, Pennington CR, Hartmann H, Pownall M, Schmidt K, Elsherif M, Breznau N, Robertson O, Kalandadze T, Yu S, Baker BJ, O'Mahony A, Olsnes JØS, Shaw JJ, Gjoneska B, Yamada Y, Röer JP, Murphy J et al (2023) The replication crisis has led to positive structural, procedural, and community changes. Commun Psychol 1(1):3. https://doi.org/10.1038/s44271-023-00003-2

Kornhuber HH (1978) Blickmotorik. In: Gauer OHK, Jung K, K. (eds) Physiologie des Menschen, vol 13. Urban & Schwarzenberger, pp 357–426

Kostrubiec V, Zanone PG (2002) Memory dynamics: distance between the new task and existing behavioural patterns affects learning and interference in bimanual coordination in humans. Neurosci Lett 331(3):193–197. https://doi.org/10.1016/S0304-3940(02)00878-9

Kostrubiec V, Zanone PG, Fuchs A, Kelso JAS (2012) Beyond the blank slate: routes to learning new coordination patterns depend on the intrinsic dynamics of the learner – experimental evidence and theoretical model [Hypothesis and theory]. Front Hum Neurosci 6. https://doi.org/10.3389/fnhum.2012.00222

Krauss P, Metzner C, Schilling A, Schütz C, Tziridis K, Fabry B, Schulze H (2017) Adaptive stochastic resonance for unknown and variable input signals. Sci Rep 7(1):2450. https://doi.org/10.1038/s41598-017-02644-w

Kugler PN, Scott Kelso JA, Turvey MT (1980) 1 on the concept of coordinative structures as dissipative structures: I. Theoretical lines of convergence**this work was supported by NIH grants HD 01994, NS 13617 and AM 25814. In: Stelmach GE, Requin J (eds) Advances in psychology, vol 1. North-Holland, pp 3–47. https://doi.org/10.1016/S0166-4115(08)61936-6

Kümmel J, Kramer A, Giboin LS, Gruber M (2016) Specificity of balance training in healthy individuals: a systematic review and meta-analysis. Sports Med 46(9):1261–1271. https://doi.org/10.1007/s40279-016-0515-z

Kunze G (1970) Programmiertes Lehren und Lernen im Sport – eine Taxonomie. Die Leibeserziehung 19(9):7

Kurz D, Fritz T, Tscherpel R (2008) Der MOBAQ-Ansatz als Konzept für Mindeststandards für den Sportunterricht? In: Oesterhelt V, Hofmann J, Schimanski M, Scholz M, Altenberger H (eds) Sportpädagogik im Spannungsfeld gesellschaftlicher Erwartungen, wissenschaftlicher Ansprüche und empirischer Befunde, pp 97–106

Lackner JR (1985) Human sensory-motor adaptation to the terrestrial force environment. In: Ingle DJ, Jeannerod M, Lee DN (eds) Brain mechanisms and spatial vision. Springer, Dordrecht, pp 175–209. https://doi.org/10.1007/978-94-009-5071-9_8

Lacourse MG, Orr EL, Cramer SC, Cohen MJ (2005) Brain activation during execution and motor imagery of novel and skilled sequential hand movements. NeuroImage 27(3):505–519. https://doi.org/10.1016/j.neuroimage.2005.04.025

Lambert TE, Harvey LA, Avdalis C, Chen LW, Jeyalingam S, Pratt CA, Tatum HJ, Bowden JL, Lucas BR (2017) An app with remote support achieves better adherence to home exercise programs than paper handouts in people with musculoskeletal conditions: a randomised trial. J Physiother 63(3):161–167. https://doi.org/10.1016/j.jphys.2017.05.015

Lanciego JL, Luquin N, Obeso JA (2012) Functional neuroanatomy of the basal ganglia. Cold Spring Harb Perspect Med 2(12):a009621. https://doi.org/10.1101/cshperspect.a009621

Lashley KS (1933) Integrative functions of the cerbral cortex. Physiol Rev 13(1):1–42. https://doi.org/10.1152/physrev.1933.13.1.1

Lashley KS (1951) The problem of serial order in behavior. In: Cerebral mechanisms in behavior; the Hixon symposium. Wiley, pp 112–146

Lauber B, Keller M, Leukel C, Gollhofer A, Taube W (2013) Specific interpretation of augmented feedback changes motor performance and cortical processing. Exp Brain Res 227(1):31–41. https://doi.org/10.1007/s00221-013-3482-8

Lee TD, Magill RA (1983) The locus of contextual interference in motor-skill acquisition. J Exp Psychol Learn Mem Cogn 9(4):730–746. https://doi.org/10.1037/0278-7393.9.4.730

Lee TD, Magill RA (1985) Can forgetting facilitate skill acquisition? In: Goodman D, Wilberg RB, Franks LM (eds) Differeing perspectives in motor learning, memory, and control. North-Holland, pp 3–22

Lee TD, Swanson LR, Hall AL (1991) What is repeated in a repetition? Effects of practice conditions on motor skill acquisition. Phys Ther 71(2):150–156. https://doi.org/10.1093/ptj/71.2.150

Lee AM, Keh NC, Magill RA (1993) Instructional effects of teacher feedback in physical education. J Teach Phys Educ 12(3):228–243. https://doi.org/10.1123/jtpe.12.3.228

Lee TD, Wulf G, Winstein CJ, Zelaznik HN (2016) In memoriam: Richard Allen Schmidt (1941-2015). J Mot Behav 48(1):1–4. https://doi.org/10.1080/00222895.2016.1124687

Lesinski M, Hortobágyi T, Muehlbauer T, Gollhofer A, Granacher U (2015) Effects of balance training on balance performance in healthy older adults: a systematic review and meta-analysis. Sports Med 45(12):1721–1738. https://doi.org/10.1007/s40279-015-0375-y

Letzelter M (1978) Trainingsgrundlagen. Rowohlt

Levi-Montalcini R, Hamburger V (1951) Selective growth stimulating effects of mouse sarcoma on the sensory and sympathetic nervous system of the chick embryo. J Exp Zool 116(2):321–361. https://doi.org/10.1002/jez.1401160206

Levitin DJ, Grahn JA, London J (2018) The psychology of music: rhythm and movement. Annu Rev Psychol 69:51–75. https://doi.org/10.1146/annurev-psych-122216-011740

Lewin K (1935) A dynamic theory of personality – selected papers. Lewin Press

Lewin K (1947) Frontiers in group dynamics: concept, method and reality in social science; social equilibria and social change. Hum Relat 1(1):5–41. https://doi.org/10.1177/001872674700100103

Li B, Todo Y, Tang Z (2022) Artificial visual system for orientation detection based on Hubel–Wiesel model. Brain Sci 12(4):470. https://www.mdpi.com/2076-3425/12/4/470

Lin CJ, Yang HC, Knowlton BJ, Wu AD, Iacoboni M, Ye YL, Huang SL, Chiang MC (2018) Contextual interference enhances motor learning through increased resting brain connectivity during memory consolidation. NeuroImage 181:1–15. https://doi.org/10.1016/j.neuroimage.2018.06.081

Liu Y, Cao C, Yan JH (2013) Functional aging impairs the role of feedback in motor learning. Geriatr Gerontol Int 13(4):849–859. https://doi.org/10.1111/ggi.12013

Lobo L, Heras-Escribano M, Travieso D (2018) The history and philosophy of ecological psychology. Front Psychol 9:2228. https://doi.org/10.3389/fpsyg.2018.02228

Lotze M, Montoya P, Erb M, Hülsmann E, Flor H, Klose U, Birbaumer N, Grodd W (1999) Activation of cortical and cerebellar motor areas during executed and imagined hand movements: an fMRI study. J Cogn Neurosci 11(5):491–501. https://doi.org/10.1162/089892999563553

Macpherson JM (1991) How flexible are muscle synergies? In: Humphrey DRF, HJ (eds) Motor control concepts and issues. Wiley

Magill RA (1983) Insights into memory and control in motor behavior through the study of context effects: a discussion of Mathews et al. and Shea and Zimny. In: Magill RA (ed) Memory and control of action, vol 12. North-Holland, pp 367–376. https://doi.org/10.1016/S0166-4115(08)61999-8

Magill RA, Hall KG (1990) A review of the contextual interference effect in motor skill acquisition. Hum Mov Sci 9(3–5):241–289. https://doi.org/10.1016/0167-9457(90)90005-X

Mahlo F (1965) Theoretische Probleme der taktischen Ausbildung in den Sportspielen. Theor Prax Korperkult 14(9):809–815

Malak B, Celichowski J, Drzymała-Celichowska H (2023) The influence of temperature on contractile properties of motor units in rat medial gastrocnemius. J Electromyogr Kinesiol 68:102738. https://doi.org/10.1016/j.jelekin.2022.102738

Marineau E, Ducas J, Mathieu J, Rodriguez AP, Descarreaux M, Abboud J (2024) From novice to expert: how expertise shapes motor variability in sports biomechanics-a scoping review. Scand J Med Sci Sports 34(8):e14706. https://doi.org/10.1111/sms.14706

Marquardt C, Diaz Meyer M, Schneider M, Hilgemann R (2016) Learning handwriting at school—a teachers' survey on actual problems and future options. Trends Neurosci Educ 5(3):82–89. https://doi.org/10.1016/j.tine.2016.07.001

Martin D, Carl K, Lehnertz K (1991) Handbuch Trainingslehre. Hofmann

Matveev LP (1964) Problem of periodization of the sport training (in Russian). FiS Publisher

Matveev LP (1981) Fundamentals of sports training. Progress Publishers

Maxwell JP, Masters RSW, Kerr E, Weedon E (2001) The implicit benefit of learning without errors. Q J Exp Psychol A 54A(4):1049–1068. https://doi.org/10.1080/02724980143000073

Mayne R (1974) A system concept of the vestbular organs. In: Kornhuber HH (ed) Handbook of sensory physiology, Vestibular system. Springer, pp 494–573

McCloskey DI (1993) Detection and execution of movements. Psychol Res 55(2):139–143. https://doi.org/10.1007/BF00419645

McCraty R (2003) The energetic heart: bioelectromagnetic interactions within and between people. The Neuropsychotherapist 6(1):1–20. https://doi.org/10.12744/tnpt(6)022-043

McCraty R (2022) Following the rhythm of the heart: HeartMath institute's path to HRV biofeedback. Appl Psychophysiol Biofeedback 47(4):305–316. https://doi.org/10.1007/s10484-022-09554-2

McCraty R, Childre D (2010) Coherence: bridging personal, social, and global health. Altern Ther Health Med 16(4):10–24

McCraty R, Atkinson M, Stolc V, Alabdulgader AA, Vainoras A, Ragulskis M (2017) Synchronization of human autonomic nervous system rhythms with geomagnetic activity in human subjects. Int J Environ Res Public Health 14(7). https://doi.org/10.3390/ijerph14070770

McCulloch WS, Pitts W (1943) A logical calculus of the ideas immanent in nervous activity. Bull Math Biophys 5(4):115–133. https://doi.org/10.1007/BF02478259

McDaniel LV (1968) Programmed instruction for aides in physical therapy. Final report. https://eric.ed.gov/?id=ED029110

McDonnell MD, Stocks NG, Pearce CEM, Abbott D (2008) Stochastic resonance: from suprathreshold stochastic resonance to stochastic signal quantization. Cambridge University Press. https://doi.org/10.1017/CBO9780511535239

McKay B, Corson AE, Seedu J, De Faveri CS, Hasan H, Arnold K, Adams FC, Carter MJ (2024) Reporting bias, not external focus: a robust Bayesian meta-analysis and systematic review of the external focus of attention literature. Psychol Bull 150(11):1347–1362. https://doi.org/10.1037/bul0000451

Mechling H, Roth K (1992) Movement theory: motor behavior. In: Haag H, Grupe O, Kirsch A (eds) Sport science in Germany: an interdisciplinary anthology. Springer, Berlin/Heidelberg, pp 201–222. https://doi.org/10.1007/978-3-642-77630-4_10

Mechsner F, Kerzel D, Knoblich G, Prinz W (2001) Perceptual basis of bimanual coordination. Nature 414(6859):69–73. https://doi.org/10.1038/35102060

Mechsner F, Knoblich G, Mechsner F (2004) Do muscles matter for coordinated action? J Exp Psychol Hum Percept Perform 30(3):490–503. https://doi.org/10.1037/0096-1523.30.3.490

Meijer OG, Roth K (1988) Complex movement behaviour: 'the' motor-action controversy. Elsevier

Meinel K (1960) Bewegungslehre. Volk und Wissen. Volkseigener Verlag

Mendoza L (1993) Biomechanisch gestützte Techniksteuerung im Hochleistungssport. Sportbuch Strauß

Mendoza L, Schöllhorn WI (1990) Technical training in the field of high performance athletes with a biomechanical feedback system. In: Brüggemann GP, Rühl JK (eds) Techniques in athletics. Sport Buch Strauß, pp 412–419

Mendoza L, Schöllhorn W (1993) Training of the sprint start technique with biomechanical feedback. J Sports Sci 11(1):25–29. https://doi.org/10.1080/02640419308729959

Merzenich MM, Nelson RJ, Stryker MP, Cynader MS, Schoppmann A, Zook JM (1984) Somatosensory cortical map changes following digit amputation in adult monkeys. J Comp Neurol 224(4):591–605. https://doi.org/10.1002/cne.902240408

Merzenich M, Wright B, Jenkins W, Xerri C, Byl N, Miller S, Tallal P (1996) Cortical plasticity underlying perceptual, motor, and cognitive skill development: implications for neurorehabilitation. Cold Spring Harb Symp Quant Biol 61:1–8. https://doi.org/10.1101/SQB.1996.061.01.003

Michaels, C. F., & Carello, C. (1981). Direct Perception. Englewoodcliffs, NJ: Printicehall.

Miglino O, Lund HH, Nolfi S (1995) Evolving mobile robots in simulated and real environments. Artif Life 2(4):417–434. https://doi.org/10.1162/artl.1995.2.4.417

Milanese C, Facci G, Cesari P, Zancanaro C (2008) "Amplification of error": a rapidly effective method for motor performance improvement. Sport Psychol 22(2):164–174. https://doi.org/10.1123/tsp.22.2.164

Milanese C, Corte S, Salvetti L, Cavedon V, Agostini T (2016) Correction of a technical error in the golf swing: error amplification versus direct instruction. J Mot Behav 48(4):365–376. https://doi.org/10.1080/00222895.2015.1102699

Miller GA (1956) The magical number seven, plus or minus two: some limits on our capacity for processing information. Psychol Rev 63(2):81–97. https://doi.org/10.1037/h0043158

Miller GA, Bruner JS, Postman L (1954) Familiarity of letter sequences and tachistoscopic identification. J Gen Psychol 50(1):129–139. https://doi.org/10.1080/00221309.1954.9710109

Miller GA, Galanter E, Pribram KH (1960) Plans and the structure of behavior. Henry Holt. https://doi.org/10.1037/10039-000

Milsum JH (1966) Biological control systems analysis. McGraw-Hill

Mitaim S, Kosko B (1998) Adaptive stochastic resonance. Proc IEEE 86(11):2152–2183. https://doi.org/10.1109/5.726785

Möhler F, Fadillioglu C, Stein T (2021) Fatigue-related changes in spatiotemporal parameters, joint kinematics and leg stiffness in expert runners during a middle-distance run. Front Sports Act Living 3:634258. https://doi.org/10.3389/fspor.2021.634258

Mörike KB, Mergenthaler E, W. (1991) Biologie des Menschen. Quelle & Meyer

Mosston M (1966) Teaching physical education: from command to discovery. C. E. Merrill Books

Mountcastle VB, Poggio GF, Werner G (1963) The relation of thalamic cell response to peripheral stimuli varied over an intensive continuum. J Neurophysiol 26:807–834. https://doi.org/10.1152/jn.1963.26.5.807

Müller H, Sternad D (2003) A randomization method for the calculation of covariation in multiple nonlinear relations: illustrated with the example of goal-directed movements. Biol Cybern 89(1):22–33. https://doi.org/10.1007/s00422-003-0399-5

Naber M, Frässle S, Einhäuser W (2011) Perceptual rivalry: reflexes reveal the gradual nature of visual awareness. PLoS One 6(6):e20910. https://doi.org/10.1371/journal.pone.0020910

Nelson WL (1983) Physical principles for economies of skilled movements. Biol Cybern 46(2):135–147. https://doi.org/10.1007/bf00339982

Neuman MC, Singer RN (1968) A comparison of traditional versus programed methods of learning tennis. Res Q 39(4):1044–1048

Newell ARP (1981) Mechanisms of skill acquisition and the law of practice. In: Anderson JR (ed) Cognitive skills and their acquisition. Hillsdale, pp 1–55

Newell KM (1986) Constraints on the development of coordination. In: Wade MG, Whiting HTA (eds) Motor development in children: aspects of coordination and control. Martinus Nijhoff, pp 341–360

Newell KM, Corcos DM (1993) Variability and motor control. Human Kinetics

Newell KM, Molenaar PCM (1998) Applications of nonlinear dynamics to developmental process modeling. Lawrence Erlbaum Associates

Newell KM, Rovegno I (2021) Teaching children's motor skills for team games through guided discovery: how constraints enhance learning. Front Psychol 12:724848. https://doi.org/10.3389/fpsyg.2021.724848

Newell KM, Kugler PN, Van Emmerik REA, McDonald PV (1989) Search strategies and the acquisition of coordination. In: Wallace SA (ed) Advances in psychology, vol 61. North-Holland, pp 85–122. https://doi.org/10.1016/S0166-4115(08)60019-9

Newell KM, Liu YT, Mayer-Kress G (2001) Time scales in motor learning and development. Psychol Rev 108(1):57–82. https://doi.org/10.1037/0033-295x.108.1.57

Nitsch JR, Hackfort D (2016) Chapter 2 – theoretical framework of performance psychology: an action theory perspective. In: Raab M, Lobinger B, Hoffmann S, Pizzera A, Laborde S (eds) Performance psychology. Academic Press, pp 11–29. https://doi.org/10.1016/B978-0-12-803377-7.00002-8

Nocks L (2007) The robot: the life story of a technology. Bloomsbury Academic

Nudo RJ (2006) Plasticity. NeuroRx 3(4):420–427. https://doi.org/10.1016/j.nurx.2006.07.006

Nudo RJ, Plautz EJ, Frost SB (2001) Role of adaptive plasticity in recovery of function after damage to motor cortex. Muscle Nerve 24(8):1000–1019. https://doi.org/10.1002/mus.1104

Oberauer K (2009) Design for a working memory. In: The psychology of learning and motivation, vol 51. Elsevier Academic Press, pp 45–100. https://doi.org/10.1016/S0079-7421(09)51002-X

Oftadeh S, Bahram A, Yaali R, Ghadiri F, Schöllhorn WI (2021) External focus or differential learning: is there an additive effect on learning a futsal goal kick? Int J Environ Res Public Health 19(1). https://doi.org/10.3390/ijerph19010317

Oliver M (2005) The problem with affordance. E-Learning and Digital Media 2(4):402–413. https://doi.org/10.2304/elea.2005.2.4.402

Ollis S, Button C, Fairweather M (2005) The influence of professional expertise and task complexity upon the potency of the contextual interference effect. Acta Psychol 118(3):229–244. https://doi.org/10.1016/j.actpsy.2004.08.003

Oppici L, Dix A, Narciss S (2024) When is knowledge of performance (KP) superior to knowledge of results (KR) in promoting motor skill learning? A systematic review. Int Rev Sport Exerc Psychol 17(1):182–207. https://doi.org/10.1080/1750984X.2021.1986849

Osgood CE (1949) The similarity paradox in human learning: a resolution. Psychol Rev 56(3):132–143. https://doi.org/10.1037/h0057488

Palyulin VV, Chechkin AV, Metzler R (2014) Lévy flights do not always optimize random blind search for sparse targets. Proc Natl Acad Sci 111(8):2931–2936. https://doi.org/10.1073/pnas.1320424111

Paschen K (1961) Didaktik der Leisbeserziehung, 1st edn. Wilhelm Limpert Verlag

Pask G (1975) Cybernetic theory of cognition and learning. Journal of Cybernetics 5(1):1–90. https://doi.org/10.1080/01969727508546082

Pask G (1992) Introduction different kinds of cybernetics. In: van de Vijver G (ed) New perspectives on cybernetics: self-organization, autonomy and connectionism. Springer, Dordrecht, pp 11–31. https://doi.org/10.1007/978-94-015-8062-5_1

Pavlyukevich I (2007) Lévy flights, non-local search and simulated annealing. J Comput Phys 226(2):1830–1844. https://doi.org/10.1016/j.jcp.2007.06.008

Peirce CS (1991) On the nature of signs. In: Hoopes J (ed) Peirce on signs. University of North Carolina Press, pp 141–143. http://www.jstor.org/stable/10.5149/9781469616810_hoopes.12

Penman KA (1968) Physical education for college students: programed instruction, 2nd edn. Mosby
Pestalozzi JH (1781–1787) Lienhard und Gertrud. Ein Buch für das Volk, vol. 1–4. Georg Jakob Decker
Phan KL, Wager T, Taylor SF, Liberzon I (2002) Functional neuroanatomy of emotion: a meta-analysis of emotion activation studies in PET and fMRI. NeuroImage 16(2):331–348. https://doi.org/10.1006/nimg.2002.1087
Phan KL, Taylor SF, Welsh RC, Decker LR, Noll DC, Nichols TE, Britton JC, Liberzon I (2003) Activation of the medial prefrontal cortex and extended amygdala by individual ratings of emotional arousal: a fMRI study. Biol Psychiatry 53(3):211–215. https://doi.org/10.1016/s0006-3223(02)01485-3
Pin-Barre C, Laurin J (2015) Physical exercise as a diagnostic, rehabilitation, and preventive tool: influence on neuroplasticity and motor recovery after stroke. Neural Plast 2015(1):608581. https://doi.org/10.1155/2015/608581
Polak P, Shefi O (2015) Nanometric agents in the service of neuroscience: manipulation of neuronal growth and activity using nanoparticles. Nanomedicine 11(6):1467–1479. https://doi.org/10.1016/j.nano.2015.03.005
Popper K (1935) Logik der Forschung. Springer
Porter JM, Magill RA (2010) Systematically increasing contextual interference is beneficial for learning sport skills. J Sports Sci 28(12):1277–1285. https://doi.org/10.1080/02640414.2010.502946
Prigogine I, Nicolis G (1971) Biological order, structure and instabilities. Q Rev Biophys 4(2):107–148. https://doi.org/10.1017/s0033583500000615
Prinz W (1990) A common coding approach to perception and action. In: Neumann O, Prinz W (eds) Relationships between perception and action: current approaches. Springer, Berlin/Heidelberg, pp 167–201. https://doi.org/10.1007/978-3-642-75348-0_7
Prinz W (1997) Perception and action planning. Eur J Cogn Psychol 9(2):129–154. https://doi.org/10.1080/713752551
Proctor RW, Miles JD (2014) Chapter six – does the concept of affordance add anything to explanations of stimulus–response compatibility effects? In: Ross BH (ed) Psychology of learning and motivation, vol 60. Academic Press, pp 227–266. https://doi.org/10.1016/B978-0-12-800090-8.00006-8
Prokopenko M (2013) Guided self-organization: inception. Springer, Berlin/Heidelberg
Quartz SR, Sejnowski TJ (1997) The neural basis of cognitive development: a constructivist manifesto. Behav Brain Sci 20(4):537–556; discussion 556–596. https://doi.org/10.1017/s0140525x97001581
Ramírez-Ruiz J, Grotsky D, Maestro Giuseppe C. et al. (2024) Complex behavior from intrinsic motivation to occupy future action-state path space. Nat Commun 15:6368. https://doi.org/10.1038/s41467-024-49711-1
Ranatunga KW, Sharpe B, Turnbull B (1987) Contractions of a human skeletal muscle at different temperatures. J Physiol 390:383–395. https://doi.org/10.1113/jphysiol.1987.sp016707
Rapoport A (1966) A study of a multistage decision making task with an unknown duration. Hum Factors 8(1):54–61. https://doi.org/10.1177/001872086600800106.
Rayleigh L (1916) LIX. On convection currents in a horizontal layer of fluid, when the higher temperature is on the under side. Philos Mag Ser 1(32):529–546
Reeve J, Lee W (2019) A neuroscientific perspective on basic psychological needs. J Pers 87(1):102–114. https://doi.org/10.1111/jopy.12390
Riley MA, Turvey MT (2002) Variability and determinism in motor behavior. J Mot Behav 34(2):99–125. https://doi.org/10.1080/00222890209601934
Ritter H, Martinetz T, Schulten K (1992) Neural computation and self-organizing maps; an introduction. Addison-Wesley Longman
Rizzolatti G, Fadiga L, Gallese V, Fogassi L (1996) Premotor cortex and the recognition of motor actions. Cogn Brain Res 3(2):131–141. https://doi.org/10.1016/0926-6410(95)00038-0
Rockmann-Rüger U (1991) Zur Gestaltung von Übungsprozessen von Bewegungstechniken. Harry Deutsch
Roland PE (1981) Somatotopical tuning of postcentral gyrus during focal attention in man. A regional cerebral blood flow study. J Neurophysiol 46(4):744–754. https://doi.org/10.1152/jn.1981.46.4.744
Roland PE, Larsen B, Lassen NA, Skinhøj E (1980) Supplementary motor area and other cortical areas in organization of voluntary movements in man. J Neurophysiol 43(1):118–136. https://doi.org/10.1152/jn.1980.43.1.118
Rosen R (1988) Similarity and dissimilarity: a partial overview. Hum Mov Sci 7(2):131–153. https://doi.org/10.1016/0167-9457(88)90010-3
Rosenbaum DA (1991) Human motor control. Academic Press
Rosenbaum DA (1998) Is dynamical systems modeling just curve fitting? Mot Control 2(2):101–104. https://doi.org/10.1123/mcj.2.2.101
Rosenblatt F (1958) The perceptron: a probabilistic model for information storage and organization in the brain. Psychol Rev 65(6):386–408. https://doi.org/10.1037/h0042519
Roth G (1991) Neuronale Grundlagen des Lernens und des Gedächtnisses. In: Schmidt SJ (ed) Gedächtnis. Suhrkamp, pp 127–158
Rousseau JJ (1762) Emile, Ou De L' Education. Menard Et Desenne, Fils, Paris
Rubinstein S (1968) Grundlagen der allgemeinen Psychologie: Volk und Wissen. Volkseigener Verlag
Ruhenstroth-Bauer G, Günther W, Hantschk I, Klages U, Kugler J, Peters J (1993) Influence of the earth's magnetic field on resting and activated EEG mapping in normal subjects. Int J Neurosci 73(3–4):195–201. https://doi.org/10.3109/00207459308986669

Rumelhart DE, Hinton GE, Williams RJ (1986) Learning representations by back-propagating errors. Nature 323(6088):533–536. https://doi.org/10.1038/323533a0

Russell CT (2000) The solar wind interaction with the Earth's magnetosphere: a tutorial. IEEE Trans Plasma Sci 28(6):1818–1830. https://doi.org/10.1109/27.902211

Rutschky K (ed) (1977) Schwarze Pädagogik. Quellen zur Naturgeschichte der bürgerlichen Erziehung. Ullstein.

Saladin KS (2011) Human anatomy. McGraw-Hill

Salmoni AW, Schmidt RA, Walter CB (1984) Knowledge of results and motor learning: a review and critical reappraisal. Psychol Bull 95(3):355–386. https://doi.org/10.1037/0033-2909.95.3.355.

Scemma A (2020) Il Profe che insegnava a sabagliare. Fuorionda

Schmidt, R. F. (1972). Propriozeptoren in Muskeln und Sehnen. In Gauer KJOH Kramer, R. (Ed.), Physiologie des Menschen – Somatische Sensibilität, Geruch und Geschmack (11, pp. 157–169). Urban Schwarzenberger.

Schmidt RA (1975) A schema theory of discrete motor skill learning. Psychol Rev 82:225–260. https://doi.org/10.1037/h0076770.

Schmidt RF (1985) In: Schmidt RF (ed) Grundriß der Sinnesphysiologie. Springer

Schmidt RF (1987) Physiologie des Menschen, 23rd edn. Springer

Schmidt RA (1988) Chapter 1 motor and action perspectives on motor behaviour. In: Meijer OG, Roth K (eds) Advances in psychology, vol 50. North-Holland, pp 3–44. https://doi.org/10.1016/S0166-4115(08)62551-0

Schmidt S (1992) Die Selbstorganisation des Sozialsystems Literatur im 18. Jahrhundert. Suhrkamp.

Schmidt RA (2003) Motor schema theory after 27 years: reflections and implications for a new theory. Res Q Exerc Sport 74(4):366–375. https://doi.org/10.1080/02701367.2003.10609106

Schmidt RA, Bjork RA (1992) New conceptualizations of practice: common principles in three paradigms suggest new concepts for training. Psychol Sci 3(4):207–218. https://doi.org/10.1111/j.1467-9280.1992.tb00029.x

Schneider K, Zernicke RF (1989) Jerk-cost modulations during the practice of rapid arm movements. Biol Cybern 60(3):221–230. https://doi.org/10.1007/bf00207290

Schneider K, Zernicke RF, Schmidt RA, Hart TJ (1989) Changes in limb dynamics during the practice of rapid arm movements. J Biomech 22(8):805–817. https://doi.org/10.1016/0021-9290(89)90064-X

Schöllhorn WI (1993a) Biomechanische Einzelfallanalyse im Diskuswurf. Prozess- und produktorientierte Technikanalyse mechanischer Energieformen, vol. 19. Harri Deutsch Verlag.

Schöllhorn WI (1993b) Process-oriented analysis of movement patterns. In: XIVth Congress of International Society of Biomechanics, Paris.

Schöllhorn WI (1995) Time course oriented analysis of biomechanical movement patterns by means of orthogonal reference functions. In: XVth congress of the international society of biomechanics, Jväskylä

Schöllhorn WI (1997) Komplexe Bewegungskoordination systemdynamisch betrachtet (Complex movement coordination from a system dynamic perspective). In Hirtz P, NSF (eds) Bewegungskoordination und sportliche Leistung integrativ betrachtet – 2. Bernstein-Konferenz. Czwalina, pp. 66–75

Schöllhorn WI (1998) Systemdynamische Betrachtung komplexer Bewegungsmuster im Lernprozeß: Prozeßorientierte Strukturierung der Entwicklung eines Bewegungsablaufs (Dynamic system approach for the learning process of complex movement patterns). Peter Lang GmbH

Schöllhorn WI (1999a) Holistic versus elementaristic movement pattern recognition by means of artificial neural nets. In: II International motor control conference August 19–22, 1999, State College, Pennsylvania.

Schöllhorn WI (1999b) Individualität – ein vernachlässigter Parameter. Leistungssport 29(2):5–12

Schöllhorn WI (1999c) Pracitcal consequences of biomechanically determined individuality and fluctuations on motor learning. In: XVIIth Congress of the International Society of Biomchanics, Calgary, Canada.

Schöllhorn WI (2000) Applications of system dynamic principles to technique and strength training. Acta Academiae Qlympiquae Estoniae 8:67–85

Schöllhorn WI (2003) Coordination dynamics and its consequences on sports. Int J Comput Sci Sport 2(2):40–46

Schöllhorn WI (2005) Differenzielles Lehren und Lernen von Bewegung – Durch veränderte Annahmen zu neuen Konsequenzen. In: Gabler H, Göhner U, Schiebl F (eds) Zur Vernetzung von Forschung und Lehre in der Biomechanik, Sportmotorik und Trainingswissenschaft. DVS Symposium Tübingen 2004. Czwalina

Schöllhorn WI (2016) Invited commentary: differential learning is different from contextual interference learning. Hum Mov Sci 47:240–245. https://doi.org/10.1016/j.humov.2015.11.018

Schöllhorn WI, Bauer HU (1997) Linear versus nonlinear classification of complex time course patterns. In: 2nd Conference of European College of Sport Science, Copenhagen

Schöllhorn WI, Bauer H-U (1998a) Assessment of running patterns using neural networks. In: Mester J, Perl J (eds) Sport und Informatik. Sport Buch Strauss, pp 169–176

Schöllhorn WI, Bauer HU (1998b) Identifying individual movement styles in high performance sports by means of self- organizing Kohonen maps. In: 16 International symposium on biomechanics in sports. Konstanz. https://ojs.ub.uni-konstanz.de/cpa/article/view/1556

Schöllhorn WI, Bauer HU (1998c) Erkennung von individuellen Laufmustern mit Hilfe von neuronalen Netzen Informatik im Sport. Computer Science in Sport. Bericht ueber das Internationale Symposium vom 12.-14. Juni 1997 in Koeln, Cologne. https://www.bisp--surf.de/Record/PU199809304244

Schöllhorn WI, Stefanyshyn D, Nigg BM, Liu W (1999) Recognition of individual walking patterns by means of artificial neural nets. Gait Posture 9:1

Schöllhorn WI, Müller E, Lindinger S, Raschner C, Schwameder H (2001a) Individuality and generality in ski turning techniques. In: Müller E, Schwameder H, Raschner C, Lindinger S, Kornexl E (eds) Second international congress on science and skiing II. Dr. Kovac, pp 69–83

Schöllhorn WI, Röber F, Jaitner T, Hellstern W, Käubler W (2001b). Discrete and continuous effects of traditional and differential sprint training. In: 6th Annual Congress of the European College of Sport Science: perspectives and profiles Cologne. https://www.ecss.mobi/DATA/EDSS/C06/06-0311.pdf

Schöllhorn WI, Nigg BM, Stefanyshyn DJ, Liu W (2002) Identification of individual walking patterns using time discrete and time continuous data sets. Gait Posture 15(2):180–186. https://doi.org/10.1016/s0966-6362(01)00193-x

Schöllhorn WI, Beckmann H, Michelbrink M, Sechelmann M, Trockel M, Davids K (2006) Does noise provide a basis for the unification of motor learning theories? Int J Sport Psychol 37(2–3):186–206

Schöllhorn WI, Mayer-Kress G, Newell KM, Michelbrink M (2009) Time scales of adaptive behavior and motor learning in the presence of stochastic perturbations. Hum Mov Sci 28(3):319–333. https://doi.org/10.1016/j.humov.2008.10.005

Schöllhorn WI, Henz D, Horst F (2017) Differenzielles Lernen als Turbo für Körper und Gehirn. Teil 1: Eine Zwischenbilanz. Leistungssport 47(1):6

Schöllhorn WI, Rizzi N, Slapšinskaitė-Dackevičienė A, Leite N (2022) Always pay attention to which model of motor learning you are using. Int J Environ Res Public Health 19(2). https://doi.org/10.3390/ijerph19020711

Scholz JP, Kelso JAS, Schöner G (1987) Nonequilibrium phase transitions in coordinated biological motion: critical slowing down and switching time. Phys Lett A 123(8):390–394. https://doi.org/10.1016/0375-9601(87)90038-7

Schöner G (1989) Learning and recall in a dynamic theory of coordination patterns. Biol Cybern 62(1):39–54. https://doi.org/10.1007/bf00217659

Schöner G (1990) A dynamic theory of coordination of discrete movement. Biol Cybern 63(4):257–270. https://doi.org/10.1007/bf00203449

Schöner G, Kelso JA (1988a) A synergetic theory of environmentally-specified and learned patterns of movement coordination. I. Relative phase dynamics. Biol Cybern 58(2):71–80. https://doi.org/10.1007/bf00364153

Schöner G, Kelso JAS (1988b) A dynamic pattern theory of behavioral change. J Theor Biol 135(4):501–524. https://doi.org/10.1016/S0022-5193(88)80273-X

Schöner G, Haken H, Kelso JA (1986) A stochastic theory of phase transitions in human hand movement. Biol Cybern 53(4):247–257. https://doi.org/10.1007/bf00336995

Schöner G, Jiang WY, Kelso JA (1990) A synergetic theory of quadrupedal gaits and gait transitions. J Theor Biol 142(3):359–391. https://doi.org/10.1016/s0022-5193(05)80558-2

Schöner G, Zanone PG, Kelso JA (1992) Learning as change of coordination dynamics: theory and experiment. J Mot Behav 24(1):29–48. https://doi.org/10.1080/00222895.1992.9941599

Schönherr T, Schöllhorn WI (2003). Differential learning in basketball. In: Schöllhorn WI, Bohn C, Jäger JM, Schaper A, Alichmann M (eds) European workshop on movement science. Book of Abstracts (pp. 58 f.). Köln: Sport & Buch Strauß

Schorer J, Baker J, Fath F, Jaitner T (2007) Identification of interindividual and intraindividual movement patterns in handball players of varying expertise levels. J Mot Behav 39(5):409–421. https://doi.org/10.3200/jmbr.39.5.409-422

Schreiner CE, Read HL, Sutter ML (2000) Modular organization of frequency integration in primary auditory cortex. Annu Rev Neurosci 23:501–529. https://doi.org/10.1146/annurev.neuro.23.1.501

Schwartz AB, Kettner RE, Georgopoulos AP (1988) Primate motor cortex and free arm movements to visual targets in three-dimensional space. I. Relations between single cell discharge and direction of movement. J Neurosci 8(8):2913–2927. https://doi.org/10.1523/jneurosci.08-08-02913.1988

Schütz-Bosbach S, Prinz W (2007) Perceptual resonance: action-induced modulation of perception. Trends Cogn Sci 11(8):349–55. https://doi.org/10.1016/j.tics.2007.06.005

Severinsen MCK, Pedersen BK (2020) Muscle-organ crosstalk: the emerging roles of myokines. Endocr Rev 41(4):594–609. https://doi.org/10.1210/endrev/bnaa016

Shanahan LK, Gottfried JA (2014) Olfactory insights into sleep-dependent learning and memory. Prog Brain Res 208:309–343. https://doi.org/10.1016/b978-0-444-63350-7.00012-7

Shannon CE, Weaver W (1949) The mathematical theory of communication. University of Illinois Press

Sharma V, Estes Z (2024) Seeing is smelling: pictures improve product evaluations by evoking olfactory imagery. Int J Res Mark 41(2):282–307. https://doi.org/10.1016/j.ijresmar.2024.02.001

Shaw RE, Kinsella-Shaw JM, Mace WM (2019) Affordance types and affordance tokens: are Gibson's affordances trustworthy?†. Ecol Psychol 31(1):49–75. https://doi.org/10.1080/10407413.2018.1508353

Shea JB, Morgan RL (1979) Contextual interference effects on the acquisition, retention, and transfer of a motor skill. J Exp Psychol Hum Learn Mem 5(2):179–187. https://doi.org/10.1037/0278-7393.5.2.179
Shea C, Zimny ST (1983) Context effects in memory and learning moivement information. In: Magill RA (ed) Memory and control of action. North Holland, pp 345–366
Shen L, Hu X, Yacoub E, Ugurbil K (1999) Neural correlates of visual form and visual spatial processing. Hum Brain Mapp 8(1):60–71. https://doi.org/10.1002/(SICI)1097-0193(1999)8:1%3C60::AID--HBM5%3E3.0.CO;2-6
Silbernagl SDA (1979) Taschenatlas der Physiologie. Thieme
Silverman S, Tyson L, Krampitz J (1992) Teacher feedback and achievement in physical education: interaction with student practice. Teach Teach Educ 8(4):333–344. https://doi.org/10.1016/0742-051X(92)90060-G
Simon HA (1962) The architecture of complexity. Proc Am Philos Soc 106(6) https://www.jstor.org/stable/985254
Simon B (1999) Why no pedagogy in England? In: Leach J, Moon B (eds) Learners & pedagogy. Sage, pp 34–45
Simon JR, Rudell AP (1967) Auditory S-R compatibility: the effect of an irrelevant cue on information processing. J Appl Psychol 51(3):300–304. https://doi.org/10.1037/h0020586
Singer W (1988) Pattern recognition and self-organization in biological systems. In: Marko HH, Struppler GA (eds) Processing structures for perception and action. Final report of the Sonderforschungsbereich "Kybernetik" 1969–1983. VCH, pp 11–18
Singer W (1989) The brain, a self-organizing learning system. In: Klivington KA (ed) The science of mind. MIT Press, pp 174–179
Singer W (1991a) Die Entwicklung kognitiver Strukturen-ein selbstreferentieller Lernprozeß. In: Schmidt SJ (ed) Gedächtnis—Probleme und Perspektiven der interdisziplinären Gedächtnisforschung. Suhrkamp, pp 96–125
Singer W (1991b) Zur Selbstorganisation kognitiver Strukturen. In: Pöppel E (ed) Gehirn und Bewußtsein. VCH-Verlagsgesellschaft, pp 45–59
Singh H, Wulf G (2022) Mind over body: creating an external focus for sport skills. Eur J Sport Sci 22(4):610–616. https://doi.org/10.1080/17461391.2021.1887367
Skyttner L (1996) General systems theory: an introduction. Macmillan Press
Slifkin AB, Newell KM (1999) Noise, information transmission, and force variability. J Exp Psychol Hum Percept Perform 25(3):837–851. https://doi.org/10.1037/0096-1523.25.3.837
Slifkin AB, Newell KM (2000) Variability and noise in continuous force production. J Mot Behav 32(2):141–150. https://doi.org/10.1080/00222890009601366
Smeeton NJ, Ward P, Williams AM (2004) Do pattern recognition skills transfer across sports? A preliminary analysis. J Sports Sci 22(2):205–213. https://doi.org/10.1080/02640410310001641494
Smirnov AA (1973) Conditions for retroactive inhibition. In: Problems of the psychology of memory. Springer, pp 279–298. https://doi.org/10.1007/978-1-4684-1968-9_10
Smith AW (1974) Information theory and cybernetics. J Cybernetics 4(3):1–5. https://doi.org/10.1080/01969727408621678
Smith PJ, Taylor SJ, Withers K (1997) Applying bandwidth feedback scheduling to a golf shot. Res Q Exerc Sport 68(3):215–221. https://doi.org/10.1080/02701367.1997.10608000
Smuts JC (1926) Holism and evolution. Macmillan
Snoddy GS (1926) Learning and stability: a psychophysiological analysis of a case of motor learning with clinical applications. J Appl Psychol 10(1):1–36. https://doi.org/10.1037/h0075814
Snoswell CL, North JB, Caffery LJ (2020) Economic advantages of telehealth and virtual health practitioners: return on investment analysis. JMIR Perioper Med 3(1):e15688. https://doi.org/10.2196/15688
Sokal AD (2000) The Sokal Hoax: the sham that shook the academy. University of Nebraska Press
Sokal AD, Bricmont J (1999) Fashionable nonsense: postmodern intellectuals' abuse of science. St Martins Press (NY)
Sontag ED, Sussmann HJ (1989) Backpropagation can give rise to spurious local minima even for networks without hidden layers. Complex Syst 3(1) http://www.complex-systems.com/abstracts/v03_i01_a07.html
Spearman C (1904) 'General intelligence,' objectively determined and measured. Am J Psychol 15(2):201–293. https://doi.org/10.2307/1412107
Stachowiak H (1973) Allgemeine Modell theorie (General model theory). Springer
Stam J, Speelman HD, van Crevel H (1989) Tendon reflex asymmetry by voluntary mental effort in healthy subjects. Arch Neurol 46(1):70–73. https://doi.org/10.1001/archneur.1989.00520370072022
Stergiou N (2004) Innovative analyses of human movement. Human Kinetics
Stergiou N, Decker LM (2011) Human movement variability, nonlinear dynamics, and pathology: is there a connection? Hum Mov Sci 30(5):869–888. https://doi.org/10.1016/j.humov.2011.06.002
Stevens SS (1970) Neural events and the psychophysical law. Science 170(3962):1043–1050. https://doi.org/10.1126/science.170.3962.1043
Strogatz S (1994) Nonlinear dynamics and chaos: With applications to physics, biology, chemistry and engineering perseus. Boca Raton. https://doi.org/10.1201/9780429492563
Stroop JR (1935) Studies of interference in serial verbal reactions. J Exp Psychol 18(6):643–662. https://doi.org/10.1037/h0054651
Suppes P (1992) Estes' statistical learning theory: past, present, and future. In: Healy AFK, Shiffrin SMRM (eds) From learning theory to connectionist theory,

vol 1, 1st edn. Psychology Press, p 20. https://doi.org/10.4324/9780203763162
Tackett JL, Brandes CM, King KM, Markon KE (2019) Psychology's replication crisis and clinical psychological science. Annu Rev Clin Psychol 15:579–604. https://doi.org/10.1146/annurev-clinpsy-050718-095710
Tani G, Corrêa UC, Basso L, Benda RN, Ugrinowitsch H, Choshi K (2014) An adaptive process model of motor learning: insights for the teaching of motor skills. Nonlinear Dynamics Psychol Life Sci 18(1):47–65
Taylor E (2015) An explication of emergence. Philos Stud 172(3):653–669. http://www.jstor.org/stable/24704091
Ten Bruggencate G (1980) Allgemeine Sinnesphysiologie. In: Gauer OHK, Jung K, R. (eds) Physiologie des Menschen – Allgemeine Neurophysiologie, vol 10. Urban & Schwarzenberger
Ten Bruggencate G (1984) Medizinische Neurophysiologie. Thieme
Thelen E, Smith LB (1994) A dynamic systems approach to the development of cognition and action. MIT
Thelen E, Corbetta D, Kamm K, Spencer JP, Schneider K, Zernicke RF (1993) The transition to reaching: mapping intention and intrinsic dynamics. Child Dev 64(4):1058–1098
Thompson RF (1990) Das Gehirn. Spektrum der Wissenschaft.
Thurstone, LL (1919) Psychological monographs 26(3): i–51. https://doi.org/10.1037/h0093187.
Tolman EC (1956) Egon Brunswik: 1903-1955. Am J Psychol 69(2):315–324. http://www.jstor.org/stable/1418173
Tolman EC, Brunswik E (1935) The organism and the causal texture of the environment. Psychol Rev 42(1):43–77. https://doi.org/10.1037/h0062156
Tranquillo J (2019) An introduction to complex systems: making sense of a changing world. Springer
Tring E, Dipoppa M, Ringach DL (2023) A power law describes the magnitude of adaptation in neural populations of primary visual cortex. Nat Commun 14(1):8366. https://doi.org/10.1038/s41467-023-43572-w
Trockel MSWI (2003) Differential learning of the goal kick in soccer. In: Mechanics, physiology, psychology. First European workshop on Movement Science, Münster, Germany.
Turvey MT (1996) Dynamic touch. American Psychologist 51(11):1134–52. https://doi.org/10.1037/0003-066X.51.11.1134.
Tudge J, Gray JT, Hogan DM (1996) Ecological perspectives in human development: a comparison of Gibson and Bronfenbrenner. In: Tudge J, Shanahan MJ, Valsiner J (eds) Comparisons in human development: understanding time and context. Cambridge University Press, pp 72–106. https://doi.org/10.1017/CBO9780511720345.004
Tuller B, Kelso JAS (1989) Phase transitions in speech production and their perceptual consequences. Attent Perform XIII
Ullman S (1980) Against direct perception. Behav Brain Sci 3(3):333–381. https://doi.org/10.1017/S0140525X0000546X.
Ungerer D (1971) Zur Theorie des sensomotorischen Lernens. K. Hofmann
van Dieën JH, Luger T, van der Eb J (2012) Effects of fatigue on trunk stability in elite gymnasts. Eur J Appl Physiol 112(4):1307–1313. https://doi.org/10.1007/s00421-011-2082-1
van Emmerik REA, den Brinker BPLM, Vereijken B, Whiting HTA (1989) Preferred tempo in the learning of a gross cyclical action. Q J Exp Psychol 41(2):251–262. https://doi.org/10.1080/14640748908402364
Vargas EA, Vargas JS (1991) Programmed instruction: what it is and how to do it. J Behav Educ 1(2):235–251. http://www.jstor.org/stable/41826789
Vehof K, Janssen D, Schöllhorn WI (2009) Handwriting acquisition in primary school by means of the differential learning approach. In: 3rd European workshop on movement science, Lisbon.
Vereijken B, Whiting HT (1990) In defence of discovery learning. Can J Sport Sci 15(2):99–106
Vereijken B, Emmerik REAV, Whiting HTA, Newell KM (1992a) Free(z)ing degrees of freedom in skill acquisition. J Mot Behav 24(1):133–142. https://doi.org/10.1080/00222895.1992.9941608
Vereijken B, Whiting HT, Beek WJ (1992b) A dynamical systems approach to skill acquisition. Q J Exp Psychol 45(2):323–344. https://doi.org/10.1080/14640749208401329
Virchow F (2006) Militär und Sport: Symbiotische Beziehungen um Nation, Leistung und Disziplin. In: Tanja T, Fabian V (eds) Banal militarism. Transcript Verlag, pp 203–222. https://doi.org/10.1515/9783839403563-011
Vitiello G (2014) On the isomorphism between dissipative systems, fractal self-similarity and electrodynamics. Toward an integrated vision of nature. Systems 2(2):203–216. https://www.mdpi.com/2079-8954/2/2/203
Viviani P, Flash T (1995) Minimum-jerk, two-thirds power law, and isochrony: converging approaches to movement planning. J Exp Psychol Hum Percept Perform 21(1):32–53. https://doi.org/10.1037/0096-1523.21.1.32
Voigt R (1933) Über den Aufbau von Bewegungsgestalten. Neue Psychologische Studien 9:1–32
von Bekesy G (1970) Physiologie der Sinneshemmung. Goldmann
von Bertalanffy L (1935) Grundzüge einer allgemeinen Biologie. Erkenntnis 5(1):368–369. https://doi.org/10.1007/BF00172328
Von Bertalanffy L (1950) The theory of open systems in physics and biology. Science 111(2872):23–29. http://www.jstor.org/stable/1676073

Von Bertalanffy L (1951a) General system theory; a new approach to unity of science. 1. Problems of general system theory. Hum Biol 23(4):302–312
Von Bertalanffy L (1951b) Problems of general system theory. Hum Biol 23(4):302–312. http://www.jstor.org/stable/41448003
Von Bertalanffy L (1951c) Towards a physical theory of organic teleology: feedback and dynamics. Hum Biol 23(4):346–361. http://www.jstor.org/stable/41448008
von Bertalanffy L (1953) Fließgleichgewicht, Homöostasis und Rückkopplung. In: von Bertalanffy L (ed) Biophysik des Fließgleichgewichts: Einführung in die Physik offener Systeme und ihre Anwendung in der Biologie. Vieweg+Teubner Verlag, pp 37–39. https://doi.org/10.1007/978-3-663-20198-4_10
von Bertalanffy L (1968) General system theory. Foundations, development, applications. George Brazillier
von Campenhausen C (1993) Die Sinne des Menschen, 2nd edn. Thieme
von Cube F (1965) Kybernetische Grundlagen des Lernens und Lehrens. E. Klett
von der Malsburg C (1981) The correlation theory of brain function. Internal report 81–2 issue.
von der Malsburg C (1987) Synaptic plasticity as basis of brain organisation. In: Changeux JPKM (ed) The neural and molecular bases of learning. Wiley
von der Malsburg CSW (1988) Principles of cortical network organisation. In: Rakic PSW (ed) The neurobiology of neocortex. Wiley, pp 69–99
von Foerster H (1960) On self-organizing systems and their environments. In: Yovitz MC, Cameron S (eds) Self-organizing systems. Pergamon Press, pp 31–50
von Foerster H (1974) Cybernetics of cybernetics (Cybernetics of Cybernetics or the Control of Control and the Communication of Communication). Issue
von Foerster H (1997) Teachers should increase the number of possibilities of their students. In: Schöllhorn WI (ed) von Foerster, Rattle Snake Hill
von Holst E, Mittelstaedt H (1950) Das Reafferenzprinzip. Naturwissenschaften 37(20):464–476. https://doi.org/10.1007/BF00622503
Wagner R (1954) Probleme und Beispiele biologischer Regelung. G. Thieme
Wagner A (2016) Pre-Gibsonian observations on active touch. Hist Psychol 19(2):93–104. https://doi.org/10.1037/hop0000028
Wagner H, Pfusterschmied J, Klous M, von Duvillard SP, Müller E (2012) Movement variability and skill level of various throwing techniques. Hum Mov Sci 31(1):78–90. https://doi.org/10.1016/j.humov.2011.05.005
Wang CX, Hilburn IA, Wu D-A, Mizuhara Y, Cousté CP, Abrahams JNH, Bernstein SE, Matani A, Shimojo S, Kirschvink JL (2019) Transduction of the geomagnetic field as evidenced from alpha-band activity in the human brain. eNeuro 6(2):ENEURO.0483-0418.2019. https://doi.org/10.1523/eneuro.0483-18.2019
Wegner DM (1997) When the antidote is the poison: ironic mental control processes. Psychol Sci 8(3):148–150. https://doi.org/10.1111/j.1467-9280.1997.tb00399.x
Wegner DM, Broome A, Blumberg SJ (1997) Ironic effects of trying to relax under stress. Behav Res Ther 35(1):11–21. https://doi.org/10.1016/s0005-7967(96)00078-2
Wegner DM, Ansfield M, Pilloff D (1998) The putt and the pendulum: ironic effects of the mental control of action. Psychol Sci 9(3):196–199. https://doi.org/10.1111/1467-9280.00037
Weik E, Lang R (2003) Selbstorganisation. In: Weik E, Lang R (eds) Moderne Organisationstheorien 2: Strukturorientierte Ansätze. Gabler Verlag, pp 243–277. https://doi.org/10.1007/978-3-322-87011-7_7
Weltner K (1970) Informationstheorie und Erziehungswissenschaft. Schnelle. Quickborn.
Weltner K, Ungerer D (1973) Programmiertes Lernen. Sport in unserer Welt—Chancen und Probleme, Berlin/Heidelberg
Wertheimer M (1912) Experimentelle Studien über das Sehen von Bewegung. J.A. Barth
Wertheimer M (1925) Über Gestalttheorie (concerning gestalt theory). Symposion 1:39–60
Westermann G, Mareschal D, Johnson MH, Sirois S, Spratling MW, Thomas MS (2007) Neuroconstructivism. Dev Sci 10(1):75–83. https://doi.org/10.1111/j.1467-7687.2007.00567.x
Whitehead M (2001) The concept of physical literacy. Eur J Phys Educ 6(2):127–138. https://doi.org/10.1080/1740898010060205
Whitehead M (2007) Physical literacy: philosophical considerations in relation to developing a sense of self, universality and propositional knowledge. Sport, Ethics Philos 1(3):281–298. https://doi.org/10.1080/17511320701676916
Wiener N (1948) Cybernetics. Sci Am 179(5):14–19. http://www.jstor.org/stable/24945913
Wiesel TN, Hubel DH (1963) Effects of visual deprivation on morphology and physiology of cells in the cats lateral geniculate body. J Neurophysiol 26:978–993. https://doi.org/10.1152/jn.1963.26.6.978
Wiesendanger M (1990) The motor cortical areas and thre problem of hierarchies. In: Jeannerod M (ed) Attention and performance XIII motor representations an control. Lawrence, pp 59–75
Willis JK, Morello A, Davie A, Rice JC, Bennett JT (2002) Forced use treatment of childhood hemiparesis. Pediatrics 110(1):94–96. https://doi.org/10.1542/peds.110.1.94
Windhorst U (1988) How brain-like is the spinal cord? Springer
Winstein CJ (1991) Knowledge of results and motor learning—implications for physical therapy. Phys Ther 71(2):140–149. https://doi.org/10.1093/ptj/71.2.140
Withagen R, de Poel HJ, Araújo D, Pepping G-J (2012) Affordances can invite behavior: reconsidering

the relationship between affordances and agency. New Ideas Psychol 30(2):250–258. https://doi.org/10.1016/j.newideapsych.2011.12.003
Wolpaw JR (2010) What can the spinal cord teach us about learning and memory? Neuroscientist 16(5):532–549. https://doi.org/10.1177/1073858410368314
Wong W (2020) On the rate coding response of peripheral sensory neurons. Biol Cybern 114(6):609–619. https://doi.org/10.1007/s00422-020-00848-4
Wood CA, Ging CA (1991) The role of interference and task similarity on the acquisition, retention, and transfer of simple motor skills. Res Q Exerc Sport 62(1):18–26. https://doi.org/10.1080/02701367.1991.10607514
Wu WF, Young DE, Schandler SL, Meir G, Judy RL, Perez J, Cohen MJ (2011) Contextual interference and augmented feedback: is there an additive effect for motor learning? Hum Mov Sci 30(6):1092–1101. https://doi.org/10.1016/j.humov.2011.02.004
Wulf G (2008) Attentional focus effects in balance acrobats. Res Q Exerc Sport 79(3):319–325. https://doi.org/10.1080/02701367.2008.10599495
Wulf G, Schmidt RA, Deubel H (1993) Reduced feedback frequency enhances generalized motor program learning but not parameterization learning. J Exp Psychol Learn Mem Cogn 19(5):1134–1150. https://doi.org/10.1037/0278-7393.19.5.1134
Wulf G, McNevin NH, Fuchs T, Ritter F, Toole T (2000) Attentional focus in complex skill learning. Res Q Exerc Sport 71(3):229–239. https://doi.org/10.1080/02701367.2000.10608903
Wulf G, Chiviacowsky S, Schiller E, Avila LT (2010) Frequent external-focus feedback enhances motor learning. Front Psychol 1:190. https://doi.org/10.3389/fpsyg.2010.00190
Wundt WM (1874) Grundzüge der physiolgischen Psychologie. Engelmann
Xiao J (2023) Thirty years of BDNF study in central myelination: from biology to therapy. J Neurochem 167(3):321–336. https://doi.org/10.1111/jnc.15968
Yamamoto K, Shinya M, Kudo K (2020) The influence of attractor stability of intrinsic coordination patterns on the adaptation to new constraints. Sci Rep 10(1):3058. https://doi.org/10.1038/s41598-020-60066-7
Yamanishi J, Kawato M, Suzuki R (1979) Studies on human finger tapping neural networks by phase transition curves. Biol Cybern 33(4):199–208. https://doi.org/10.1007/bf00337409
Yamanishi JI, Kawato M, Suzuki R (1980) Two coupled oscillators as a model for the coordinated finger tapping by both hands. Biol Cybern 37(4):219–225. https://doi.org/10.1007/BF00337040
Zanone PG, Kelso JA (1992) Evolution of behavioral attractors with learning: nonequilibrium phase transitions. J Exp Psychol Hum Percept Perform 18(2):403–421. https://doi.org/10.1037/0096-1523.18.2.403
Zanone P, Kelso JA (1994) The coordination dynamics of learning: theoretical structure and experimental agenda. In: Swinnen SP, Heuer H, Masion J, Casaer P (eds) Interlimb coordination: neural, dynamical, and cognitive constraints. Academic Press, pp 461–490
Zanone PG, Kelso JAS (1997) Coordination dynamics of learning and transfer: collective and component levels. J Exp Psychol Hum Percept Perform 23(5):1454–1480. https://doi.org/10.1037/0096-1523.23.5.1454
Zenner HP (1993) Gleichgewicht. In: Schmidt RF (ed) Neuro- und Sinnespyhsiologie. Springer
Zhou B, Wang Z, Zhu L, Huang G, Li B, Chen C, Huang J, Ma FI, Liu TC (2022) Effects of different physical activities on brain-derived neurotrophic factor: a systematic review and bayesian network meta-analysis [systematic review]. Front Aging Neurosci 14. https://doi.org/10.3389/fnagi.2022.981002
Zilles K, Rehkämper G (1993) Funktionelle Neuroanatomie. Springer
Zimmermann M (1980) Somato-viscerale Sensibilität. In: Schmidt RFTG (ed) Physiologie des Menschen. Springer, pp 209–227
Zucca S, Firrone CM (2014) Nonlinear dynamics of mechanical systems with friction contacts: coupled static and dynamic multi-harmonic balance method and multiple solutions. J Sound Vib 333(3):916–926. https://doi.org/10.1016/j.jsv.2013.09.032

Differential Learning

3

Wolfgang I. Schöllhorn

3.1 Introduction

Once two of the fundamental assumptions of classical therapy and training approaches for model- and repetition-based learning had been deconstructed and were no longer justifiable (cf. Chaps. 1 and 2), other prerequisites for more logically consistent physiotherapy and training had to be found. Mainly, three conditions were given in 1999 for finding or creating this:

- First, the transition from a holistic, static systems theory to the temporal dynamics of systems theory—particularly focusing on state transitions—presented a promising framework for further exploration.
- Second, expanding from first-order to second-order cybernetics, where the cybernetics of the learner or observer is emphasized, aligns with the reform pedagogical approach advocating for a more learner-centered educational model. This shift should be incorporated into the framework.
- Third, the integration of these two criteria must be underpinned by neurophysiological parallels and be congruent with the biomechanics of learning processes. This ensured the development of a concept that is both practical and applicable and goes beyond a mere redescription of existing approaches.

Having succeeded, contrary to Bernstein's predictions, in quantifying the movement topologies of noncyclic every day and sports movements by means of the process-oriented pattern recognition approach (Schöllhorn 1993, 1995, 1996; Schöllhorn and Bauer 1998; Schöllhorn et al. 2001a), the increased fluctuations observed in the studies of Kelso and coworkers (Kelso 1995) during phase transition could be unified with the concept of "*order through noise*" (Ashby 1947; von Foerster 1960) as a condition for self-organization. The intentional increase of fluctuations was realized by increasing the variability of movements that brought the learning system into an unstable state, which initiated a self-organization process. Without giving concrete information about a solution, the system had the opportunity to find a new stable movement and a more effective solution that was not prescribed from the outside but resonated more with the subject's own characteristics and personal possibilities. From a physicist's point of view, the addition of *noise* was directly linked to the question of the optimum amount of noise and to what extent the noise should possibly have a special color (noise can have pink, brown, etc., colors that characterize the shape of the frequency spectrum) or special characteristics. Furthermore, the use of the term "noise" did not only refer to the frequency-

W. I. Schöllhorn (✉)
Institute for Sport Science, Johannes Gutenberg-University, Mainz, Germany
e-mail: schoellw@uni-mainz.de

W. I. Schöllhorn, A. Slapšinskaitė-Dackevičienė (eds.), *Differential Learning in Physiotherapy*,
https://doi.org/10.1007/978-3-031-98787-8_3

based definition, which requires an equidistant sampling rate that is rarely given in exercise sequences, but rather in the more general sense of disturbance or interference also to keep the door open to irregular interventions and catastrophe theory (Gilmore 1981) that studies also the influence of single events.

On the one hand, the stochastic resonance model provided an approach to this problem, and on the other hand, the experience with the training of artificial neural networks (ANNs) supported the practical realization. Related to ANNs, the aim was to provide the system with so much noise that it can fall back on the process of interpolation in the application phase.

Stochastic resonance is considered a phenomenon in which an additional stochastic signal amplifies the response of a system to an input signal. The human system is an example that must recognize, process, and relay signals in a noisy environment, suggesting that it is a good candidate for the use of stochastic resonance (Schöllhorn 2003; Vázquez-Rodríguez et al. 2017). Originally, stochastic resonance meant that white noise is added to a weak (subthreshold) signal to become visible above threshold (Gammaitoni et al. 1998; Moss et al. 1994). Thus, the frequencies in the white noise that correspond to the frequencies of the original signal resonate with each other and amplify the original signal. The rest of the white noise is not amplified, which increases the signal-to-noise ratio, making the original signal more prominent. Meanwhile, the understanding of stochastic resonance has evolved significantly (Millonas 1996). For example, if one considers not only the frequencies of the noise but also the phases, then the noise can also delete the higher harmonics of the original signal at a corresponding phase, and stochastic resonance can be used as a filter (Bartussek et al. 1994; Jung and Bartussek 1996).

The original interpretation was used to enhance sensorimotor function in terms of posture by stimulating physiological sensors that were assumed to influence the control of posture in the elderly, namely, the foot soles mechanically or the vestibular organ galvanically with subthreshold stochastic noise (Collins 1999; Collins et al. 1996; Cordo et al. 1996; Dhruv et al. 2002; Gravelle et al. 2002; Priplata et al. 2002, 2003; Scinicariello et al. 2001). Instead of stimulating only parts of the sensorimotor system, such as the mechano-sensors in the foot soles or the vestibular organ while standing and walking, the idea in DL was to stimulate the whole sensorimotor system by means of additional noise consisting of variations of the to-be-learned movement. If we look at the movements performed by beginners, these are generally described as very unstable and associated with only coarse movement concepts (Fitts and Posner 1967; Meinel 1960). In this case, coarse can also be understood as a weak signal of the movement to be learned compared to the then almost dominating noise (detrimental signal-to-noise ratio). By adding noise, the weak signal (coarse movement concept) is amplified. In the case of stimulating the foot soles or the vestibular organ, this additional noise is used to provide additional information for adequately processing and filtering the disturbances to make the posture signal more stable. Transferred to the learning or therapy of a movement, the additional noise should therefore help to refine the coarse idea of the movement to be learned by "filtering" the corresponding disturbances through adequate coordination. A problem of the isolated stimulation of foot soles was their restriction to the time of stimulation. The foot sole stimulations did not show sustainable or learning effects. Whether this is changing by combining DL with foot sole stimulation could be proven by future research.

Similar indications in terms of positive effects by adding noise came from the experiments of Turvey and coworkers on the dynamic touch (Turvey 1996). The objects had to be wielded (=adding noise) to derive the mechanical properties that were held in the hand. In addition to the idea of self-organization through amplification of fluctuations, the idea of tuning the externally added noise to the signal originating from the learner was added here. Indications for a dependence of the amount of noise on the complexity of the signal were provided from a computational approach (Usher and Feingold 2000).

The connection between the externally visible and biomechanically measurable movements on the one hand and the mechano-sensors of the skin, vestibular organ, and proprioception as well as the stimulation of the muscles on the other is based on the utilization of Newton's law of motion with $F = ma$ (F: force; m: mass; a: acceleration) for linear and $D = \Theta\alpha$ (D: angular momentum; Θ: moment of inertia; α: angular acceleration) for its rotational pendant. If the law is applied to all joints, it already offers an infinite number of possibilities for variation and stimulation. A variation in "mass" can be achieved by changing the length of the levers in each joint, whereas a variation in acceleration is achieved by changing the movement speed. If we lift in an upright position, for example, one arm sideways with the elbow fully bent, the stimulus or the muscular force required for the deltoid muscle to be trained is relatively low. This already increases significantly when the elbow is extended. If the arm is then raised fast while still extended, a significantly greater force is required than in the slow movement, and the deltoid muscle is stimulated accordingly. Varying between a long and short lever, fast and slow, etc., stimulates not only the muscle accordingly but also the neural networks responsible for its adequate and versatile control. Applying this principle while walking provides the possibility to stimulate the trunk muscles dynamically as well. When we walk with more abducted arms, automatically the trunk muscles must compensate for higher angular momentums around the vertical axis, and in parallel, the stabilizing leg muscles are stimulated more. The same applies to the leg muscles, which could also be used to fine-tune rehabilitation measures for ACL rehabilitation. An extension of this approach to other senses and qualities, such as the visual, acoustic, and vestibular, is self-evident due to the neuronal anatomy of the central nervous system.

From the point of view of cybernetic pedagogy, the resonance problem with its tuning of two signals was the abstract counterpart to the setting of teacher-learner, therapist-patient, or coach-athlete interaction in the sense of second-order cybernetics, where the observer's characteristics must be considered as well. The resonance and interpolation aspects led to two consequences. On the one hand, the noise that is given by the number and frequency of variations of exercises must not be too large or too small, i.e., optimal, and on the other hand, the noise that is administered by the exercise selection may be adjusted to the learner's noise response, which can vary due to emotions, fatigue, etc., as well. Too much noise has been associated with the risk of overloading and destabilizing the system to a degree that typically leads to fear of losing control, which completely blocks the system. Too little noise means that there is not enough information available for learning, which would be necessary for progress (Newell et al. 1993). To utilize the interpolation capability, it is also necessary to apply the noise in the area where the future application area will lie. Both resonance and interpolation involve the matching of two signals, in which a signal coming from the teacher, therapist, or coach has to resonate with the signal from the learner, patient, or athlete. Therapy or training must therefore be adapted individually and situationally by the therapist with sufficient variation in the relevant area.

Quantifying the movement topologies of sports movements not only bridged the system dynamics of cyclical and ballistic whole-body movements but also connected to methodical exercise (Gaulhofer and Streicher 1924) and game series (Mahlo 1965; Mester 1959). These exercises, which consisted of different movement topologies, have been used since the 1920s, initially in gymnastics and later in team sports. As a reminder: Up to the introduction of DL in 1999, sports psychologists and movement researchers had only assumed that variation in metrics was the key to effective learning. Contextual interference (CI) learning had not been observed to have any systematic effect on sports movements until this point (Brady 1997, 2004; Magill and Hall 1990).

By quantifying the movement topologies, all motor learning approaches, including the sports pedagogical ones, could thus be summarized under the umbrella of noise (Schöllhorn 1999a, b; Schöllhorn et al. 2006a, 2009). This means that each motor learning approach proposed up to that point could be understood as an intervention measure with varying levels and structures of noise (Fig. 3.1). However, the proposed optimal curve did not account for the emerging separation between acquisition (in-session performance) and learning (retention/transfer). At the time, there were too few comparative studies across approaches to justify that distinction. From this point of view, the suggested group of curves (dotted line) could and can be rather considered a research program. The curve in Fig. 3.1 also suggests that, since even repetition-based learning (RL) always shows small deviations, we have learned all the time more from the small deviations than from the repetitive part. However, these differences seem to be too small for effective learning, unless they are performed by children or beginners. Repetitions for beginners still have so much variation that they are sufficient for learning. With increasing constancy of movement, however, the learning rate decreases accordingly. So, we have not learned despite the many mistakes, but only because of them.

More noise and thus more differences between two consecutive movements are revealed by the approaches of the methodical rows of exercise

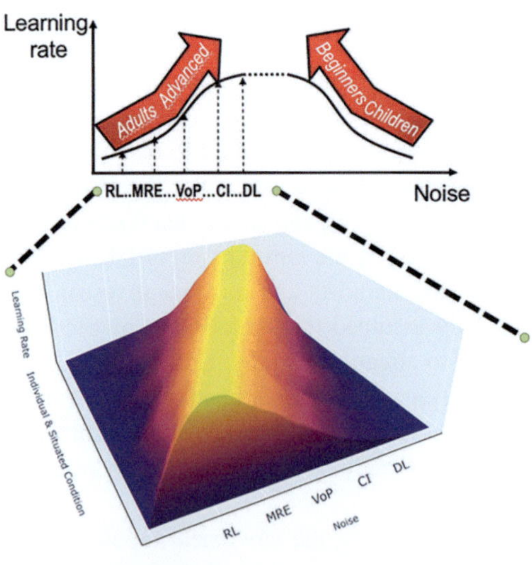

Fig. 3.1 Hypothetical graph for the unification of several motor learning approaches dependent on the individual and on the individual's situation

(MRE), variability of practice (VoP), contextual interference contextual interference (CI), and differential learning (DL). Thus, these traditional master teachings (MRE, VoP, and CI), each with a very limited scope of application (Schöllhorn et al. 2022), can be understood in the context of the stochastic resonance model as the stochastic signal from the external teacher, therapist, or trainer that dictates the exercise variation (noise) from the outside. The other internal stochastic signal represents the different responses of the learner, patient, or athlete to the different exercise varieties. Overall, the figure suggests more focus (but not exclusively) on the differences for the therapist-patient or coach-athlete interaction during learning than on repetitions (Fig. 3.1).

3.1.1 Various DL Strategies

Three strategies were considered for satisfying these assumptions related to resonance, practically all of which have already been implemented, but only one of which has been used in studies to date. Thus, in all approaches, it was essential not to provide augmented feedback to avoid counteracting self-organization on the one hand and to avoid the known problems of augmented feedback discussed in Chap. 2 on the other.

In one approach, noise in the form of stochastic perturbations is simply added to the movement to be learned to initiate self-organization. The noise can be added using different and varying approaches. Whether the noise is added by the therapist through open tasks with or without auxiliary equipment is thereby of secondary interest. Following the basic systemic idea, the noise can be applied holistically to the overall movement or partially to the subsystems (partial movements). In the case of too obviously (biomechanically) disadvantageous and persistent deviations, the noise can be focused on these subsystems but should include the surrounding areas (e.g., because of the double-jointed musculature, the interplay of muscular and passive forces (Schneider et al. 1989)), possibly persistent reflexes (e.g., primitive reflexes (Vreeling et al.

1993)), and "phylogenetic" co-activations (e.g., right wrist and left ankle or left knee and right elbow as a phylogenetic legacy of the crossover gait in quadrupedal gait, etc. (Dietz 2002; Dietz and Michel 2009; Zehr and Duysens 2004)).

Another approach is to look for the biggest anomaly or fluctuation in a single executed movement and instruct to amplify this anomaly in the next movement. This approach can be considered as using the athlete's subjective information to control the amplitude and structure of noise to keep the self-organization process running. This strategy was relying on the tradition that therapists, trainers, and teachers were trained and accustomed to looking for errors (=anomaly) in the patient's movement execution. This habit and ability were to be used, but this time not in the sense that the errors were to be eliminated or at least reduced, but rather these errors were understood as fluctuations (as a source for learning) that needed to be reinforced to allow interpolation. In this way, the therapists' and coaches' ability to see the extraordinary can be further used by increasing the fluctuation; the patients and athletes get a different chance to experience the "problem" with its consequences and with their own feedback. With the amplification of these fluctuations, other extraordinary fluctuations occurred in the next movement, which were again regarded as instability and thus as a potential source of learning and were amplified again, etc. By reinforcing a different fluctuation with each attempt, each movement (or at least after every third) is clearly different from the previous ones. Very soon, the number of changes becomes too big to remember them all and to try to correct them all. Accordingly, it becomes increasingly difficult for the patient, athlete, or learner to make conscious comparisons with previous movements or to recognize mistakes, which leads relatively quickly to a situation in which he or she concentrates only on the momentary movements and, over time, develops an attitude of "being in the moment." Whether this is causing a similar change in processing data like the ones observed in the "magic" number of 7 in chunking information (Mathy and Feldman 2012; Miller 1956) would be an interesting question for future studies. By using the information coming from the learner for the teacher's next instruction, both signals undergo a reciprocal coordination, which, in conjunction with the initiated self-organization process, enables greater consideration of the learner's characteristics.

> The term "differential" (in DL) not only referred to the difference between subsequent movements but also had a connection to various aspects of Far Eastern philosophy. First, people of different opinions A and B should not necessarily compromise, as is often recommended in Western philosophy according to Hegel's dialectic, but rather stick to their opinion so that both can also learn from the difference. The frequently used Far Eastern saying "*the path is the goal*" also takes on an additional meaning with the differences from trial to trial. The path seems to refer not only to the path to the long-term goal but also to the path of the next step of adaptation and thus points to being in the moment. Another aspect was related to the Chinese quote, "*If you want to be unhappy, just compare.*" This was another reason to do it without feedback and to change the movements as often as possible to avoid these comparisons. Meanwhile, this approach is supported by the brain activation (Dietrich 2003, 2006; Henz et al. 2018; Henz and Schöllhorn 2016), and also the error-free learning approach (Broadbent et al. 2017; Maxwell et al. 2001) follows this strategy.

Another approach relates to the effects of exercise sequences and actually corresponds to a simple prolongation of the previous time scale. Here, the sequence of exercises was selected according to the principle of optimal subjective information rate for maximal individual learning. At the beginning, only single variables related to the movement geometry were varied before the variation of two or more variables was introduced, and then proceeded with speed, acceleration, and rhythm variables to keep the subjective information rate close to the individual optimum (Fig. 3.2). This

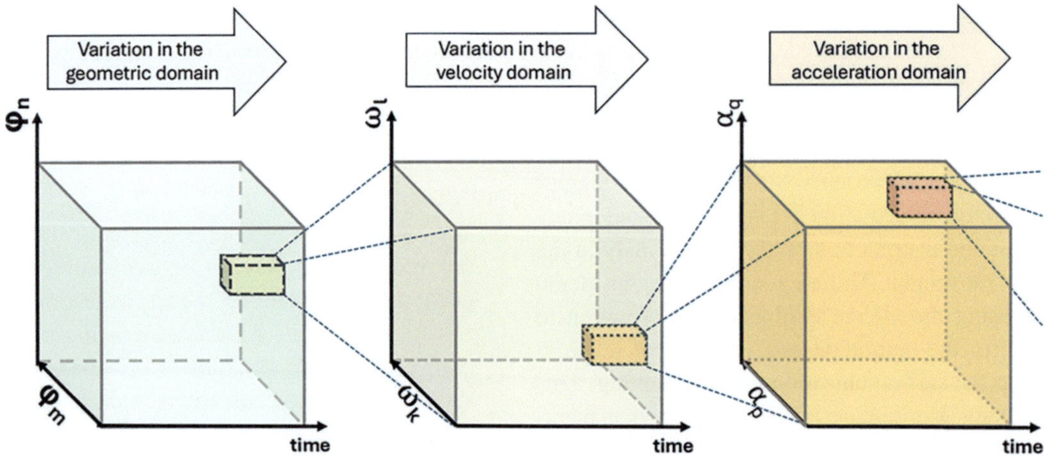

Fig. 3.2 Schematic representation of the rough procedure for DL from beginner to advanced to professional

only serves as a coarse orientation, as these variables are physically dependent on each other. The signal coming from the learner represented the mean variance across trials. If the movement instructions could all be reasonably realized, the difficulty level in the form of an increased subjective information rate was increased, either by increasing the frequency of changes or by increasing the parallel complexity of exercises. If the movements were no longer executed satisfactorily (too large deviation) over several trials or only with excessive deviations, the level of difficulty was either lowered again, or the number of repetitions was increased up to three "repetitions," short aerobic exercises for faster central nervous recovery were included or the session was terminated. The suggested maximum of three repetitions was based on the power law of adaptation, according to which the first three repetitions still contain enough noise to enable reasonable adaptation (see Sect. 2.3.4). The two last approaches are meanwhile attracting increasing interest in general under the topic of adaptive stochastic resonance and guided self-organisation (Krauss et al. 2017; Mitaim and Kosko 1998).

Irrespective of the variation strategy in practice, the exercises and exercise sequences were primarily intended to stimulate the systems that are supposed to be responsible for learning in humans via their mechano-sensors (tactile, kinesthetic, and proprioception) and neuronal network structures in conjunction with versatile muscular activation patterns in such a way that they are stimulated to self-organize (de Arcangelis et al. 2006). Since these mechanisms were already known and tested in relation to the visual system (Gray et al. 1989; Hubel and Wiesel 1964; Singer 1983; Wiesel and Hubel 1963), it was necessary to transfer the correspondences of localization, color, orientation, etc., to the sensorimotor system to subsequently extend the system to both systems together. The stimulation of the sensorimotor system was initially realized against a biomechanical background using various levers on the joints and different execution speeds, before the system was extended to movements with a stronger visual component and their diverse variation.

3.2 Initial Positive Findings Through More Variation in Movement Topology

In the following, selected studies on DL in skill acquisition are briefly presented that illustrate the key characteristics in the line of research questions and also provide concrete examples of the variety of intervention options. The list, therefore, makes no claim to completeness and is not a systematic review. Details of the studies can be found in the publications listed.

With reference to alternatives to classical hypothesis testing in the context of the replication crisis (Ioannidis 2005), the aim was rather to offer a variety of arguments (Feest 2019, 2024) that relate to the fundamental aspects of DL theory, rather than conducting the largest possible samples or meta-analyses using homogeneous experimental designs (Acree 2021; Lin et al. 2013). This variety of approaches, per se, makes it problematic for a meta-analysis in general. Neither the large sample approach nor its counterpart, the meta-analysis approach, allows for statements regarding the probability of the tested hypotheses. At best, they enable conclusions to be drawn about the data, assuming the hypothesis is true (Gigerenzer 2004, 2018). Nonetheless, in accordance with Popper, statements on probabilities can neither be verified nor falsified (Popper 1935). To be able to make statements about the probability of a hypothesis, for example, it would be helpful to have several hypotheses available at the same time. When tossing a coin or dice, the probability of a single event is given relative to the available possibilities. In the case of a coin, the probability of tails or crests is 1 out of 2 possibilities; correspondingly, in the case of a die, the probability of rolling a 3 is 1 out of 6 possibilities. How can statements be made about the probability of a single available hypothesis? The studies of one's own working group are therefore at best to be understood as coroboration (Popper 1935), and if a 5% value is reached in the sense of the original interpretation of Fisher (Fisher and Russell 1922), it is worthwhile to continue researching.

The first studies on DL were primarily aimed at improving single movement techniques, on the one hand by increasing precision and on the other hand to increase distance, height, or (running) speed. This distinction is made because in the second case of mks-sports (meter-kilogram-seconds), at least in the advanced range, a change in conditional characteristics such as strength or endurance parameters can be assumed in addition to the coordinative change, and the focus of the fluctuations must be shifted accordingly. Initial studies were carried out as part of pre-posttest designs for sprint running (Schöllhorn et al. 2001b), serve reception in volleyball (Römer et al. 2003; Schöllhorn et al. 2001c), shooting in basketball (Schönherr and Schöllhorn 2003), and soccer (scoring, passing, ball reception) (Schöllhorn et al. 2004, 2006a; Trockel and Schöllhorn 2003). While maximum speed was to be increased in sprinting, the aim of the other studies was to increase passing, shooting, and throwing accuracy. In the sprint study, many variations were used that were aimed at a faster change in the activation of agonists and antagonists to achieve increased fluctuations at the muscular level with different contraction intensities. The applied exercise variations were oriented on coaching experiences since the beginning 1980s that resulted in a book on speed training (Schöllhorn et al. 1995). In conjunction with varying movement amplitudes in the single joints, increased stretch-shortening cycles (Komi 1984) were to be activated to make the sprint stride more effective (Schöllhorn et al. 1995). As a result, the DL group achieved the highest running speed, even though they only trained twice a week for 4 months, whereas the control group trained five times a week in a model- and amount-oriented manner. In parallel, the biomechanical pattern recognition of the ground contact phase during maximum speed revealed a higher individualization in the DL group (Schöllhorn et al. 2001b).

In the volleyball study (Römer et al. 2003; Schöllhorn et al. 2001c), the fluctuations were didactically and metaphorically reinforced by asking the juveniles to name an animal before each serve in the training game, in whose style the DL group then had to play until the next point. On the one hand, this was intended to encourage creativity regarding the implementation of the open movement tasks, and on the other hand, to support an even stronger (divergent) learner centering through the choice of an animal. For example, if the elephant was named as the animal, it could happen that all ball contacts were only played with one arm. This idea was based on experiences in Far Eastern martial arts, where some fighting styles are named after animals. The result showed a statistically significant improvement in the precision of the underarm pass of the DL group after 4 weeks of training with two sessions per week. Thus, the classical group was outperformed too. Both results statistically encouraged continuing this type of research.

In the first soccer studies, goal kicking (Trockel and Schöllhorn 2003), passing (Schöllhorn et al. 2004), and ball reception (Schöllhorn et al. 2004) were examined in 4- to 6-week interventions, whereby the interventions were only allowed to be practiced twice a week for a maximum of 20–30 min, due to the coaches' skepticism. In the first two techniques, in addition to the standing leg, kicking leg, torso, arm, and head position, the approach, the balls, and the goal were also varied. The passes and shots on goal should also be aimed next to the goal or away from the pass target to keep the interpolation frame wide. When receiving the ball, the DL group's reception was varied, with different body parts moving in different directions and different balls coming from different directions at different speeds or on different surfaces. The incoming ball should also be stopped as close to the player as possible, and the ball should also be allowed to bounce further away on first contact, which is needed for direct play. Here, too, all three studies showed statistically significant advantages for the DL groups in the posttest compared to the classic training groups.

Comparable results were shown in the study on basketball free throws (Schönherr and Schöllhorn 2003), in which the DL group had to vary the throws from different positions, with different balls, with different rotations, with one hand, next to the basket, over the board, etc. Movements, targets, and balls were varied, too.

A very inspiring study with a quite different design based on the resonance idea examined how differential and variable training methods influence the quality of the handball throw, focusing on ball velocity, accuracy, and movement patterns (Wagner and Müller 2008). Using a single-case design, the authors applied a multiphase training program—predominantly based on DL principles—to foster self-organization and motor learning. The results highlight that DL significantly improves ball velocity and alters kinematic sequences, especially in high-level athletes. Importantly, the study shows that the timing and focus of differential interventions—whether aimed at accuracy or speed—affect their outcomes, suggesting that DL should be dynamically adapted depending on the velocity or accuracy improvement. A decrease in performance during the variable training phase emphasizes the importance of precision in how and when DL is applied. Overall, the research advocates for DL as a powerful tool in sports training, provided it is used with attention to the athlete's individual learning trajectory and responsiveness.

3.3 Increased Sustainability and More Consistent Movements Thanks to Increased Noise

After these initial confirmations of the predictions, the next step was to focus on the sustainability of the interventions and extend the pre-posttest design with an additional retention test at a time interval from the posttest. This was partly due to the findings of contextual interference research. These indicated that, at least in the case of fine motor skills (Magill and Hall 1990; Newell 1989; Wulf and Lee 1993; Wulf and Shea 2002), the acquisition process from the pre-test to the posttest can certainly be disadvantageous, but that this process can be reversed after a short break until the retention test. In a study on shot put (Beckmann and Schöllhorn 2003) and another one on tennis serve (Humpert and Schöllhorn 2006), one group was trained according to the DL model and the other according to the classical model and correction-oriented training. After 4 or 6 weeks of intervention twice a week, the DL group showed significantly greater increases in shot put distance performance. In the tennis study, the DL group showed greater accuracy in the serve, but this was not great enough for a statistically significant result immediately after the intervention. Interestingly, in the 6-week tennis study, an intermediate test was carried out after 4 weeks, in which differences were already apparent, which increased until the posttest. However, the differences in serve accuracy in tennis only became statistically significant in the retention test. Surprisingly, despite significantly greater variations than in CI studies, no disadvantages were observed during the recording phase, which called into question the explanation of working memory overload.

More Recent studies on the acute effects of DL during warm-up (Gaspar et al. 2019) and DL studies over a period of 3 months (Oftadeh et al. 2021) point in the same direction, that the differences to other forms of training become greater with increasing time.

Surprisingly, the shot put and tennis studies showed further increases in performance in the retention phase, i.e., after the end of the intervention and a break of at least 2 weeks, which lasted up to 4 weeks in the shot put. In the end, in the shotput experiment, the DL group achieved a performance increase of approx. 70 cm within 6 weeks, while the classic group only gained approx. 20 cm in the first 4 weeks and fell back to the initial level at the end (Fig. 3.3). The classic group in the tennis study was able to maintain the increase in performance they had achieved until the retention test. Future studies will have to show to what extent the differences between the two studies during the acquisition phase can be attributed to the different starting levels or the usual training methodology.

To determine performance consistency as an indicator of a relatively long-lasting change in behavior (=learning), not only the best shot but also the performance of three shots (Fig. 3.3) was taken into account in the shot put study (Beckmann and Schöllhorn 2003, 2006). Interestingly, the DL group also showed greater distance consistency as the performance curve increased, which improved even further up to the last retention test. Somewhat surprising was the increase in target variance in the posttest in the traditional training group, although the training exercises showed considerably less variation. Only after the variance increased did it decrease until the first retention test, only to return to the initial level on the second. The increase in variance up to the posttest, despite more constant exercise selection, indicates a certain influence of variance on learning. It seems as if the nature of variance is fighting against the model of constancy here. Regardless of this, however, the continuous reduction in variance in the DL group provided evidence for the benefit of topology variation on movement constancy on the one hand and confirmation of the predicted improvement in adaptability on the other.

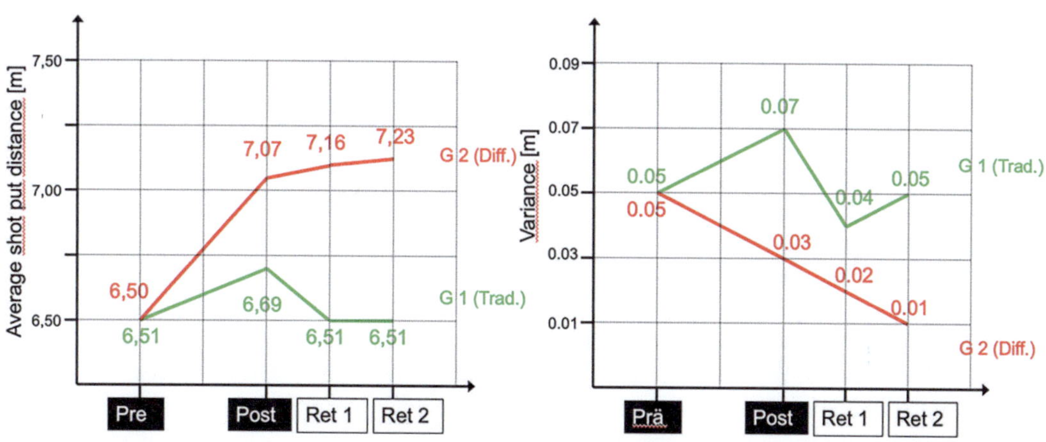

Fig. 3.3 Performance- (left) and variance-curve (right) of the shot put experiment. (Beckmann and Schöllhorn 2006)

3.4 Activities During the Retention Phase Influence the Learning Result

Several confirmations of the additional increase in performance during the break after the intervention by DL-training groups drew our attention to this phase. However, in some studies, the achieved performance gains could "only" be kept on the same level (but never decreased). This observation was often made when the subjects were pupil, and the retention phase was during their school holidays during Christmas or Easter vacation. The system dynamical analysis (Frank et al. 2008) of the DL data suggested that during the retention phase, not only does the pause in practicing the movement technique has an influence on performance development but also the amount of "*background noise*" in terms of other activities during this time. So, if activities are generally reduced during the retention phase (e.g., school vacations), this also appears to have an influence on the learning progression of the paused technique. More extensive research is needed here.

Another question was related to the extent to which this retention phase could be influenced by additional mental training. After absolute beginners in tennis had undergone 3 weeks of differential serve training, the group was randomly assigned to three different groups. One group had a break (as in the previous studies), one group was given 1 h of literature to read on the tennis serve three times a week, and the third group was given mental training three times a week for 1 h. The mental training consisted of watching videos showing their own best serve from previous training sessions, extracting key points from them, and then mentally repeating the serve movement based on these. A retention test was carried out after 3 weeks. While the group with a break showed the greatest increase in performance, as in previous studies, this was slightly lower in the literature group and, to our surprise, was even negative in the mental training group. This initial surprise quickly gave way to an extension of the DL theory, as the findings pointed to rates of change on different time scales of the subsystems. While the mind was kept in approximately the same state by the mental training, a change could be assumed for the motoric system (cf. Fig. 1.11 in Sect. 1.3.4). However, if both develop at different rates, this is of little benefit to overall performance. The continuous changes to which our body is subject, therefore, make it necessary to constantly increase or change the noise to keep pace with the changes in terms of coordination and keep the subjective information rate on the necessary level. While this is still obvious in childhood and adolescence, the growth rates make it unlikely that coordination learned at the beginning of a year will still work at the end of the year with completely different biomechanical conditions; this seems to be ignored in adulthood and even in shorter timescales of therapy and training. It would be worth considering whether this might also apply to the elderly when the body changes more quickly again. Shouldn't more variations in movement be used again to keep pace with these changes to give the human sensory-motor system more possibilities to adapt?

In the meantime, several studies have shown that movement patterns can also change significantly in adults within a few minutes and a few days without any intervention (Albrecht et al. 2014; Horst et al. 2016a, 2017a, b; Jäger et al. 2003a; Janssen et al. 2008, 2011). It seems that the arrow of time has been widely neglected in therapy and training research (Horst et al. 2023; Schöllhorn et al. 2022).

This inspired us to do another study where we explored how different types of soccer shooting training—classical repetition-based, physical differential, and mental differential—affect brain activity, measured through EEG (Henz et al. 2014b). Results showed that physical differential training significantly increased theta activity in left frontal and central areas and Mu-wave activity in motor-related regions, suggesting enhanced motor system engagement. In contrast, mental differential training led to decreased alpha activity in the left occipital region, but no increase in motor-related activity. The findings suggest that physical differential training activates the brain's motor areas more strongly than repetition-based or mental training and that kinesthetic input may play a key role in building motor working memory through differential learning.

The increase in theta waves in the frontal brain area also made DL a candidate for influencing performance in the context of choking under pressure (Henz et al. 2014a). This study investigated whether differential training in basketball free throws is more effective than classical repetition-based training in helping athletes perform under pressure. Thirty-two participants trained for 4 weeks in either method and were tested before and after training under low-pressure conditions. A follow-up test was conducted 3 weeks later under high-pressure conditions involving an audience and a jury. Results showed that while both groups improved over time, those who received differential training performed significantly better under pressure, with fewer airballs and more stable performance. The findings suggest that differential training helps athletes maintain motor performance in stressful environments, likely due to its reliance on sensorimotor-based working memory, which is less susceptible to distractions. In contrast, repetition-based training depends more on executive control, which is more easily disrupted under pressure.

3.5 From Training a Single Technique to Training Multiple Techniques

Since most people rarely learn just a single movement in everyday life, therapy, or most sports, another question arises: to what extent can the findings on the learning of single movement techniques be applied to the learning of multiple techniques? Is there a mutual inhibition, as was observed in the context of interference learning in the acquisition phase, or are there possibly even synergy effects? This issue has long been thematized in learning psychology under the terms antero- and retro-grade inhibition, but only referred to two alternating effects in each case (Smirnov 1973). A fundamental difference to the contextual inference (CI) learning approach should at least be apparent here (Schöllhorn 2016). While in CI, a limited number of precisely prescribed movements are repeated through interleaved practice, and deviations from this are not permitted (Shea and Zimny 1983), in DL, in its most extreme form, no repetitions are performed even when learning a single technique. This is continued when learning several techniques and thus also thematizes the importance of the similarities between exercises and their influence on the learning process.

An initial approach was taken in volleyball for young students with the parallel learning of two techniques, namely lower and upper passing (Schöllhorn and Paschke 2007; Schöllhorn et al. 2006b). Both techniques were trained differentially in blocks, i.e., first the DL variations in one technique and then the DL variations in the other technique. Here too, after just six training sessions over 6 weeks, the DL group showed significantly greater passing precision in both techniques in the posttest, which continued in the upper passing technique until the retention test 2 weeks later, while the increase in performance was maintained in the lower passing technique. The classically trained group was only able to improve in the upper pass, while the lower pass remained relatively unchanged in all tests. It appears that the type of learning also influences the learning of two techniques, albeit rather disadvantageously in classical repetition learning.

This approach was extended to three techniques in several studies (Apidogo et al. 2021, 2022, 2023). In volleyball, these were the serve, in addition to the overarm and underarm pass. All three techniques were trained differentially by the DL groups in a blocked manner. In one study (Apidogo et al. 2021), the DL approach was compared with blocked repetition learning, and another time (Apidogo et al. 2022) with randomized context interference learning. In both studies, a group that played general ball games served as a control group. In both studies, the DL groups were able to increase significantly in all three techniques in the posttest; in the retention test, the increases were at least maintained, whereas the changes in the comparison groups in the post-

and retention tests remained within the random range. The third study focused on the influence of the learning approaches dependent on the similarity of the exercises (Apidogo et al. 2023).

A comparison of differential and repetition-based training of three soccer techniques (dribbling, passing, and juggling) in a pre- and posttest design showed comparable performance improvements for both approaches, with slight advantages for the differential training group (Bozkurt 2018). Future studies will have to show to what extent the duration of 4 weeks for the three techniques or the high similarity of the exercises influenced the result. Unfortunately, no retention or transfer test was carried out in this study, in which differential learning has so far shown the greatest effects. However, the results confirm previous findings in the form that differential training does not perform worse than planned training.

The combined training of two shooting techniques in field hockey (flick and push) led to a first differentiation of the variation strategies of DL, which was closely linked to the question of the optimal amount of noise (Beckmann et al. 2010). For this purpose, not only were the two techniques trained differentially in blocked form for 4 weeks, but a distinction was also made between (a) variation of the movement execution, (b) variation of the target, and (c) both combined. The results for the posttests and both retention tests, 2 and 4 weeks after the intervention, did not lead to consistent results, neither in the posttests nor in the retention tests. The large scatter that occurred suggested that the optimal amount of variation needs to be examined in more detail and most probably individually.

This aspect was considered in a pilot study on the parallel training of two soccer techniques (Hegen et al. 2012; Schöllhorn et al. 2012). An additional differentiation of the variation strategy was included. There, the goal-shooting and ball-receiving exercises were trained in one experimental group in blocked form as before. The second experimental group trained, analogous to serial or randomized CI learning combined with DL (s-CI-DL or r-CI-DL), alternately on goal shooting and ball reception, but each technique was different; that is, each time, not only the technique but also the exercise was changed. Both differentially trained groups showed significantly greater performance improvements in both techniques on average than the traditionally trained group but did not differ from each other in a statistically significant way. A more detailed look at the individual results shows very different learning behavior in all three groups, where, for example, only one athlete in the s-CI-DL training group responded very strongly, whereas the others showed no changes in performance.

3.6 Variation Strategies of Differential Learning Are Reflected in Brain Activity

A further differentiation of the strategies was derived from the theory of information in time series, which can be quantified using the entropy measure (a measure of disorder) (Kantz and Schreiber 1994; Strogatz 1994). For example, the information content of a linear or sinusoidal time series has less information content and a lower entropy than a random time series, as the following value can be predicted with a high degree of probability based on the previous one. On the other hand, the entropy increases with random time series because the previous value contains no information about the subsequent one. Interestingly, our brain also releases more dopamine (Narasimhan 1998; Schultz 1998) when coping with unexpected events, which plays an important role in learning (Schultz et al. 1997; Takahashi et al. 2017). The reference to the role of prediction errors provides neurological equivalents of the common coding theory (Hommel et al. 2001; Prinz 1990).

The corresponding strategy differentiation was termed gradual and chaotic DL. In the first case, the exercises were varied so that the learner knew approximately what would come next, e.g., variation of the left ankle joint, the right ankle joint, the left knee joint, the right knee joint, etc. In the second case, on the other hand, the sequence of exercises was varied in a largely unpredictable way, e.g., variation of the right elbow, left hip, right ankle, etc. As the type of sequence has different information content, this should be most likely to be reflected in the area in which information processing takes place, which in humans should be most likely to be reflected in brain activation. In two studies, the changes in brain activation caused by different movement sequences in connection with the badminton serve were investigated using EEG (Henz et al. 2018; Henz and Schöllhorn 2016). The movement sequences followed the structure of RL (repetition of the forehand serve), serial CI learning (alternation between forehand and backhand serve), gradual DL, and chaotic DL. The changes after 10–15 min of intervention are shown in Fig. 3.4. Essentially, repetition learning did not lead to large changes in EEG; CI learning was primarily associated with an increase in beta and gamma frequencies, which are typically associated with increased attention, problem-solving, and concentration. After gradual differential learning, a stronger activation in the alpha and theta frequency range can be recognized, which are typically associated with inner attention, creativity, and memory consolidation but are also related to attention and concentration. Chaotic differential learning not only led to a higher activation of the lower alpha and theta frequencies but also to an increased activation of the higher

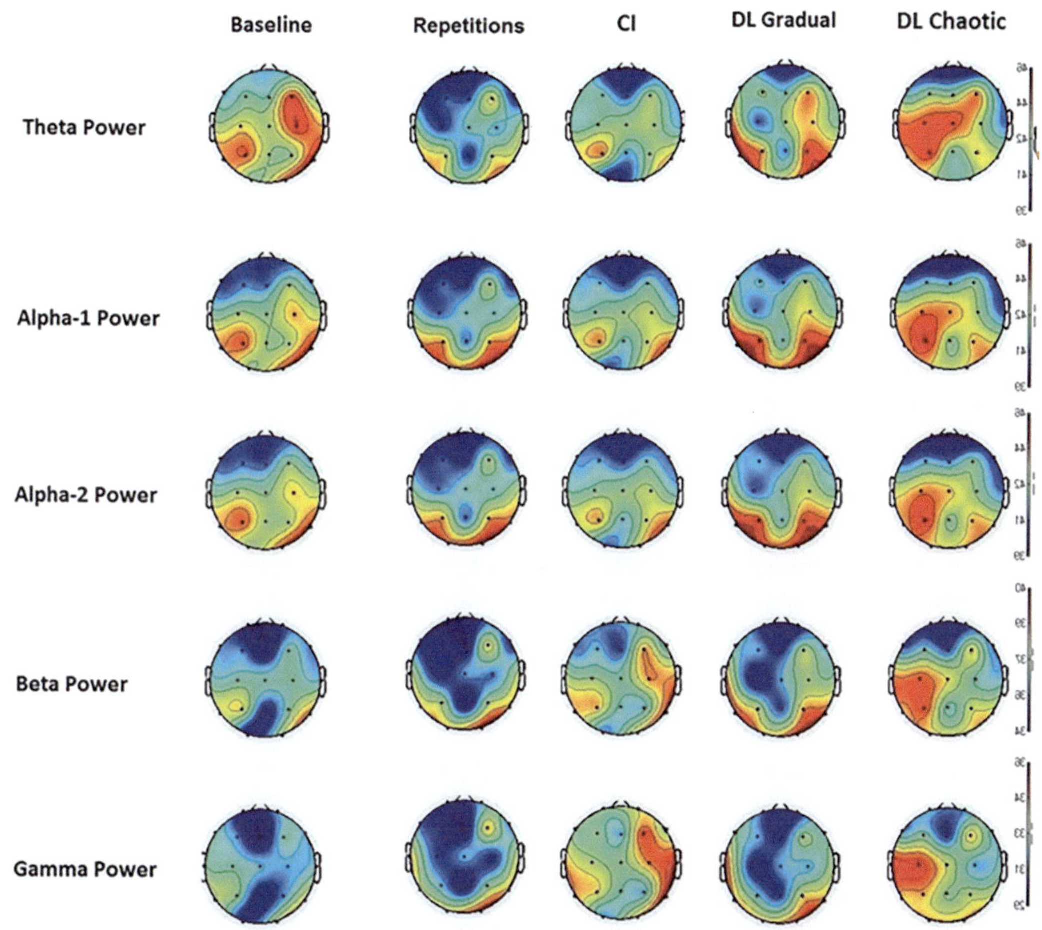

Fig. 3.4 EEG-brain activation before and after four different exercise sequences (repetition learning, contextual interference, gradual differential learning, and chaotic differential learning) of badminton serves

frequency bands. This phenomenon of an increase in all frequency bands had previously only been observed in long-term meditation practitioners and confirmed the previously mentioned parallel to the Far Eastern philosophy of "being in the moment," which is considered central for meditation (Goleman and Davidson 2017; Henz and Schöllhorn 2017a, b; Kabat-Zinn 1994).

Interestingly, an increase in theta frequencies is suspected to be associated with an increase in dopamine (Esch 2014; Kjaer et al. 2002), and if these are activated, for example, by means of 10 min of yoga a day, this can lead to structural anatomical changes that are connected to improved stress management (Hölzel et al. 2010, 2011). In this context, the question of the extent to which the increased theta frequencies also activate the parasympathetic system and thus have an influence on the immune system could be of interest for future research.

Recent studies point in a similar direction, i.e., triggering specific brain states through appropriate forms of movement. For example, jumping rope differentially three times for 1 min after mathematics lessons seems to be beneficial for learning mathematics (Burdack and Schöllhorn 2022). However, it is important to ensure that the change of jumping technique takes place at optimal intervals (John et al. 2022). The corresponding study investigated the influence of four different change frequencies when jumping rope (not at all, every 20 s, every 10 s, and every second). Switching to a different skipping technique every 10 s led to maximum interaction between the heart and brain. To what extent this behavior can be attributed to an activation of the locus coeruleus by the parallel increase in heart rate to 120 bpm and simultaneous confrontation with new jumping techniques, or to what extent this supports the production of BDNF, must be shown in future studies (John and Schöllhorn 2018; John et al. 2022). System dynamics considerations of self-organizing criticality and neuronal plasticity point in a similar direction (Carhart-Harris et al. 2014; Carhart-Harris 2018; de Arcangelis et al. 2006; Liu et al. 2012). It appears that a critical level of variable central nervous activation is necessary to initiate neuronal plasticity (Beggs and Plenz 2003; Turrigiano and Nelson 2004). This is seen as having great potential for the prevention and treatment of age-related central nervous disorders.

A more recent study challenged the prediction that had already been made in the first paper on DL (Schöllhorn 1999a, 2000). This is related to "When a certain range of variation has been applied for a certain period of time, the variation has to be varied too in order to reveal a new difference on another time scale" (Schöllhorn 2000). Beginners in Badminton were randomly assigned to three groups, who practiced the serve toward a given target in the opposite field. One group followed the RL approach, the second group the CI approach, and the third group the chaotic DL approach. Before and after 20, 40, 60, and 80 serves, brain activity was measured by means of EEG. The same procedure was repeated on two consecutive days. For the first day, the results revealed for the RL group only increases in the alpha-frequency band after 60 (Fig. 3.5). The CI group showed increases mainly in the alpha and theta frequency bands even later after 80 serves. In contrast to both other groups, the DL group displayed various increases in all frequency bands already after 20 serves, indicating high responsiveness already during the first training session. Interestingly, on the second day, the RL group showed nearly the same behavior, but the CI group now responded with more changes that were mainly related to an increase in beta frequencies, but all happened only after 60 serves. Of similar surprise was the reduction in EEG activity in the DL group but mainly in the higher beta and gamma frequency bands. In sum, the study indicates a change in responsiveness dependent on the applied learning approach, whereby the repetitive approach always showed the smallest responses. It seems that the application of a single learning method also dulls over time (e.g., DL) and points in the direction of varying the variation over time as well, whereas others increase their responsiveness. However, this is only a first pilot study that not only needs to be controlled by other populations but also related to the changes in responsiveness over several days, as well as differences in individuals. In consequence, related to therapy, this is putting into question applying the same approach to the

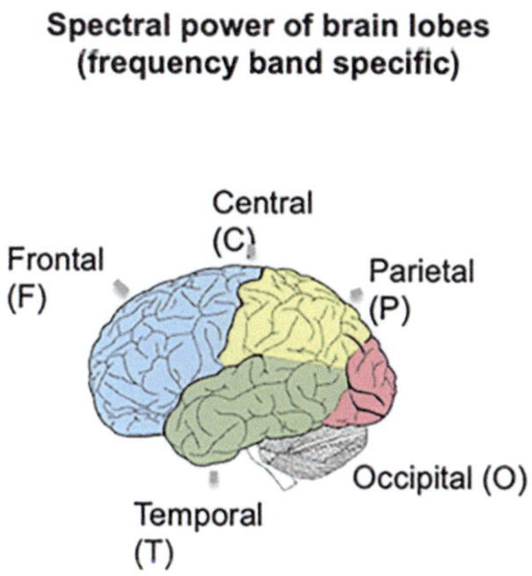

		RL		CI		DL	
		Day 1 (s 20 40 60 80)	Day 2 (s 20 40 60 80)	Day 1 (s 20 40 60 80)	Day 2 (s 20 40 60 80)	Day 1 (s 20 40 60 80)	Day 2 (s 20 40 60 80)
F	theta				+∘∘••	+∘∘••	+∘∘∘•
	alpha	+∘∘••		+∘∘••	+∘∘••	+∘•••	+∘∘••
	beta					+∘•∘•	
	gamma					+∘•∘∘	
	overall					+∘•••	
C	theta			+∘∘••	+∘∘••	+∘∘••	+∘∘••
	alpha	+∘∘••	+∘∘••	+∘∘••	+∘∘••	+∘•••	+∘•••
	beta		+∘∘∘•	+∘•∘•	+∘∘∘•	+∘•••	+∘∘∘•
	gamma					+∘•∘•	+∘∘∘•
	overall		+∘∘∘•	+∘•••	+∘∘••	+∘•••	+∘∘••
T	theta			+∘∘∘∘	+∘∘•∘	+∘∘•∘	
	alpha	+∘∘••	+∘∘••		+∘∘•∘	+∘∘••	+∘∘•∘
	beta					+∘•••	
	gamma					+∘•••	
	overall					+∘•••	+∘∘•∘
P	theta			+∘∘∘•	+∘∘••	+∘∘••	+∘∘••
	alpha	+∘∘••	+∘∘••	+∘∘∘•	+∘∘••	+∘•••	+∘•••
	beta		+∘••∘		+∘∘∘•	+∘•••	+∘∘∘•
	gamma					+••••	
	overall		+∘•••	+∘•∘•	+∘•∘•	+∘•••	+∘∘••
O	theta			+∘∘∘•	+∘∘••	+∘∘∘∘	
	alpha	+∘∘••	+∘∘••		+∘∘•∘	+∘∘∘•	+∘•••
	beta				+∘∘••	+••••	+∘∘•∘
	gamma					+••••	
	overall					+••••	+∘∘•∘
Overall	theta			+∘∘∘•	+∘∘••	+∘∘••	+∘∘••
	alpha	+∘∘••	+∘∘••	+∘∘∘•	+∘∘••	+∘∘••	+∘•••
	beta				+∘•∘•	+∘•••	+∘∘∘•
	gamma					+••••	
	overall				+∘∘∘•	+∘•••	+∘∘••

Fig. 3.5 Changes of EEG activation after 20, 40, 60, and 80 badminton serves on two consecutive days differentiated by learning approach (*RL* repetition, *CI* contextual interference, *DL* chaotic differential learning) and brain lobes

same person when coming for treatment with the same diagnosis but after several months or years.

3.7 Differential Learning and Team Tactical Behavior

Since teams could also be recognized based on their movements on the pitch with the help of process-oriented pattern recognition, and these patterns also do not have identical repetitions (Aydilek et al. 2022; Jäger and Schöllhorn 2007, 2012; Jäger et al. 2003b; Westphal and Schöllhorn 2001), the same prerequisites were given as for movement learning by means of DL. This meant that more stable and more flexible tactical behavior could be observed by means of increased fluctuations, or more noise. To reinforce the fluctuations, additional variations were proposed by means of additional coordinative tasks, changes in the shape of the playing field, different numbers and shapes of balls, number of goals, division of zones with assigned tasks, changes of tactical formation (e.g., In handball: change between 6:0, 5:1, 4:2, 3:3, or man-to-man; in soccer: change between 4-4-2, 3-4-3, 4-3-2-1, etc.), and equipment (clothing, rackets, shoes, etc.). With these findings, small sided games as developed in the 1960s, could be considered as tactical exercises with various levels of noise too. In line with the idea of systems theory, the theory should be transferable to other systems regardless of the area of application, which in this case had the same prerequisites, namely the occurrence of fluctuations with simultaneous individuality characteristics. To this end, several studies were conducted by Diogo Coutinho and Sara Santos in the field of soccer with juveniles, which showed not only the applicability of differential learning, but also its positive influence on the creativity of athletes in terms of tactical behavior (Coutinho et al. 2018; Santos et al. 2017, 2018). The fluctuations were primarily targeted through additional coordination tasks and their assignment to zones. A study in the field of basketball conducted by Nuno Leite impressively demonstrated the phenomenon of self-organization of tactical behavior (Poureghbali et al 2020). Juvenile beginners in basketball trained in eight sessions with small sided games on half the court (4 sets × 3 min + 1 min passive recovery) under randomly varying numerical conditions. Without additional help, restrictions, or instructions from outside, the players changed their behavior in the direction of professional players after only 3 weeks, with three sessions per week. A central idea for this study was again the question, "Who was the teacher of the first?" related to team tactical behavior. Thus, it is not about inventing the wheel again but rather about experiencing this "aha" effect during learning (Kounios and Beeman 2009). It is often assumed that a therapist, teacher, or coach is necessary to learn something. There is no doubt about the possible supportive influence of a therapist, coach, or teacher. However, their necessity is called into question when it comes to the question of the very first beginnings themselves. And interestingly, it was often the first ones who did not know about the limitations and latent assumptions and simply did it. And people are actually "aware" of this when they learn to crawl, walk, run, etc., in their earliest childhood. The main motivation for this and for the development of humankind was and is the natural curiosity to discover something new. Sometimes it simply helps just to arouse curiosity instead of making the patient, athlete, or learner dependent on constant instructions and feedback.

3.8 Applying Differential Learning in the Conditional Area

For the transfer of system-theoretical laws to other areas, the abstraction of the original qualities was identified in Sect. 2.4 as the first step to assign foreign qualities to the variables in a second step and to interpret them in the original sense of the process of the system. In this case, a transfer to the conditional area no longer means paying attention to the similarity of the kinematics but to the parameters of strength and endurance training. In the area of strength training, this would correspond to the biomechanical parameters of starting power, explosive power, maximum power, and speed. Transferring these two forms of movement, such as jumps and sprints, would shift the focus to joint moment progressions in combination with stretch-shortening cycles. In the endurance area, parameters known as critical thresholds would most likely be used, as these offer the system the opportunity to compare upper and lower threshold states with each other to switch to possible alternatives. The study situation in the area of differential strength training is by no means as favorable as that in the endurance area (see Chap. 8).

The first studies on the specific development of jumping power were carried out in handball jump training (Jaitner and Pfeiffer 2003). For this purpose, a women's first league handball team was randomly divided into two groups, of which the classic group performed blocked two-legged jump training over obstacles, and the differential group performed the same number of two-legged jumps, but the height and distance of the obstacles were constantly changed. After 5 weeks and 10 training sessions, both groups showed significant increases in drop-jump performance, but only the differential training group also showed significant increases in jump height in the handball jump throw. The second finding in particular indicates an improvement in adaptability under new conditions. Fuchs et al. (2020a) conducted a similar intervention with first division volleyball players over a period of six weeks during the season. While performance in the control group declined by approximately 5%, the DL group was able to increase their jumping performance by an average of approximately 12%. Motor tests conducted in parallel indicate additional preventive effects of differential jump training (Fuchs et al. 2020b).

Several studies in the area of strength training (Budija et al. 2017; Hegen 2018; Hegen et al. 2015; Horst et al. 2016b; Tug et al. 2017) provided evidence of the same increases in performance with differential strength training at only 60% of the maximum external load as with repetition-based training with up to 100% external load and less production of creatine kinase, which is typically associated as a measure for the damage of skeletal muscle, heart, or brain tissue. The studies were conducted in the bench press and squat areas. For example, the upward and downward movements, speeds, symmetry, etc., were varied during the bench press. The barbell was shifted to the left when going down and to the right when pressing up; the left arm was bent first and then the right and symmetrically stretched, symmetrically bent and stretched to the right first and then to the left; the barbell was lowered to chest height but pressed up again at neck or navel height, etc. The same procedure was used for squats with a long barbell. The squats with the barbell were performed in the same way. It was interesting to note that the differentially trained groups had no failures due to injury, whereas the repetition-based groups had between 10% and 20% failures due to injury each time. Similar tendencies to utilize different levers can now also be observed in newer fashion sports such as calisthenics.

The earlier-mentioned study on jumping rope was a first step toward addressing another direction of research. The question of the effects of DL when learning movements with a stronger conditional component in conjunction with a high parallel coordination component was pursued. Within the framework of the rope skipping study, the interaction between endurance and complex parallel coordination (in contrast to sequential complexity) was to be investigated (John and Schöllhorn 2018; John et al. 2022). As part of a study on Olympic weightlifting, we investigated the interaction of complex coordination and strength in relation to four different learning approaches in beginners. In addition to an altered brain activation through DL, the study interestingly showed that even absolute beginners had very characteristic barbell time courses (Ammar et al. 2024a, b, c). This not only indicates earlier discussed individual movement patterns but also individual responses to comparable interventions. In this area, too, the first studies led to more questions than answers.

After the first publication of the DL, a significant expansion and tolerance for diversity of practice was observable in therapy, sport, and also in the area of music. The ideas of DL quickly spread under various names such as life kinetics (Lutz 2008 (the original work was based on an article of Beck (2008) on a possible neurophysiological explanation of DL), nonlinear pedagogy (Chow et al. 2006), and constraints-led approach (Davids et al. 2008) (– K. Davids and D. Araujo were introduced into DL in 2001 and 2003—although the constraints-based learning term was applied by Newell in 1986 to summarize existing approaches, the content changed drastically after 2003)), the athletic skills model (Wormhoudt et al. 2018), (– G. Savelsbergh was introduced into DL in 2004), the Frans Bosch (introduced in 2005) training method, or creative training as a modification of life kinetics (Nowak and Seewald 2017; Voglsinger et al. 2023), and multiple other interpretations. Most of these authors received personal introductions to DL. Unfortunately, the new names given and their interpretation often reflect a cultural background that widely neglected reform pedagogical ideas in the concepts of kindergarten (Froebel 1826), learner-centered teaching (Basedow 1774; GutsMuths 1796; Pestalozzi 1781–1787; Steiner 1907), and problem-based teaching (Dewey 1903; Kerschensteiner 1912) and had been transferred to sports pedagogy in the 60s and 70s in mainland Europe (Arbeitsgruppe 1982; Brodtmann and Frankfurter Arbeitsgruppe 1982).

Ongoing research is attempting to combine the DL approach with models based on individuality per se, e.g. the ActionType System approach developed by Ralph Hyppolite and Bertrand Theraulaz (Theraulaz and Hyppolite 2021), which establishes a clear link between individual motor preferences and the Jung typology, or

Magnetic field dependent approach where neuronal growth during embryonic phase depends on the fluctuations of the earth magnetic field (Schöllhorn et al 2022). Both are expected to assist in specifying the noise applied depending on the person and the situation.

In sum, the studies on differential learning from a systems dynamics perspective merely indicate the potential of its scope and are probably no more than a drop in the ocean at the moment. Nevertheless, the many positive and varied indications encourage further studies from a different perspective. This primarily involves a more differentiated approach to the problem of learning in general and that of therapy in particular as a phase transition in connection with individuality and situatedness.

Overall, although the differential learning strategies that were mainly developed in the field of sports due to their general basis in system dynamics, neurophysiology, biomechanics, and artificial neural net theory, the findings have similar consequences for therapy.

In general, varying movement execution and unpredictability in training can significantly impact brain activity and learning processes. In particular:

A. Fluctuations in movement patterns can lead to more stable and flexible motor behavior, or tactical learning in sports. Physiotherapists can take advantage of variability to improve patients' adaptability in rehabilitation.
B. Different people respond differently to movement variation, and this is changing over time. In consequence, rehabilitation exercises should be tailored to each patient's needs.
C. Adjusting exercise conditions—such as changing equipment, surfaces, or movement constraints—can encourage patients to explore and develop new movement strategies.
D. Allowing patients to self-organize their movement patterns by increasing variability and overloading the control-related brain structures, rather than relying solely on external instructions and repetition-without-repetition, can foster problem-solving, independence, and long-term learning.
E. Encouraging curiosity and exploration in rehabilitation may enhance motor recovery by leveraging natural learning processes, much like early childhood development.
F. Gradual variation provides predictability, while chaotic variation introduces randomness—both can enhance neural activation and learning in different ways.
G. Movement variation influences brain waves linked to attention, memory, and creativity. This suggests that integrating varied and unpredictable exercises may improve motor learning and recovery.
H. Strategies like differential movement training and controlled variation in exercise frequency may have benefits for neurological rehabilitation and preventing age-related cognitive decline.

In practice, these aspects can be applied for therapy by incorporating structured yet variable movement patterns in patients' rehabilitation programs to optimize motor learning and recovery. They can be applied by configuring therapy sessions that integrate structured yet varied movement tasks, helping patients regain function more effectively. Examples of specific applications of DL in areas of physiotherapy are reported in the following chapters.

Questions

1. What are the fundamental differences between traditional repetition-based training and the Differential Learning approach?
2. How does the concept of stochastic resonance contribute to motor learning and skill acquisition?
3. What role does movement variability play in enhancing adaptability and self-organization in motor learning?
4. Which biomechanically based interventions lead to central nervous stimulation and self-organization?
5. What experimental evidence from sports supports the effectiveness of movement variability in learning and performance?

6. How can the stochastic resonance model be transferred to the training of endurance sports?
   A. By adding white-noise audio during warm-up only.
   B. By periodically altering cadence, gradient, body-/extremity-posture, footwear hardness, etc., so that moderate biomechanical noise enhances proprioceptive sensitivity and aerobic efficiency.
   C. By holding speed constant and minimizing variability in stride.
   D. By replacing outdoor runs with treadmill sessions at fixed incline.
   E. By masking all sensory input with earplugs and blindfolds.
7. In what ways can the principles of movement variability and self-organisation be applied to physiotherapy and rehabilitation?
   A. By prescribing one error-free movement and having the patient repeat it 200 times.
   B. By using robotic exoskeletons that lock joints into a single trajectory.
   C. By designing tasks that systematically vary load, direction and timing so the patient's nervous system explores alternative coordinations and selects the momentarily most functional.
   D. By eliminating any unpredictable surface or perturbation.
   E. By instructing the patient to observe but never perform the task.
8. What are the potential risks of too much or too little variability in training, and how can they be managed?
   A. Excessive variability guarantees injury; zero variability guarantees mastery.
   B. Too little variability can lead to over-use syndromes and stagnation, whereas too much can cause chaos and inconsistent performance; regulating noise intensity and monitoring fatigue keeps variability in a beneficial window.
   C. High variability always improves motivation, so it carries no risk.
   D. Low variability accelerates learning for all athletes.
   E. Risks are irrelevant because the nervous system self-protects automatically.
9. How does the research presented in this chapter lay the groundwork for the application of DL in physiotherapy, as discussed in later chapters?
   A. By proving that repetition is indispensable for neural recovery.
   B. By demonstrating that only visual feedback drives cortical change.
   C. By showing that spinal reflexes cannot be modified in adults.
   D. By documenting neurophysiological and biomechanical evidence that variable, noise-rich practice reorganizes central pathways, a principle later translated into patient-specific therapy protocols.
   E. By concluding that movement variability is detrimental to motor relearning.
10. How does DL challenge conventional assumptions about error correction and feedback in learning?
   A. It requires continuous real-time verbal corrections from the coach.
   B. It replaces physical practice with mental imagery alone.
   C. It argues that external error correction can be counter-productive because amplified intrinsic variability already supplies sufficient information for self-optimization, reducing the need for augmented feedback.
   D. It keeps the traditional hierarchy but adds vibration to each joint.
   E. It views errors as pathological noise that must be eliminated immediately.

References

Acree MC (2021) The myth of statistical inference. Springer Nature, Cham. https://doi.org/10.1007/978-3-030-73257-8

Albrecht S, Janssen D, Quarz E, Newell KM, Schöllhorn WI (2014) Individuality of movements in music—finger and body movements during playing of the flute. Hum Mov Sci 35:131–144. https://doi.org/10.1016/j.humov.2014.03.010

Ammar A, Boujelbane MA, Simak M, Fraile-Fuente I, Rizz N, Washif J, Zmijewski P, Jahrami H, Schöllhorn

WI (2024a) Unveiling the acute neurophysiological responses to strength training: an exploratory study on novices performing weightlifting bouts with different motor learning models. Biol Sport 41:249. https://doi.org/10.5114/biolsport.2024.133481

Ammar A, Salem A, Simak M, Horst F, Schöllhorn WI (2024b) Acute effects of motor learning models on technical efficiency in strength-coordination exercises: a comparative analysis of Olympic snatch biomechanics in beginners. Biol Sport:151–161. https://doi.org/10.5114/biolsport.2025.141662

Ammar A, Simak ML, Salem A, Horst F, Schöllhorn WI (2024c) Unveiling individuality in the early phase of motor learning: a machine learning approach for analysing weightlifting technique in novices. Front Bioeng Biotechnol 12:1426058. https://doi.org/10.3389/fbioe.2024.1426058

Apidogo JB, Burdack J, Schöllhorn WI (2021) Repetition without repetition or differential learning of multiple techniques in volleyball? Int J Environ Res Public Health 18(19). https://doi.org/10.3390/ijerph181910499

Apidogo JB, Burdack J, Schöllhorn WI (2022) Learning multiple movements in parallel-accurately and in random order, or each with added noise? Int J Environ Res Public Health 19(17). https://doi.org/10.3390/ijerph191710960

Apidogo JB, Ammar A, Salem A, Burdack J, Schöllhorn WI (2023) Resonance effects in variable practice for handball, basketball, and volleyball skills: a study on contextual interference and differential learning. Sports (Basel) 12(1). https://doi.org/10.3390/sports12010005

Arbeitsgruppe Frankfurt (1982) Offener Sportunterricht. Rowohlt, Reinbek

Ashby WR (1947) Principles of the self-organizing dynamic system. J Gen Psychol 37(2):125–128. https://doi.org/10.1080/00221309.1947.9918144

Aydilek E, Jäger K, Xhaxho K, Akdas R, Wallbach M, Wulf G, Brökers N (2022) Hypernatriämie und Polyurie bei einer Patientin mit Erstdiagnose einer sekundären akuten myeloischen Leukämie [Hypernatremia and polyuria in a female patient with an initial diagnosis of secondary acute myeloid leukemia]. Inn Med (Heidelb) 63(11):1194–1199. https://doi.org/10.1007/s00108-022-01381-1

Bartussek R, Hänggi P, Jung P (1994) Stochastic resonance in optical bistable systems. Phys Rev E 49(5):3930–3939. https://doi.org/10.1103/PhysRevE.49.3930

Basedow JB (1774) Das in Dessau errichtet Philantropinum. Crusius, Leipzig

Beck F (2008) Sportmotorik und Gehirn. Sportwiss 38: 423–450. https://doi.org/10.1007/BF03217046.

Beckmann H, Schöllhorn WI (2003) Differencial learning in shot put mechanics, physiology. Psychology – first European workshop on movement science, Münster, Germany, 22–24 May 2003

Beckmann H, Schöllhorn WI (2006) Differenzielles Lernen im Kugelstoßen. Leistungssport 36(4):44–50

Beckmann H, Winkel C, Schöllhorn WI (2010) Optimal range of variation in hockey technique training. International Journal of Sport Psychology 41(4, Suppl):5–45.

Beggs JM, Plenz D (2003) Neuronal avalanches in neocortical circuits. J Neurosci 23(35):11167–11177. https://doi.org/10.1523/jneurosci.23-35-11167.2003

Bozkurt S (2018) The effects of differential learning and traditional learning trainings on technical developemnt of football players. J Educ Train Stud 6(4):25–29

Brady F (1997) Contextual interference and teaching golf skills. Percept Mot Skills 84(1):347–350. https://doi.org/10.2466/pms.1997.84.1.347

Brady F (2004) Contextual interference: a meta-analytic study. Percept Mot Skills 99(1):116–126. https://doi.org/10.2466/pms.99.1.116-126

Broadbent DP, Causer J, Williams AM, Ford PR (2017) The role of error processing in the contextual interference effect during the training of perceptual-cognitive skills. J Exp Psychol Hum Percept Perform 43(7):1329–1342. https://doi.org/10.1037/xhp0000375

Brodtmann DD, Frankfurter Arbeitsgruppe K (1982) Offener Sportunterricht: analysieren und planen. Rowohlt, Reinbek

Budija N, Hegen P, Schöllhorn WI (2017) Differential training applied in strength training for woman. 22nd annual congress of the European College of Sport Science (ECSS): 5–8 July 2017, MetropolisRuhr, Germany

Burdack J, Schöllhorn WI (2022) Cognitive enhancement through differential rope skipping after math lesson. Int J Environ Res Public Health 20(1). https://doi.org/10.3390/ijerph20010205

Carhart-Harris RL (2018) The entropic brain – revisited. Neuropharmacology 142:167–178. https://doi.org/10.1016/j.neuropharm.2018.03.010

Carhart-Harris R, Leech R, Hellyer P, Shanahan M, Feilding A, Tagliazucchi E, Chialvo D, Nutt D (2014) The entropic brain: a theory of conscious states informed by neuroimaging research with psychedelic drugs [hypothesis and theory]. Front Hum Neurosci 8. https://doi.org/10.3389/fnhum.2014.00020

Chow JY, Davids K, Button C, Shuttleworth R, Renshaw I, Araújo D (2006) Nonlinear pedagogy: a constraints-led framework for understanding emergence of game play and movement skills. Nonlinear Dynamics Psychol Life Sci 10(1):71–103

Collins JJ (1999) Fishing for function in noise. Nature 402(6759):241–242. https://doi.org/10.1038/46179

Collins JJ, Imhoff TT, Grigg P (1996) Noise-enhanced tactile sensation. Nature 383(6603):770. https://doi.org/10.1038/383770a0

Cordo P, Inglis JT, Verschueren S, Collins JJ, Merfeld DM, Rosenblum S, Buckley S, Moss F (1996) Noise in human muscle spindles. Nature 383(6603):769–770. https://doi.org/10.1038/383769a0

Coutinho D, Santos S, Gonçalves B, Travassos B, Wong DP, Schöllhorn W, Sampaio J (2018) The effects of an enrichment training program for youth football attackers. PLoS One 13(6):e0199008. https://doi.org/10.1371/journal.pone.0199008

Davids K, Button C, Bennett S (2008) Dynamics of skill acquisition: A constraints-led approach. Human Kinetics, Champaign

de Arcangelis L, Perrone-Capano C, Herrmann HJ (2006) Self-organized criticality model for brain plasticity. Phys Rev Lett 96(2):028107. https://doi.org/10.1103/PhysRevLett.96.028107

Dewey J (1903) Democracy and education. Elem School Teach 4:193

Dhruv NT, Niemi JB, Harry JD, Lipsitz LA, Collins JJ (2002) Enhancing tactile sensation in older adults with electrical noise stimulation. Neuroreport 13(5):597–600. https://doi.org/10.1097/00001756-200204160-00012

Dietrich A (2003) Functional neuroanatomy of altered states of consciousness: the transient hypofrontality hypothesis. Conscious Cogn 12(2):231–256. https://doi.org/10.1016/S1053-8100(02)00046-6

Dietrich A (2006) Transient hypofrontality as a mechanism for the psychological effects of exercise. Psychiatry Res 145(1):79–83. https://doi.org/10.1016/j.psychres.2005.07.033

Dietz V (2002) Do human bipeds use quadrupedal coordination? Trends Neurosci 25(9):462–467. https://doi.org/10.1016/s0166-2236(02)02229-4

Dietz V, Michel J (2009) Human bipeds use quadrupedal coordination during locomotion. Ann N Y Acad Sci 1164:97–103. https://doi.org/10.1111/j.1749-6632.2008.03710.x

Esch T (2014) Die neuronale Basis von Meditation und Achtsamkeit. SUCHT 60(1):21–28. https://doi.org/10.1024/0939-5911.a000288

Feest U (2019) Why replication is overrated. Philos Sci 86(5):895–905. https://doi.org/10.1086/705451

Feest U (2024) What is the replication crisis a crisis of? Philos Sci 91(5):1361–1371. https://doi.org/10.1017/psa.2024.2

Fisher RA, Russell EJ (1922) On the mathematical foundations of theoretical statistics. Philos Trans R Soc Lond Ser A Contain Papers Math Phys Character 222(594–604):309–368. https://doi.org/10.1098/rsta.1922.0009

Fitts PM, Posner MI (1967) Human performance. Brooks/Cole, Pacific Grove

Frank TD, Michelbrink M, Beckmann H, Schöllhorn WI (2008) A quantitative dynamical systems approach to differential learning: self-organization principle and order parameter equations. Biol Cybern 98(1):19–31. https://doi.org/10.1007/s00422-007-0193-x

Froebel FWA (1826) Die Menschenerziehung, die Erziehungs- Unterrichts- und Lehrkunst, angestrebt in der allgemeinen deutschen Erziehungsanstalt zu Keilhau. (Human education, the art of education, instruction and teaching, pursued in the general German educational institution at Keilhau). Wiebrad, Munich

Fuchs PX, Fusco A, Bell JW, von Duvillard SP, Cortis C, Wagner H (2020a) Effect of differential training on female volleyball spike-jump technique and performance. Int J Sports Physiol Perform 15(7):1019–1025. https://doi.org/10.1123/ijspp.2019-0488

Fuchs PX, Fusco A, Cortis C, Wagner H (2020b) Effects of differential jump training on balance performance in female volleyball players. Appl Sci 10:5921. https://doi.org/10.3390/app10175921

Gammaitoni L, Hänggi P, Jung P, Marchesoni F (1998) Stochastic resonance. Rev Mod Phys 70(1):223–287. https://doi.org/10.1103/RevModPhys.70.223

Gaspar A, Santos S, Coutinho D, Gonçalves B, Sampaio J, Leite N (2019) Acute effects of differential learning on football kicking performance and in countermovement jump. PLoS One 14(10):e0224280. https://doi.org/10.1371/journal.pone.0224280

Gaulhofer K, Streicher M (1924) Grundzüge des Österreichischen Schulturnens. Deutscher Verlag für Jugend und Volk, Wien

Gigerenzer G (2004) Mindless statistics. J Socio-Econ 33(5):587–606. https://doi.org/10.1016/j.socec.2004.09.033

Gigerenzer G (2018) Statistical rituals: the replication delusion and how we got there. Adv Methods Pract Psychol Sci 1(2):198–218. https://doi.org/10.1177/2515245918771329

Gilmore R (1981) Catastrophe theory for scientists and engineers. Wiley, New York

Goleman D, Davidson RJ (2017) Altered traits: science reveals how meditation changes your mind, brain, and body. Penguin, London

Gravelle DC, Laughton CA, Dhruv NT, Katdare KD, Niemi JB, Lipsitz LA, Collins JJ (2002) Noise-enhanced balance control in older adults. Neuroreport 13(15):1853–1856. https://doi.org/10.1097/00001756-200210280-00004

Gray CM, König P, Engel AK, Singer W (1989) Oscillatory responses in cat visual cortex exhibit intercolumnar synchronization which reflects global stimulus properties. Nature 338(6213):334–337. https://doi.org/10.1038/338334a0

GutsMuths JCF (1796) Spiele zur Übung und Erholung des Körpers und Geistes: gesammelt und bearbeitet für die Jugend, ihre Erzieher und alle Freunde unschuldiger Jugendfreuden. Buchahndlung der Erziehungsanstalt, Schnepfenthal

Hegen P (2018) Krafttraining auf der Basis systemdynamischer Prinzipien. Kovacz, Dr. Verlag, Hamburg

Hegen P, Schöllhorn W (2012) Lernen an Unterschieden und nicht durch Wiederholung – Über ‚Umwege' schneller zur besserenTechnik: Differenzielles Lernen im Fußball. fussballtraining 30–37

Hegen P, Polywka G, Schöllhorn WI (2015) The differential learning approach in strength training. 20th annual congress of the european college of sport science, Malmö, Sweden, 24–27 June 2015

Henz D, Schöllhorn WI (2016) Differential training facilitates early consolidation in motor learning. Front Behav Neurosci 10:199. https://doi.org/10.3389/fnbeh.2016.00199

Henz D, Schöllhorn WI (2017a) EEG brain activity in dynamic health qigong training: same effects for mental practice and physical training? Front Psychol 8:154. https://doi.org/10.3389/fpsyg.2017.00154

Henz D, Schöllhorn WI (2017b) Temporal courses in EEG theta and alpha activity in the dynamic health Qigong techniques Wu Qin Xi and Liu Zi Jue. Front Psychol 8:2291. https://doi.org/10.3389/fpsyg.2017.02291

Henz D, Lattwein M, Schöllhorn WI (2014a) Differential training as an intervention strategy to prevent choking under pressure in basketball freethrow. 19th annual congress of the European College of Sport Science, Amsterdam, 2–5 July

Henz DL, Leinberger O, Schöllhorn WI (2014b). EEG brain activation patterns in differential and mental differential soccer shooting training. 19th annual congress of the European College of Sports Science, Amsterdam, The Netherlands

Henz D, John A, Merz C, Schöllhorn WI (2018) Post-task effects on EEG brain activity differ for various differential learning and contextual interference protocols. Front Hum Neurosci 12:19. https://doi.org/10.3389/fnhum.2018.00019

Hölzel BK, Carmody J, Evans KC, Hoge EA, Dusek JA, Morgan L, Pitman RK, Lazar SW (2010) Stress reduction correlates with structural changes in the amygdala. Soc Cogn Affect Neurosci 5(1):11–17. https://doi.org/10.1093/scan/nsp034

Hölzel BK, Carmody J, Vangel M, Congleton C, Yerramsetti SM, Gard T, Lazar SW (2011) Mindfulness practice leads to increases in regional brain gray matter density. Psychiatry Res 191(1):36–43. https://doi.org/10.1016/j.pscychresns.2010.08.006

Hommel B, Müsseler J, Aschersleben G, Prinz W (2001) The theory of event coding (TEC): a framework for perception and action planning. Behav Brain Sci 24(5):849–878; discussion 878–937. https://doi.org/10.1017/s0140525x01000103

Horst F, Kramer F, Schäfer B, Eekhoff A, Hegen P, Nigg BM, Schöllhorn WI (2016a) Daily changes of individual gait patterns identified by means of support vector machines. Gait Posture 49:309–314. https://doi.org/10.1016/j.gaitpost.2016.07.073

Horst F, Rupprecht C, Schmitt M, Hegen P, Schöllhorn WI (2016b) Muscular activity in conventional and differential back squat exercise. 21th annual congress of the European College of Sport Science (ECSS), Vienna, Austria, 6–9 July 2016

Horst F, Eekhoff A, Newell KM, Schöllhorn WI (2017a) Intra-individual gait patterns across different time-scales as revealed by means of a supervised learning model using kernel-based discriminant regression. PLoS One 12(6):e0179738. https://doi.org/10.1371/journal.pone.0179738

Horst F, Mildner M, Schöllhorn WI (2017b) One-year persistence of individual gait patterns identified in a follow-up study – a call for individualised diagnose and therapy. Gait Posture 58:476–480. https://doi.org/10.1016/j.gaitpost.2017.09.003

Horst F, Slijepcevic D, Simak M, Horsak B, Schöllhorn WI, Zeppelzauer M (2023) Modeling biological individuality using machine learning: a study on human gait. Comput Struct Biotechnol J 21:3414–3423. https://doi.org/10.1016/j.csbj.2023.06.009

Hubel DH, Wiesel TN (1964) Effects of monocular deprivation in kittens. Naunyn Schmiedebergs Arch Exp Pathol Pharmakol 248:492–497. https://doi.org/10.1007/bf00348878

Humpert, V & Schöllhorn, WI (2006). Vergleich von Techniktrainingsansätzen zum Tennisaufschlag. In A. Ferrauti & H. Rcmmcrt (Hrsg.). Trainingswissenschaft im Freizeitsport (S. 121-124). Hamburg: Czwalina.

Ioannidis JPA (2005) Why most published research findings are false. PLoS Med 2(8):e124. https://doi.org/10.1371/journal.pmed.0020124

Jäger JM, Schöllhorn WI (2007) Situation-orientated recognition of tactical patterns in volleyball. J Sports Sci 25(12):1345–1353. https://doi.org/10.1080/02640410701287230

Jäger JM, Schöllhorn WI (2012) Identifying individuality and variability in team tactics by means of statistical shape analysis and multilayer perceptrons. Hum Mov Sci 31(2):303–317. https://doi.org/10.1016/j.humov.2010.09.005

Jäger JM, Alichmann M, Schöllhorn WI (2003a) Erkennung von Ermüdungszuständen anhand von Bodenreaktionskräften. In: Brüggemann GP, Morey-Klapsing G (eds) Biologische Systeme. Czwalina, Hamburg, pp 179–183

Jäger JM, Schöllhorn WI, Schwerdfeger B (2003b) A pattern recognition approach for an opponent specific classification of tactical moves in team sports. Proceedings of the 8th annual congress of the European College of Sport Science, Salzburg

Jaitner T, Pfeiffer M (2003) Developing jumping strength based on system dynamics principles. European workshop on movement science – "Mechanics, physiology, psychology", Münster

Janssen D, Schöllhorn WI, Lubienetzki J, Fölling K, Kokenge H, Davids K (2008) Recognition of emotions in gait patterns by means of artificial neural nets. J Nonverbal Behav 32(2):79–92. https://doi.org/10.1007/s10919-007-0045-3

Janssen D, Schöllhorn WI, Newell KM, Jäger JM, Rost F, Vehof K (2011) Diagnosing fatigue in gait patterns by support vector machines and self-organizing maps. Hum Mov Sci 30(5):966–975. https://doi.org/10.1016/j.humov.2010.08.010

John A, Schöllhorn WI (2018) Acute effects of instructed and self-created variable rope skipping on EEG brain activity and heart rate variability. Front Behav Neurosci 12:311. https://doi.org/10.3389/fnbeh.2018.00311

John AT, Barthel A, Wind J, Rizzi N, Schöllhorn WI (2022) Acute effects of various movement noise in differential learning of rope skipping on brain and heart recovery analyzed by means of multiscale fuzzy measure entropy. Front Behav Neurosci 16:816334. https://doi.org/10.3389/fnbeh.2022.816334

Jung P, Bartussek R (1996) Generation of higher harmonics in noisy nonlinear systems. In: Millonas M (ed) Fluctuations and order: the new synthesis. Springer, pp 35–52. https://doi.org/10.1007/978-1-4612-3992-5_3

Kabat-Zinn J (1994) Wherever you go, there you are: mindfulness meditation in everyday life. Hachette Books, New York

Kantz H, Schreiber T (1994) Nonlinear time series analysis, 1st edn. Cambridge University Press, Cambridge

Kelso JAS (1995) Dynamic patterns: the self-organization of brain and behavior. MIT Press, Cambridge

Kerschensteiner G (1912) Begriff der Arbeitsschule n der Pädagogik. Teubner, Leipzig

Kjaer TW, Bertelsen C, Piccini P, Brooks D, Alving J, Lou HC (2002) Increased dopamine tone during meditation-induced change of consciousness. Brain Res Cogn Brain Res 13(2):255–259. https://doi.org/10.1016/s0926-6410(01)00106-9

Komi PV (1984) Physiological and biomechanical correlates of muscle function: effects of muscle structure and stretch-shortening cycle on force and speed. Exerc Sport Sci Rev 12:81–121

Kounios J, Beeman M (2009) The Aha! Moment: the cognitive neuroscience of insight. Curr Dir Psychol Sci 18(4):210–216. https://doi.org/10.1111/j.1467-8721.2009.01638.x

Krauss P, Metzner C, Schilling A, Schütz C, Tziridis K, Fabry B, Schulze H (2017) Adaptive stochastic resonance for unknown and variable input signals. Sci Rep 7(1):2450. https://doi.org/10.1038/s41598-017-02644-w

Lin M, Lucas HC, Shmueli G (2013) Research commentary—too big to fail: large samples and the p-value problem. Inf Syst Res 24(4):906–917. https://doi.org/10.1287/isre.2013.0480

Liu YT, Luo ZY, Mayer-Kress G, Newell KM (2012) Self-organized criticality and learning a new coordination task. Hum Mov Sci 31(1):40–54. https://doi.org/10.1016/j.humov.2011.06.005

Lutz H (2008) Life Kinetik®: Gehirntraining durch Bewegung. Gräfe und Unzer Verlag GmbH, München

Magill RA, Hall KG (1990) A review of the contextual interference effect in motor skill acquisition. Hum Mov Sci 9(3–5):241–289. https://doi.org/10.1016/0167-9457(90)90005-X

Mahlo F (1965) Theoretische Probleme der taktischen Ausbildung in den Sportspielen. Theor Prax Korperkult 14(9):809–815

Mathy F, Feldman J (2012) What's magic about magic numbers? Chunking and data compression in short-term memory. Cognition 122(3):346–362. https://doi.org/10.1016/j.cognition.2011.11.003

Maxwell JP, Masters RSW, Kerr E, Weedon E (2001) The implicit benefit of learning without errors. Q J Exp Psychol A Hum Exp Psychol 54A(4):1049–1068. https://doi.org/10.1080/02724980143000073

Meinel K (1960) Bewegungslehre. Volk und Wissen. Volkseigener Verlag, Berlin

Mester L (1959) Gemeinschaftserziehung und Mannschaftsspiel. Das Spiel: Kongress für Leibeserziehung, Osnabrück, Germany, 3–5 Oktober 1958

Miller GA (1956) The magical number seven, plus or minus two: Some limits on our capacity for processing information. Psychol Rev 63(2):81–97. https://doi.org/10.1037/h0043158

Millonas M (1996) Fluctuation and order – the new synthesis. Springer. https://doi.org/10.1007/978-1-4612-3992-5

Mitaim S, Kosko B (1998) Adaptive stochastic resonance. Proc IEEE 86(11):2152–2183. https://doi.org/10.1109/5.726785

Moss F, Pierson D, O'Gorman D (1994) Stochastic resonance: tutorial and update. Int J Bifurc Chaos 4(6):1383–1397. https://doi.org/10.1142/s0218127494001118

Narasimhan K (1998) Unexpected rewards. Nat Neurosci 1(4):265–265. https://doi.org/10.1038/1076

Newell KM (1989) On task and theory specificity. J Mot Behav 21(1):92–96. https://doi.org/10.1080/00222895.1989.10735467

Newell KM, van Emmerik REA, Sprague RL (1993) Stereotypy and varaibility. In: Newell KM, Corcos DM (eds) Varaibility and motor control. Human Kinetics, Champaign, pp 475–496

Nowak M, Seewald J (2017) Beweg dein Hirn: Das tägliche 10-Minuten-Programm für mehr Potenzial, Kreativität und Lebensqualität. Gräfe und Unzer Verlag GmbH, München

Oftadeh S, Bahram A, Yaali R, Ghadiri F, Schöllhorn WI (2021) External focus or differential learning: is there an additive effect on learning a futsal goal kick? Int J Environ Res Public Health 19(1). https://doi.org/10.3390/ijerph19010317

Pestalozzi JH (1781–1787) Lienhard und Gertrud. Ein Buch für das Volk, vol 1-4. Georg Jakob Decker, Berlin

Popper K (1935) Logik der Forschung. Springer, Berlin

Poureghbali S, Arede J, Rehfeld K, Schöllhorn W, Leite N. Want to Impact Physical, Technical, and Tactical Performance during Basketball Small-Sided Games in Youth Athletes? Try Differential Learning Beforehand. Int J Environ Res Public Health. 2020;17(24):9279. https://doi.org/10.3390/ijerph17249279

Prinz W (1990) A common coding approach to perception and action. In: Neumann O, Prinz W (eds) Relationships between perception and action: current approaches. Springer, Berlin/Heidelberg, pp 167–201. https://doi.org/10.1007/978-3-642-75348-0_7

Priplata A, Niemi J, Salen M, Harry J, Lipsitz LA, Collins JJ (2002) Noise-enhanced human balance control. Phys Rev Lett 89(23):238101. https://doi.org/10.1103/PhysRevLett.89.238101

Priplata AA, Niemi JB, Harry JD, Lipsitz LA, Collins JJ (2003) Vibrating insoles and balance control in elderly people. Lancet 362(9390):1123–1124. https://doi.org/10.1016/s0140-6736(03)14470-4

Römer J, Schöllhorn WI, Jaitner T, Preuss R (2003) Differenzielles Lernen bei der Aufschlagannahme im Volleyball Messplätze, Messplatztraining, motorisches Lernen: ausgewählte Beiträge; 5. gemeinsames Symposium der dvs-Sektionen Biomechanik, Sportmotorik und Trainingswissenschaft, Leipzig, 19–21 Sept 2002

Santos S, Coutinho D, Goncalves B, Schöllhorn WI, Sampaio J, Leite N (2017) Exploring the differential learning routes on creative and tactical behaviour in association football players. Complex systems in sport, International congress linking theory and practice, Barcelona

Santos S, Coutinho D, Gonçalves B, Schöllhorn W, Sampaio J, Leite N (2018) Differential learning as a key training approach to improve creative and tactical behavior in soccer. Res Q Exerc Sport 89(1):11–24. https://doi.org/10.1080/02701367.2017.1412063

Schneider K, Zernicke RF, Schmidt RA, Hart TJ (1989) Changes in limb dynamics during the practice of rapid arm movements. J Biomech 22(8):805–817. https://doi.org/10.1016/0021-9290(89)90064-X

Schöllhorn WI (1993) Biomechanische Einzelfallanalyse im Diskuswurf. Prozess- und produktorientierte Technikanalyse mechanischer Energieformen, vol 19. Harri Deutsch Verlag, Frankfurt am Main

Schöllhorn WI (1995) Time course oriented analysis of biomechanical movement patterns by means of orthogonal reference functions. XVth congress of the international society of biomechanics, Jväskylä

Schöllhorn WI (1996) Topology and metrics of a ballistic grossmotor movement during a learning process. First conference on bernsteins traditions in motor control, University Park, PA, USA

Schöllhorn WI (1999a) Individualität – ein vernachlässigter Parameter. Leistungssport, 29 (2), 5–12.

Schöllhorn WI (1999b) Pracitcal consequences of biomechanically determined individuality and fluctuations on motor learning. XVIIth congress of the International Society of Biomchanics, Calgary, Canada

Schöllhorn WI (2000) Applications of system dynamic principles to technique and strength training. Acta Academiae Qlympiquae Estoniae 8:67–85

Schöllhorn WI (2003) Coordination dynamics and its consequences on sports. Int J Comput Sci Sport 2(2):40–46

Schöllhorn WI (2016) Invited commentary: differential learning is different from contextual interference learning. Hum Mov Sci 47:240–245. https://doi.org/10.1016/j.humov.2015.11.018

Schöllhorn WI, Bauer HU (1998) Identifying individual movement styles in high performance sports by means of self-organizing Kohonen maps. 16th international symposium on biomechanics in sports, 1998, Konstanz. https://ojs.ub.uni-konstanz.de/cpa/article/view/1556

Schöllhorn WI, Paschke M (2007) Differenzielles Training. Volleyballmagazin 12:28–36

Schöllhorn WI, Hurth P, Mendoza L (1995) Schnelligkeitstraining: die Sprint- und Laufschule für alle Sportarten. Rowohlt, Reinbek

Schöllhorn WI, Müller E, Lindinger S, Raschner C, Schwameder H (2001a) Individuality and generality in ski turning techniques. In: Müller E, Schwameder H, Raschner C, Lindinger S, Kornexl E (eds) Second international congress on science and skiing II. Dr. Kovac, Hamburg, pp 69–83

Schöllhorn WI, Röber F, Jaitner T, Hellstern W, Käubler W (2001b) Discrete and continuous effects of traditional and differential sprint training. 6th annual congress of the european college of sport science: perspectives and profiles Cologne. https://www.ecss.mobi/DATA/EDSS/C06/06-0311.pdf

Schöllhorn WI, Römer J, Jaitner T (2001c) Comparing three volleyball spiking techniques by means of a process oriented pattern recognition approach. XVIIIth congress of the International Society of Biomechanics Zürich, Switzerland

Schöllhorn WI, Sechelmann M, Trockel M, Westers R (2004) Nie das Richtige trainieren, um richtig zu spielen [Never do the right thing in training to play correctly]. Leistungssport 34(5):13–17. https://www.iat.uni-leipzig.de/datenbanken/iks/open_archive/ls/lsp04_05_13_17.pdf?

Schöllhorn WI, Beckmann H, Michelbrink M, Sechelmann M, Trockel M, Davids K (2006a) Does noise provide a basis for the unification of motor learning theories? Int J Sport Psychol 37(2–3):186–206

Schöllhorn WI, Paschke M, Beckmann H (2006b) Differenzielles Training im Volleyball beim Erlernen von zwei Techniken. In: Langolf K, Roth R (eds) Volleyball 2005—Beach-WM. Czwalina, Hamburg, pp 97–105

Schöllhorn WI, Mayer-Kress G, Newell KM, Michelbrink M (2009) Time scales of adaptive behavior and motor learning in the presence of stochastic perturbations. Hum Mov Sci 28(3):319–333. https://doi.org/10.1016/j.humov.2008.10.005

Schöllhorn WI, Hegen P, Davids K (2012) The nonlinear nature of learning - A differential learning approach. Open Sports Sci J 5:100–112. https://doi.org/10.2174/1875399X01205010100

Schöllhorn WI, Rizzi N, Slapšinskaitė-Dackevičienė A, Leite N (2022) Always pay attention to which model of motor learning you are using. Int J Environ Res Public Health 19(2). https://doi.org/10.3390/ijerph19020711

Schönherr T Schöllhorn WI (2003) Differencial learning in Basketball. European workshop on movements science, Münster, Germany, 22–24 May 2003

Schultz W (1998) Predictive reward signal of dopamine neurons. J Neurophysiol 80(1):1–27. https://doi.org/10.1152/jn.1998.80.1.1

Schultz W, Dayan P, Montague PR (1997) A neural substrate of prediction and reward. Science 275(5306):1593–1599. https://doi.org/10.1126/science.275.5306.1593

Scinicariello AP, Eaton K, Inglis JT, Collins JJ (2001) Enhancing human balance control with galvanic vestibular stimulation. Biol Cybern 84(6):475–480. https://doi.org/10.1007/pl00007991

Shea C, Zimny ST (1983) Context effects in memory and learning moivement information. In: Magill RA (ed) Memory and control of action. North Holland, Amsterdam, pp 345–366

Singer W (1983) Neuronal activity as a shaping factor in the self-organization of neuron assemblies. Synergetics of the brain, Berlin, Heidelberg

Smirnov AA (1973) Conditions for retroactive inhibition. In: Problems of the psychology of memory. Springer, pp 279–298. https://doi.org/10.1007/978-1-4684-1968-9_10

Steiner R (1907) Die Erziehung des Kindes: vom Gesichtspunkte der Geisteswissenschaft. Rudolf Steiner Verlag, Basel

Strogatz S (1994) Nonlinear dynamics and chaos with applications to physics, biology, chemistry and engineering. Perseus, New York

Takahashi YK, Batchelor HM, Liu B, Khanna A, Morales M, Schoenbaum G (2017) Dopamine neurons respond to errors in the prediction of sensory features of expected rewards. Neuron 95(6):1395–1405.e1393. https://doi.org/10.1016/j.neuron.2017.08.025

Theraulaz B, Hyppolite R (2021) LA BIBLE DES PREFERENCES MOTRICES: ACTION TYPES. Amphora

Trockel M, Schöllhorn WI (2003) Differential learning of the goal kick in soccer mechanics, physiology, psychology. First European workshop on movement science, Münster, Germany, 22–24 May 2003

Tug S, Tross AK, Hegen P, Neuberger EWI, Helmig S, Schöllhorn W, Simon P (2017) Acute effects of strength exercises and effects of regular strength training on cell free DNA concentrations in blood plasma. PLoS One 12(9):e0184668. https://doi.org/10.1371/journal.pone.0184668

Turrigiano GG, Nelson SB (2004) Homeostatic plasticity in the developing nervous system. Nat Rev Neurosci 5(2):97–107. https://doi.org/10.1038/nrn1327

Turvey MT (1996) Dynamic touch. Am Psychol 51(11):1134–1152. https://doi.org/10.1037/0003-066x.51.11.1134

Usher M, Feingold M (2000) Stochastic resonance in the speed of memory retrieval. Biol Cybern 83(6):L11–L16. https://doi.org/10.1007/pl00007974

Vázquez-Rodríguez B, Avena-Koenigsberger A, Sporns O, Griffa A, Hagmann P, Larralde H (2017) Stochastic resonance at criticality in a network model of the human cortex. Sci Rep 7(1):13020. https://doi.org/10.1038/s41598-017-13400-5

Voglsinger D, Nowak M, Vestberg T, Schack T (2023) Creative game forms in soccer. game intelligence & creativity. Independently Published

von Foerster H (1960) On self-organizing systems and their environments. In: Yovitz MC, Cameron S (eds) Self-organizing systems. Pergamon Press, pp 31–50

Vreeling FW, Verhey FR, Houx PJ, Jolles J (1993) Primitive reflexes in Parkinson's disease. J Neurol Neurosurg Psychiatry 56(12):1323–1326. https://doi.org/10.1136/jnnp.56.12.1323

Wagner H, Müller E (2008) The effects of differential and variable training on the quality parameters of a handball throw. Sports Biomech 7(1):54–71. https://doi.org/10.1080/14763140701689822

Westphal N, Schöllhorn WI (2001) Identifying volleyball teams by their tactical moves. 6th annual congress of the European College of Sport Science: perspectives and profiles, Cologne

Wiesel TN, Hubel DH (1963) Effects of visual deprivation on morphology and physiology of cells in the cats lateral geniculate body. J Neurophysiol 26:978–993. https://doi.org/10.1152/jn.1963.26.6.978

Wormhoudt R, Savelsbergh GJP, Teunissen JW, Davids K (2018) Athletic skills model: optimizing talent delvelopment through movement education. Taylor & Francis, London

Wulf G, Lee TD (1993) Contextual interference in movements of the same class: differential effects on program and parameter learning. J Mot Behav 25(4):254–263. https://doi.org/10.1080/00222895.1993.9941646

Wulf G, Shea CH (2002) Principles derived from the study of simple skills do not generalize to complex skill learning. Psychon Bull Rev 9(2):185–211. https://doi.org/10.3758/bf03196276

Zehr EP, Duysens J (2004) Regulation of arm and leg movement during human locomotion. Neuroscientist 10(4):347–361. https://doi.org/10.1177/1073858404264680

Part II

Application of DL in Physiotherapeutic Fields

4 Differential Learning in Musicians' Rehabilitation: Focal Dystonia as an Example

Jaume Rosset-Llobet

4.1 Introduction

Injuries result from a loss of body function or structural integrity when a musician's system is unable to adapt to changing internal and/or external demands. For example, a sudden increase in practice time can lead to tendon sheath friction that exceeds the tissue's capability to compensate through increased blood flow, collagen synthesis, inflammatory response, and cellular changes (Thorpe 2015). Similarly, when an automated movement needs to adapt to a new requirement—such as playing a new instrument—and the neural network fails to adjust, a dysfunctional pattern can emerge, which leads to either injuries or reduced performance in the long term (Sadnicka and Rosset-Llobet 2019). The intensity or degree of these demands is a relatively visible determinant of injury, but the system's capacity to respond is equally crucial, albeit less perceptible. A rigid and less adaptive system, with poor, slow, or inefficient adjustments to changes, is more prone to injury (Bartlett et al. 2007).

From this perspective, an injury is the result of two factors: (1) the demands placed on a certain part of the system and (2) the system's capability to adjust. To prevent musicians' injuries, we can either focus on controlling and reducing these demands—reducing the absolute load or the load per time by carefully programming changes to minimize the need for adaptation—or work on making the musician's system more adaptable to these demands. However, for many years, efforts have primarily focused on the first approach. This is why therapists have advised musicians—both in treating injuries and promoting health—to better organize their work, reduce postural loads, improve ergonomics, optimize biomechanics, and enhance body balance and musculoskeletal tolerance. While these recommendations are beneficial, they are often challenging to implement, and the results do not always justify the effort.

The second factor, increasing the system's adaptability, has been largely overlooked, partly because its importance was not recognized and partly because healthcare professionals lacked knowledge of how to effectively improve it. This is particularly critical for musicians, given the nature of their work and, more importantly, how they practice. As happens in sports, learning musical practice often relies on the repetition of a predefined model or template, particularly during the initial phases. This practice has become a standard in teaching movement techniques (Albrecht et al. 2014). This widespread approach, which prioritizes the imitation of established models in movement learning, often overlooks the scientific evidence that suggests a marked individuality in people's movement patterns and their link to the risk of injury.

J. Rosset-Llobet (✉)
Institut de l'Art. Medicina i Fisiologia, Terrassa, Barcelona, Spain

W. I. Schöllhorn, A. Slapšinskaitė-Dackevičienė (eds.), *Differential Learning in Physiotherapy*,
https://doi.org/10.1007/978-3-031-98787-8_4

4.1.1 Concepts of Individuality, Variability, and Flexibility

These concepts have been extensively studied in the context of athletic performance. The concept of *individuality in human movement* emphasizes that each person exhibits unique patterns, even when performing identical tasks. This can be seen, for example, in gait patterns during running and walking (Schöllhorn et al. 2002) or in throwing patterns in different sports (Andrews et al. 2024; Bauer 1997). This body of research challenges the notion of a singular optimal technique.

Variability refers to the natural fluctuations in movement patterns that occur during performance. While an athlete may exhibit distinctive individual patterns, these patterns will inevitably show some degree of variability when observed at different times. Rather than being an error to be minimized, as was interpreted in the past, variability is essential as it allows athletes to explore different ways of performing tasks, fostering the flexibility needed for effective adaptation (van Emmerik and van Wegen 2000). Contrary to traditional learning theories, this variability in movement patterns helps athletes, such as cricket fast bowlers, maintain consistent results by allowing them to make crucial adjustments during their performance. This ensures that, despite changes or challenges, the outcome—like the speed of the ball in cricket—remains constant (Andrews et al. 2024). Moreover, Phillips (2012) demonstrated that as athletes gain experience, they further refine their ability to strategically vary their movements while still achieving consistent outcomes.

Flexibility refers to an athlete's ability to adapt their movements in response to changing and unpredictable conditions or task demands. It highlights how effectively an athlete can modify their actions to achieve optimal performance in varying situations. Importantly, flexibility should not be perceived as a loss of stability but rather as an indication of adaptability (Van Emmerik 2005). This adaptability enables athletes to maintain stability when necessary and at the same time react flexibly to situational requirements (Ranganathan and Newell 2010; Bernstein 1935). In his research, Stergiou and Decker (2011) found evidence that supports the necessity of an optimal state of variability for health and functional movement.

4.1.2 What About the Musicians?

Much like in sports, most musicians initially learn to play their instrument by imitating a model that is typically their teacher. This approach assumes that the teacher's model represents the "correct" way to play. However, this notion conflicts with the idea of individuality in music. Although this aspect has not been as extensively studied in musicians as it has in athletes, there is growing scientific evidence supporting individuality also in musicians.

Using an artificial lip, Almeida (2013) illustrates how clarinet players can achieve the same acoustic output through different combinations of blowing pressure, lip position, reed hardness, and lip force. Similarly, Velut (2015) investigates the various control parameters used by brass instrument players to produce sound. The study reveals that while there are commonalities in how musicians control their instruments, significant individual differences also exist. These differences can be attributed to each musician's unique characteristics (Turner et al. 2022), but there are a great number of internal and external variables that come into play. For example, Bertsch (1997) identifies over 80 musician-dependent factors (such as dental configuration, muscle thickness, mouthpiece pressure, diaphragm movement, instrument position, age, or motivation), 35 instrument-related factors (including instrument material, mouthpiece shape and dimensions, and instrument imperfections), and numerous external factors (such as temperature, hall acoustics, and the presence of other musicians) that impact the final sound produced by a trumpet player. This complexity underscores that each musician's approach is inherently individualized, making it impossible to establish a singular "correct" way to play an instrument. Moreover, this individuality is so important that it is possible to identify a flutist with high accuracy (up to 100%

for finger movements and 94% for body movements) based on their unique movement patterns (Albrecht et al. 2014). This phenomenon has also been observed in pianists, where more experienced individuals exhibit more consistent movement patterns (Bella and Palmer 2011).

Variability in musicians' movements has also been demonstrated in several studies. Albrecht (2014) found that flute key movement parameters—such as distance, maximum stroke, and velocity—varied within individuals across different performances. Bella and Palmer (2011) observed that pianists adjust their unique movement patterns according to the execution tempo. These variations stem from the musician's need to adapt their movements to changing conditions, optimize performance, prevent fatigue, and achieve the desired musical expression (Furuya and Altenmüller 2013). Adaptation can also be influenced by unexpected factors. For instance, pianists with a late chronotype—those who naturally prefer to stay up late and wake up later—exhibited more stable timing (less trial-to-trial variability) when playing in the evening compared to the morning. Conversely, early chronotype pianists showed no significant difference in timing stability between morning and evening performances (Van Vugt et al. 2013).

Uehara (2023) measured flexibility using electroencephalography by analyzing how synchronizations between different brain areas evolve as the brain prepares to play a note. The greater the changes observed during the initiation phase, the more flexible the brain is considered. Notably, Uehara also found that brass musicians with higher brain flexibility tend to produce long notes with greater timbral quality and precision, suggesting that this flexibility is linked to superior musical ability.

Flexibility is not only essential in physical execution but also in maintaining the freshness of musical performance. Demos (2016) explores how practice influences performance stability and reveals a counterintuitive finding: the most repeated passages did not always become more stable. In some cases, increased practice led to greater variability in performance. This challenges the traditional view that more practice would inevitably lead to automaticity and consistency. Instead, it suggests that flexibility allows musicians to keep their performances engaging and dynamic, even after extensive practice. This balance between automaticity and creative expression is a hallmark of professional musicianship, where the ability to adapt and inject variability into performances ensures that each rendition of a piece remains vibrant and unique.

All these findings suggest, as it happens with athletes, that musicians possess unique physical and technical attributes, leading them to develop personalized methods of sound production, with some degree of variability in how they execute the same task. This variability not only allows them to adapt flexibly to changing parameters but also plays a crucial role in shaping their unique identity and style.

4.1.3 What Reduces Musicians' System Flexibility?

Musicians, like athletes and other performance-driven professionals, face a range of factors that impact their adaptability. While some of these factors are shared across different fields, others are unique to musicians due to the nature of their practice and performance. Both direct research on musicians and insights transferred from other disciplines provide valuable understanding of the contributors to the loss of flexibility in musicians.

4.1.3.1 Type of Practice

Many musicians tend to establish work routines that they repeat, sometimes without any variation, day after day. They use the same warm-up routines with the same exercises. They approach learning a piece using the same strategies and order. Intuitively, one might assume that while this way of working is effective and provides the musician with a sense of security, it also likely leads to a lack of flexibility in the system. This is supported by several studies that show that rigid practice, focused on a single "ideal" coordination pattern, limits the development of motor equivalence—the ability of a system to perform the same function in different ways (Bernstein 1935, Lashley 1933; Seifert et al. 2016). This reduction in movement variability can hinder a musician's ability to adapt flexibly to new or continuously changing conditions, ultimately reducing flexibility. In contrast, Herholz and Zatorre (2012) concluded that multimodal and varied practice, which engages different sensory and motor systems (such as auditory, visual, and motor systems) simultaneously, promotes the system's flexibility by encouraging the exploration of multiple movement solutions. This diversity in practice indicates fostering a more adaptive system.

4.1.3.2 Personality

A musician's personality and emotional state can significantly affect their motor precision and adaptability. Ferrari and Mautz (1997) shows that perfectionism leads to low attitudinal flexibility, and self-oriented perfectionism is related to greater motor-cognitive rigidity. This means that highly perfectionistic individuals tend to be less flexible in their thoughts and behaviors, especially when imposing high standards on themselves.

Butković (2021) studied this in musicians and found that maladaptive perfectionism (referring to the tendency to set excessively high standards, being overly self-critical when these are not met, and constantly worrying about mistakes and criticism) is associated with a lack of flexibility, difficulties in adapting to changing circumstances, or managing setbacks efficiently.

Kotani and Furuya (2018) found that performance anxiety can diminish motor precision by disrupting finger coordination and causing timing errors in musical execution. But the consequences of stress extend beyond immediate performance. Williamon (2013) observed that during high-stress conditions, such as live performances, musicians exhibit a decrease in physiological complexity. This reduction indicates a less flexible autonomic nervous system, impairing the body's ability to adapt to stressors and potentially leading to long-term health issues. On the other hand, Betzel (2017) found that a positive mood is associated with increased brain flexibility, demonstrating that emotional state plays a crucial role in a musician's adaptability.

Ioannou (2016) found striking evidence for a connection between perfectionism and a lack of adaptive flexibility in musicians with focal dystonia. It was observed that patients with high levels of perfectionism also tend to have more difficulty adapting flexibly to situations, as their personalities are strongly oriented toward control and the demand for perfect performance. This can increase neurological rigidity, leading to a poorly adaptable motor response to stress, contributing to the onset or worsening of dystonia. They also found that perfectionistic patients tend to develop dystonia about 10 years earlier than those with a less perfectionistic personality, suggesting that perfectionistic traits may accelerate the processes of neural maladaptation.

4.1.3.3 Level of Expertise

A musician's degree of proficiency can also affect their sensorimotor flexibility. Pfordresher and Chow (2019) demonstrated that while piano training enhances the rapid learning of new pieces, it also reduces sensorimotor flexibility. Pianists develop strong sensorimotor associations that, while improving skilled performance, limit their ability to adapt to new or altered feedback environments. For instance, pianists in the study made more errors when the pitch assignment for keys was inverted compared to non-pianists. Albrecht (2014) similarly noted that professional musicians exhibit less movement variability than semi-professional musicians. While this consistency can reflect mastery, it also indicates a loss of flexibility, as seen when expert athletes adapt more slowly to changes in tasks than novices (Kast and Leukel 2016.

4.1.3.4 Injuries

Injuries play a critical role in reducing motor variability and, consequently, adaptability. Côté (2014) analyzed the bidirectional relationship between injuries and motor variability: injuries reduce variability, making individuals more prone to further injuries, and reduced variability increases the risk of injury. This creates a vicious circle that can lead to chronic pain and persistent damage. Van Emmerik (2005) expanded on this by showing that individuals with conditions like patellofemoral pain syndrome often display reduced joint coordination variability, resulting in more rigid movement patterns that exacerbate stress on tissues and contribute to further trauma. Interestingly, Madeleine et al. (2008) suggests that acute pain can initially increase motor variability as the body searches for new movement strategies, but chronic pain leads to a persistent loss of flexibility over time.

4.1.3.5 Fatigue

Fatigue also reduces system adaptability by decreasing response variability. Shine (2016) found that fatigue and sleepiness are associated with less flexible brain states, impairing the brain's ability to adapt. Conversely, muscle responses with greater variability have been shown to better resist fatigue. Fedorowich (2013) observed that women exhibit greater initial muscle variability, which is linked to increased resistance to fatigue. This gender difference may help explain varying incidences of musculoskeletal problems, particularly in the neck and shoulders, across different populations.

4.1.3.6 Age

Age is another critical factor affecting adaptability, with older musicians often experiencing a decline in flexibility. Baugh (2009) demonstrated that aging individuals exhibit a significant loss of adaptability when performing visuo-motor tasks under altered conditions, highlighting a decline in cognitive and motor flexibility. Wilson et al. (2016) further supported this finding, showing that seniors displayed more variability in power output (outcome variability) and had less variability in joint coordination (technique variability), which could increase injury risk. Manor (2010) emphasized that aging leads to a reduction in physiological complexity, reducing the body's ability to adapt to stressors and increasing the risk of falls or other complications. Beckers (2006) highlighted the decline in nonlinear heart rate variability indices with aging, indicating a reduction in heart rate complexity and a decreased ability to adapt to physiological stressors. Furuya (2023) further explored this decline in adaptability using a hand exoskeleton robot to study pianists, finding that adolescent pianists showed greater adaptability to passive somatosensory training than adults. Although it is not possible to determine whether this is due to age-related physiological shifts or lifestyle changes, the results show that neuroplasticity diminishes with age, further reducing adaptability.

4.1.4 Why DL for Musicians?

We have seen that various factors contribute to musicians developing a more rigid and less adaptable system, which can lead to decreased performance and a heightened risk of injury. Enhancing system flexibility in musicians is an important strategy for both preventing injuries and potentially improving performance.

When we attend to a musician, it is usually because they are in pain or injured. We have previously seen that these conditions further exacerbate rigidity. Therefore, it is highly probable that these musicians have even less flexibility than their already rigid peers. Additionally, when certain components of a system lose function due to injury, other components adjust to maintain overall functionality—a process described as synergy (Haken 1983; Latash 2007). These compensatory mechanisms enable the system to keep functioning temporarily, but they can persist even after the injury has healed. This persistence often makes the system less efficient and less adaptable, ultimately increasing the risk of future injuries (Hodges 2011). Thus, improving system flexibility is key not only for recovery but also for restoring full functionality.

Recognizing this, we began exploring strategies to enhance system flexibility, not only to prevent injuries in those who have not yet experienced problems, but also to aid in recovery and help musicians regain high-performance efficiency while reducing the risk of future injuries.

When we first encountered DL, we immediately realized its potential. The core idea of DL is to intentionally introduce small variations or "errors" into tasks to encourage individuals to adapt and find more effective, individualized solutions. From a traditional perspective, these movement variations may appear as the training of inadequate movements. This induces system fluctuations, enhancing adaptability and allowing the system to self-organize (Schöllhorn 2000). Originally developed for athletes, DL has proven effective in rehabilitation settings as well (Schöllhorn 2010; Repšaitė et al. 2015). While the detailed principles of DL are covered in other chapters of this book, we want to emphasize its remarkable potential to restore or enhance system flexibility. More importantly, it offers a way to restructure more flexible automatisms—a crucial need when addressing musician's dystonia (MD). Once we realized its effectiveness, we quickly saw that this approach could be an exceptionally powerful tool for the musicians we treat at our Institute.

4.2 Differential Learning for Musicians

In 2009, we first became aware of the effects of DL on athletes' performance. We quickly realized its potential to improve the treatment of musician's dystonia (MD). At the time, we already had an effective treatment for this condition, but there were areas in need of improvement, such as shortening the treatment duration (which typically exceeds 18 months) and, most importantly, providing supplementary tools for those patients who did not respond well to the available strategies. This led us to explore the potential of DL with our patients.

In an effectiveness analysis conducted 9 years later, we found that the percentage of fully cured patients rose from 50% to 76% after implementing this strategy (Rosset-Llobet and Fàbregas-Molas 2018). We have also progressively used DL for the recovery process of a wide range of other conditions affecting performing artists (from postural issues to tendinitis). We also aimed to identify the factors that predict whether this approach will be more or less beneficial for each of our patients, and to determine which is the best way to implement the strategy.

4.2.1 What Is Musician's Dystonia (MD)?

MD is characterized by difficulty, slowness, loss of motor control, or tension that affects specific parts of the body during music performance. Some of its most distinctive features are task specificity and the presence of sensory tricks. Task specificity means that up to 60% of affected musicians experience involuntary movements or difficulties only while playing their instrument, and these issues may only affect certain movements but not others (Rosset-Llobet et al. 2007). For example, a guitarist with hand dystonia might struggle with ascending arpeggios but manage descending ones, or a clarinet player may experience mouth difficulties when playing the soprano saxophone but not the baritone. Sensory tricks are stimuli, usually proprioceptive, that can temporarily alleviate or reduce symptoms. For example, wearing a latex glove on the affected hand or touching the back of the hand can provide temporary relief for some musicians (Paulig et al. 2014).

4.2.1.1 What Causes Musician's Dystonia?

The exact cause of MD remains unclear. However, research indicates that there is no evidence of structural brain damage in these patients. Instead, the disorder appears to be linked to organizational and functional changes within neuronal networks. These changes include alterations in inhibitory circuits, sensory processing, sensory motor integration, and motor planning in various regions such as the cortex, brainstem, and spinal cord (Berardelli 1998; Ridding 1995; Butefisch 2005; Elbert 1998; Pujol 2000; Bara-Jimenez 1998; McKenzie 2003; Quartarone 2006; Tamura 2009). While there are some common disruptions, MD does not follow a uniform pattern across all patients. In other words, individuals with MD do not always share the same characteristics. For example, there are different psychological profiles among patients (Ioannou and Altenmüller 2014), and they display varying behaviors in several aspects, such as their response to sensory tricks, genetic predispositions, biomechanical limitations, or hormonal status (Rosset-Llobet et al. 2009; Rosset-Llobet et al. 2012; Lohmann 2014; Paulig et al. 2014). Therefore, considering a single pathophysiological model or a one-size-fits-all therapeutic strategy is unlikely to be the wisest approach.

From our experience, having treated over a thousand musicians with MD, there is a direct relationship between the onset of dystonia and the rigidity of the system. This disorder tends to emerge when a highly trained brain (thus, it is most seen in advanced-level musicians) is confronted with situations that demand adaptation from its neuronal networks (such as a change in teacher, modifications in the instrument's characteristics, technical changes, injuries, economic problems, emotional conflicts, or increased motor control demands). When the brain's capacity to adapt is exceeded, maladaptive changes occur, leading to the development of a motor dysfunctional response. The more rigid the system is, the more vulnerable it becomes. As we have previously analyzed, factors such as reliance on stereotyped models, perfectionism, poor stress responses, and unresolved injuries further contribute to this rigidity.

Given that these dysfunctional changes primarily affect motor automatisms, the maladaptive response will inevitably occur whenever the system recognizes the trained task, meaning every time the musician plays. Since the brain cannot cancel this response, it consciously or unconsciously tries to improve the dysfunctional reaction but cannot prevent its manifestation. This leads to compensatory mechanisms that typically only increase involuntary tensions, difficulties, and the intensity of symptoms (Sadnicka and Rosset-Llobet 2019).

4.2.1.2 How Is Musician's Dystonia Typically Treated?

Until the 1980s, MD was often misunderstood as a mental illness, akin to conversion hysteria, believed to stem from feelings of guilt and repressed hostilities. Treatments during this period were primarily based on psychoanalysis or behavioral therapies, which sometimes included aversive electric shocks applied whenever the dysfunctional movement occurred, with the aim of extinguishing the maladaptive behavior (Cleveland 1959; Gibson 1972).

When the condition was later recognized as a neurological disorder, treatment approaches shifted toward the use of anticholinergic drugs and neuromodulators. However, these treatments were purely symptomatic and offered only limited benefits (Sheehy and Marsden 1982).

As research into the disorder progressed, neurological abnormalities associated with MD were identified. Some researchers focused on addressing these specific neurological alterations, such as employing sensory retraining to correct the blurred cortical representation of the affected fingers (Byl 2000). Although this approach led to some improvement and normalization of certain brain changes, which correlated with clinical benefits, none of these protocols resulted in a complete and definitive resolution of the condition (Byl 2000; McKenzie 2009; Rosenkranz 2009; Buttkus 2010).

The first therapeutic strategy to show clear improvements was a retraining program described by Tubiana and Chamagne (1983). This program aimed to reeducate the muscles of the hand, forearm, shoulder, neck, and trunk, enhancing body awareness of gravity, joint pressures, and muscular balance. Many patients were able to return to their professional roles after undergoing this treatment. However, consistent replication of these results has been challenging, likely due to the lack of a standardized protocol, with therapists applying it mostly based on their expertise.

The first structured approach was developed by Victor Candia in the 1990s. His technique, known as sensory motor retuning (SMR), aimed to change the brain's perception of the task through proprioceptive modifications. Originally, this was done by placing one or more fingers in a more extended position using splints. However, since the goal was to alter perception rather than merely restrict movement, other methods were also employed, such as using rubber bands to introduce forced finger flexion or placing weights at various points on the fingers. Musicians would perform exercises on their instruments or, in more advanced stages, play pieces while using these tools. We began using this strategy in 1999, replicating the successful results of its creator. More details can be found in a previous publication by our team (Rosset-Llobet and Fàbregas-Molas 2013). Our success rate with SMR alone was 50%. These patients achieve complete recovery, free from dystonia symptoms, without requiring ongoing preventive exercises or avoiding certain musical techniques (Rosset-Llobet and Fàbregas-Molas 2018).

There are other retraining approaches, some of which may be useful, but there is no scientific publication detailing their rationale, methodology, and results, making them impossible to replicate.

Two other notable therapies for MD are botulinum toxin injections and stereotactic brain surgery. Botulinum toxin works by blocking acetylcholine release at the neuromuscular junction, temporarily paralyzing muscles and reducing involuntary contractions. The leading center for botulinum toxin treatment for musicians is in Hannover, renowned for its extensive expertise in customizing treatments to meet the specific needs of individual musicians needs. Their reports indicate that 69% of musicians experience symptom improvement, with 36% achieving long-term benefits in their performance (Schuele et al. 2005). However, only 15–20% are able to return to professional-level performance (Jabusch and Altenmüller 2006). Stereotactic ventro-oral thalamotomy, a procedure that involves inserting an electrode into the brain to create a small, precise lesion in the thalamus, has shown impressive results, with 93% of patients experiencing significant improvements in motor control and some returning to professional activity. These benefits typically last an average of 2.5 years (Horisawa et al. 2013). However, despite its effectiveness, neurosurgeons in Western countries seldom perform this procedure due to its potential risks.

4.2.2 How Does Our Protocol Treat the Musician's Dystonia?

To begin the treatment, the musician will work at our center for five consecutive days, with sessions lasting 2–3 h per day. A physiotherapist will administer the treatment under the supervision of our team, which includes a doctor and four physiotherapists. During these days, the treatment protocol will be defined, the necessary tools will be created, and the customized design will be tested to ensure it suits the patient. The therapy, its goals, and the patient's role in achieving them will be thoroughly explained to patient. Additionally, this period will be used to assess whether the patient needs any supplementary support in areas such as physical conditioning, posture, ergonomics, emotional well-being, or behavior.

Following this initial phase, musicians are instructed to continue the exercises independently at home, dedicating approximately 90 min per day to their practice.

Our protocol incorporates three key strategies that will be implemented during the first days: SMR, DL, and second task (ST) exercises. For most patients, the treatment will involve all three strategies; however, for those with mild dystonia symptoms affecting only specific movements, the treatment may begin with just DL and ST exercises.

4.2.2.1 Sensory Motor Retuning (SMR)

The main goal is to alter the proprioception of the task, making the system perceive that it is not playing the instrument while it actually is. The method involves using splints to immobilize one or more non-dystonic fingers, allowing the dystonic finger to perform controlled, repetitive movements without interference from compensatory finger actions. The first step is to identify the focal dystonic finger, which exhibits involuntary movements, and determine which other fingers contribute to compensatory movement patterns. The therapy then targets these compensatory movements by immobilizing the compensating finger(s), isolating the dystonic finger for practice (see Rosset-Llobet et al. 2012 for detailed procedure).

Customized splints are used to slightly adjust the position of specific non-dystonic fingers during therapy, altering hand proprioception and facilitating the development of new motor programs. For instance, if the dystonic finger is the ring finger, a splint may be applied to the middle or little finger, which typically compensates for the abnormal movement.

Each day, the patient performs two series of splint exercises with a 10–15 min rest between them. Each series consists of seven different exercises, lasting 3 min per exercise, with 1 min of rest between each. The musician performs basic technical movements (e.g., scales, arpeggios) using the non-splinted fingers.

Following the splint exercises, task execution work is introduced. Initially, this lasts only a few minutes but progressively increases to up to 60 min as the patient improves. This phase involves repetitive practice of the musician's specific task (e.g., piano or guitar playing) without the splints. Both the difficulty and duration of task execution are gradually adjusted to prevent dystonic responses.

Patients are reviewed monthly to assess progress and adjust the therapy accordingly. Exercises are designed to progressively challenge the musician's motor skills by varying the speed and complexity of movements based on their ongoing improvement.

4.2.2.2 Differential Learning (DL)

The main objective is to regain flexibility and adaptability by inducing system fluctuations. A musician must introduce noise to musical instrument practice or SMR exercises by means of doing "wrong" things. DL also calls this a variation in its original sense. But, as a variation in music is typically known as a modification of the tune that already sounds good, we must explain to the musician that this is closer to a mistake rather than a variation. He must introduce a variation every 5–15 s, approximately. Each musician will require a different degree of variation to create enough system fluctuation without causing excessive discomfort. The challenge should be big enough to destabilize but not collapse the performer.

The aim is not to look for solutions (a way to play where dystonia symptoms improve or where the patient feels more comfortable) but to introduce noise (different ways to play, it does not matter if they are more functional than the original one or not; it does not matter whether they have a biomechanical or technical purpose or not; it does not matter if the final sound is good or not). In fact, the final way the musician will play after the treatment is unpredictable. It can be close to the original one or not. Neither the musician nor the therapist must decide in advance how to play. The system itself will reorganize after being destabilized by means of these variations.

Variations can affect many things like body posture, the instrument position or configuration, the interaction between the instrument and the body, the way movements are done, the musical execution, adding a physical object that alters proprioception, balance, tactile feedback, or otherwise interferes with the execution of the musical gesture, modifying how the score is played, or how practice is organized. We can combine variations to create a new one. For instance, if you place a weight at the tip of a finger, this is one variation. But probably it will be difficult to change this weight every 5–15 s. But you can do wrist variations for 1 min, and then do the same wrist variations while you have the weight in your finger. This is still something new for your system.

It is important to understand that variations should be intrusive, interfering with the task. For example, grasping the violin bow at the middle part of the stick rather than the frog is clearly destabilizing. It is important to notice that variations are not equally disturbing for every instrument or musician. Moving the head could be very annoying for a flute player, but perhaps not so much for a pianist. Moreover, sometimes it can be not obvious, but already intrusive. For example, many players tend to move a specific part of their body when playing certain types of notes (Moura et al. 2023). So, if you notice the saxophonist flexing their knee while playing high register notes, a variation, in accordance with the stochastic resonance principle of DL theory (Schöllhorn 2005; Schöllhorn et al. 2009), could be to reverse this action by flexing the knee during low register notes and extending it for the high ones. You can refer to different examples in Tables 4.1, 4.2, 4.3 and 4.4 but do not hesitate to be creative—and more importantly, encourage

Table 4.1 Body position/action examples

Wrist	Bend	To the maximum, in a middle position. Relaxed or with tension
	Extend	
	Ulnar deviation	
	Radial deviation	
	Pronation	
	Supination	
	Move from flexion to extension	Move slowly or quickly; advance slowly and return rapidly; pause at intermediate positions; incorporate a shaking motion. Alternate between large and small movements. Add rebounds at the end of each motion. Combine different directions with varying speeds; adjust speed or direction midway through the movement; change starting or ending points
	Move from ulnar to radial	
	From pronation to supination	
	Circle to the right	
	Circle to the left	
Shoulder	Up	Determine 3 degrees of movement (e.g., position 0 = starting point, 1 = slightly up, 2 = moderately up, 3 = fully up), and randomly place the shoulder in the different positions, holding each for a few seconds. Combine positions (e.g., up and forward)
	Down	
	Forward	
	Backward	
	Up and down	Straight, in S shape; continuously moving or stopping briefly at the end of the movement; stop long; stop short; move to the maximum or an intermediate position with small movements; pause at the midpoint, return to the starting position, and then proceed to the maximum position
	Back and forth	
	Circle forward	
	Circle backward	
	Drawing geometrical figures	Imagine a pencil is attached to the shoulder, pointing up, forward, backward, or to the side. Use it to "draw" letters, words, or numbers. Keep in mind that if the exercise is so difficult, it will become a second task, as it will need the musician's attention
Body	Seated	To the back of the chair, the middle, the edge, almost falling to the right or left side. Sitting on only the right or left ischium, with one ischium at the back of the chair and the other toward the front. Rise on foot from the floor
	Standing up	Tilt the pelvis forward or backward; bend both knees or just one; stand on tiptoes, or balance with one foot on tiptoes and the other on the heel. Lame foot; lame foot and move the other in circles, or draw words
	Leaning against the wall	Place feet slightly away from or farther from the wall. Rest only on the right or left shoulder blade, or lean sideways on the right or left shoulder. Try lifting one foot. Move the pelvis
	Walking	Slowly, fast, backward, sideways. Hold the knee up for a few seconds with each step. Walk like a soldier, or like an elderly person, or like an elephant
	Sitting on a stability ball or wobbling chair	Move the pelvis in different directions; make shapes or letters. Bounce on the ball; make the bounces on the ball go in different directions. Keep one leg extended; move the leg while it is extended; tilt the body to one side; rotate the torso

(continued)

Table 4.1 (continued)

Mouth and face (wind instruments)	Face	Make different facial expressions: Smile, blow a kiss, lower the corners of the mouth, puff out the cheeks, puff out only one cheek, puff out the upper or lower lip. Tense one part of the face. Pull with only one side
	Mandibula	Move it forward, backward, to one side or the other; move it right and left; move it forward slowly and backward quickly. Separate the teeth widely, then close them
	Tongue	Articulate with different consonants (T, C, K, Z, G…). Change the point where the tongue strikes to articulate; change the part of the mouthpiece the tongue touches when articulating; change where the tongue is placed when playing legato. Place the tongue on the upper right canine or the lower left molars; curl the tongue, flatten it, or even bite it. Vary the tongue's position in a specific sequence
	Throat	Change the throat configuration while playing, imitating the shape used for different sounds. Sing the note at the same moment it is played with the instrument; sing the same note all the time, even while playing a different one

Table 4.2 Instrument examples

Position	Change the instrument position	Examples for different instruments: Lift the bell of the trombone Hold the violin as if it were a cello Tilt the guitar forward or lay it flat on the lap Turn the clarinet to the right For instruments that cannot be moved, such as the piano, make the musician move (e.g., stand very close to the piano, far away, to the side, sit on the floor, stand up, etc.)
	Incorporate movement	Examples for different instruments: Draw numbers with the tip of the flute. At the beginning of each line of the staff, place the double bass tilted to the left, gradually turning it fully to the right by the end of the line. While playing, change the point where the bow touches the cello string
For wind musicians	Mouthpiece	Move it slightly in different directions; significantly shift it. Apply very light pressure; apply considerable pressure; change the pressure during the execution of each note. Apply the opposite pressure to what is typically expected (more pressure on the low notes and less on the high notes). Apply lip balm and continuously slide the mouthpiece from one position to another
	Reed	Use a broken reed; position it incorrectly, in different positions. Play with a reed that is thicker or thinner than usual. Insert the reed deeper or more shallowly in the mouth than usual

Table 4.3 Music examples

Score	Change fingering	If an arpeggio is played as 1-3-5 or index-middle-ring, play it as 5-2-3 or middle-index-ring
	Change the rhythm	Swap the duration of the first and second notes of each measure; double the length of the shortest note in the measure; make all the notes in the measure equal in duration
	Change the dynamics and the expression markings	Make the second note of each measure pianissimo and the last note forte. Then, invert the dynamics. In each measure, play one note forte followed by one note piano. Reverse the direction of the expression markings
	Order changes	Play the piece or exercises in reverse, starting with the last measure, then the second-to-last, third-to-last, and so on. Only play the even-numbered measures (without pausing between them). Play only the even-numbered lines of the score. Change the order of every two lines of the score (so play line two first, then line one, line four, then line three, and so on). Change the order of the warm-up exercises. Start from different sections of the piece. Play the sections of the piece in a different order
	Others	Change the legato to staccato. Always play the second note of each measure staccato. Play everything staccato. Alternate between playing one measure legato and the next staccato. Play the even-numbered measures a whole tone (or a third, or an octave) higher than written in the score. In piano players, reverse the pedal markings on the piano. Apply the pedal to alternate measures. For bowed instruments, switch bowing techniques (e.g., change legato to détaché, or staccato to spiccato)
Changes	Each time a specific note is played, perform a particular action	Always raise the second note by a semitone. Each time a D appears, either skip the note, sing it without playing, or sing it a tone higher. Skip all sixteenth notes; play them pianissimo; or play them an octave lower or higher
	Each time a specific finger is used, perform a particular action	Do the opposite dynamic. Extend the finger. Play the note twice. Do not press the note but sing it. Do not press but extend the finger. Press the note; extend the finger; and press the note again
	Each time a certain note appears, perform a specific action	Skip the note; do not play it, but sing it; extend the finger from the previous note, or move a specific part of the body. Play a random note, a specific note, or a note above. Make it more complex by choosing two notes and assigning different actions to each
	Others	During arpeggio exercises, accentuate the first note, then the second, then the third, and then both the first and third. Every time the ring finger plays, execute it with a slow extension movement; then with a slow flexion; then alternate between slow extension with the ring finger and fast flexion with the middle finger. Change where the finger touches/presses the string—then a bit to the right, then to the left. After every note played with the index finger, extend it. Then apply the same process to the middle or ring finger, or combine different fingers for variation

Table 4.4 Intrusive objects

	Ball	Place a ball (varying in size and material, such as plastic, foam, glass, or metal) in various positions that create discomfort, such as under the armpit, between the chin and chest, in the palm of the hand, between the fingers, and other strategic spots
	Weight	Tie a weight to different parts of the body that interfere with performance. Sports stores sell weights of various sizes that can easily be strapped to the wrist, elbow, or forearm. Fishing weights can also be used and placed on different parts of the fingers. Tie a weight to a string, attach the other end to the wrist or elbow, and allow the weight to move freely, adding further instability and challenge to the movements Additionally, attach weights to different parts of the instrument or the bow, and keep moving them to different locations. Remember that any interference that is difficult to change every 5–15 s can be combined with other variations to ensure it remains destabilizing
	Others	Incorporate additional elements such as elastic bands, pencils, a book, Velcro, sponge, foam, clay, magnets, or gloves. It is also useful to place objects like paper clips, pieces of cotton, lentils, or rice inside the glove for added texture and sensation. Experiment with clothespins, foam pieces, or elastic tape around the abdomen or chest (especially useful for wind musicians) to introduce new physical challenges that disrupt typical movements and sensations
For wind musicians	The bell	Cover the bell with plastic wrap or aluminum foil, place a piece of paper, foil, a ball, or a cloth inside the bell. For instruments where the bell can be removed, take it off
	The holes	Cover one or more of the instrument's holes either fully or partially. Place foam pieces of varying thicknesses on the keys to alter the height of the finger placement
	Modify the face	Apply adhesive tape to different areas of the face, including the point where the mouthpiece or reed rests. Use both short and long strips. Make the tape pull or tense a specific part of the face. Apply several strips for additional restriction. Use elastic tape to slightly restrict jaw movement or cheek expansion Rubber bands can also be useful.
	Inside the mouth	With a ball (large or heavy enough—made of glass, for example—To avoid swallowing), move it around different places in the mouth. You can do the same with pieces of foam. Place foam or similar materials between the teeth to create thickness. Stick gum in different spots inside the mouth. Unbend a paperclip so that it does not press as hard, and place it on the tongue. Use other materials like cotton balls, a piece of fabric, cork, sports dental guard

the musician to do the same. It is surprising to observe how musicians, who can be highly imaginative when performing or composing, often struggle to be equally creative when inventing variations within Differential Learning. Some musicians can create variations on the fly, making a new one every 5–15 s, with very little repetition. For others, it is so difficult that they need to decide and plan them before starting the exercises or playing. In these cases, we often recommend making a list as long as possible and, from that list, select the variations for the next exercise. It may be helpful to choose the variations randomly. For example, by assigning numbers to the variations and using a random number generator—numerous apps or websites can do this—or by writing each variation on a small piece of paper, mixing them up, and drawing them randomly.

It may also be useful to create various audio tracks that call out variations every 10 s. If you always use the same audio, it will no longer be destabilizing. It is also helpful for the audio to be longer than the exercises. This way, you can start the audio at different points, thus adding more variety as well.

A good way for musicians to explore different variations is by asking them to change the way they press the keys or buttons or grasp the instrument. Fingers can be fully bent or completely extended, and they can press by sliding in flexion or extension. They might approach the instrument with vertical fingers or play from the side. They can also change where they press or grip the keys, strings, or bow, using different parts of the finger (the pad, side, tip, joint, or even the back). They can look for different ways of obtaining a bad or muted sound. These altered movements can involve one or several fingers, switching as needed.

Figure 4.1 shows a potential series of variations, with each variation performed by the pianist every 10–15 s.

4.2.2.3 Second Task

The goal of the second task (ST) is to engage musicians in one of several simultaneous activities during instrument practice that captures as much of their attention as possible. For musicians with Dystonia, compensatory movements are often used to improve musical performance (Rosset-Llobet and Fàbregas-Molas 2013). For therapy, these compensations will be a hindrance as they add tensions that further draw the patient's attention to the task. By shifting most or all of the musician's focus to the ST, these compensatory movements can be reduced or even eliminated. Buy the other hand, one of the core principles of DL is to allow the system to reorganize itself naturally by overloading the declarative working memory that is considered to limit motor learning and control processes (Schöllhorn et al. 2022). Therefore, it is crucial not to interfere by dictating how things should be done during exercises. Since the musician is highly trained and accustomed to controlling the entire process, the ST serves as a tool to prevent interference with this self-reorganization.

There are countless STs that can be used, but not all will suit every musician. If the task is too difficult, it may cause frustration, making it impossible for the musician to perform both the exercises and play the instrument simultaneously. In such cases, dependent on the musician, the difficulty of the task can be adjusted, or a new task should be selected that better suits the musician's specific needs. Similarly, the complexity of the music being practiced should also be adjusted to avoid any hindrance in performance. Over time, as the musician becomes accustomed to the tasks, they must be reassessed and adjusted to maintain their effectiveness.

Some examples of ST include performing coordinated sequences with the feet (e.g., two taps with the right toe, one with the left heel, two with the left toe, and one with the right heel), reading a book, reciting words containing a specific letter, chaining words together, performing arithmetic calculations, solving logic puzzles on a smart device, or mentally walking through a familiar route (such as from home to work) while recalling the names of streets or shops along the way.

As you can imagine, many exercises can simultaneously serve as variations and ST. For example, a musician could play a score, but each time they encounter a note F, they would move the neck of the guitar forward; for a G, they would move it backward; for a D, they would move it upward; and for a B, they would move it downward. This exercise introduces variation in how the task is performed, while also acting as a ST since the musician must be aware of the next note and remember whether it triggers a change in the guitar's neck position and, if so, which direction to move.

4.2.2.4 How Is This Organized?

The daily work routine for musicians with dystonia begins with 10 min of preparatory exercises. The goal is to create a relaxation and attentional state that facilitates the neurorehabilitation program. Typically, we ask the musician to perform either the dynamic Wu Qin Xi (five animals play) Qigong routine, High-Intensity Interval Training exercises, or coordination exercises.

The dynamic Wu Qin Xi routine imitates the movements and energies of five different animals, each of which, based on Traditional Chinese Medicine, is associated with specific health benefits and aspects of the body's energy flow. It has been demonstrated that this practice activates certain brain patterns, similar to those achieved with DL, that facilitate learning (Henz and Schöllhorn 2018). High-Intensity Interval Training is a workout method that often includes movements like sprinting, jumping, or bodyweight exercises that alternate short bursts of intense exercise with brief periods of rest or lower-intensity exercise. Although the aim is to

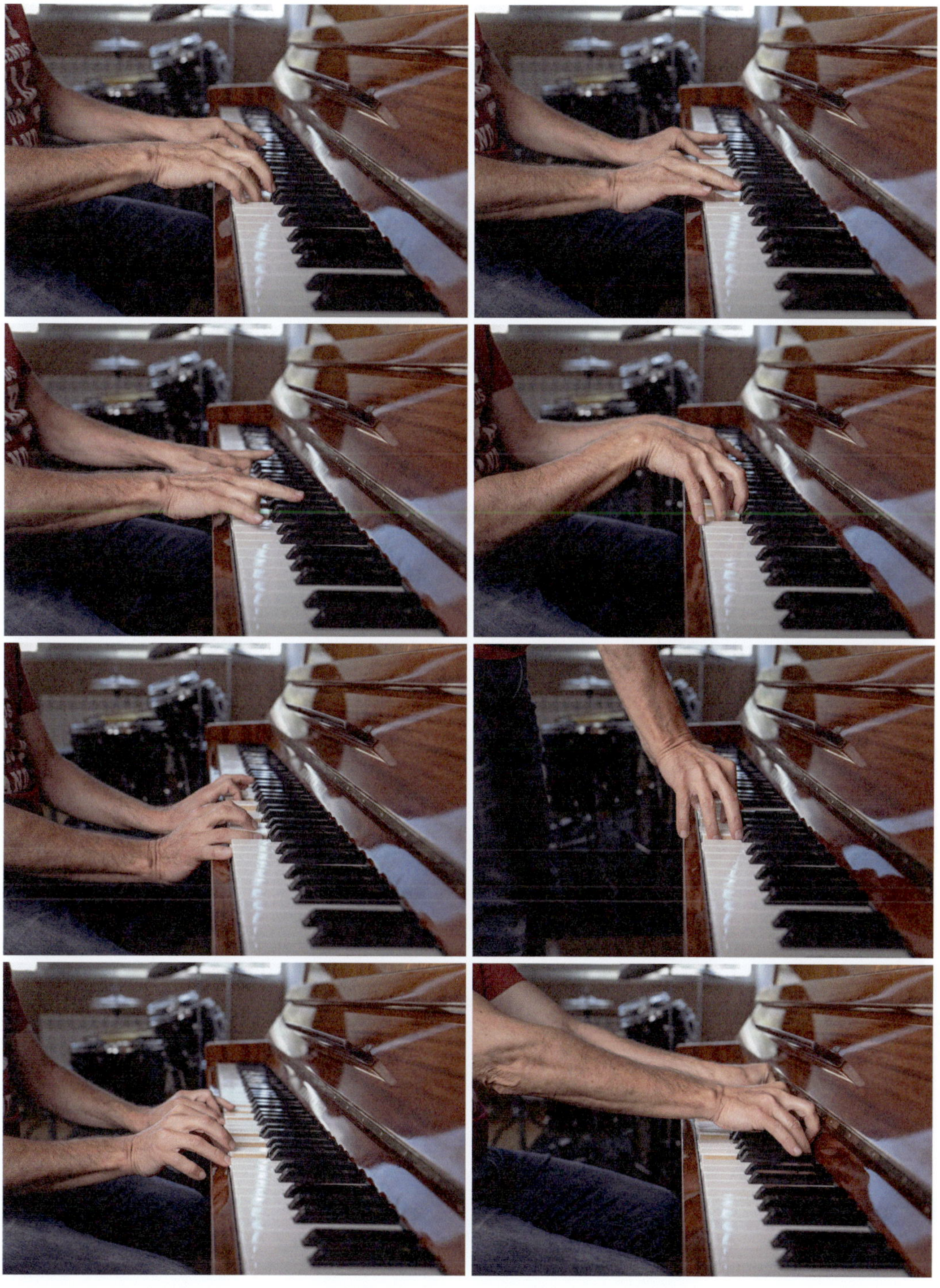

Fig. 4.1 (1) Normal playing, (2) Straight fingers, (3) Middle and ring straight, (4) Wrists up, (5) Wrists down, (6) From the top, (7) At the edge of the keys, (8) At the root of the keys, (9) From the left, (10) From the right, (11) Close to the piano, (12) Away from the piano, (13) Left arm up, right wrist down, (14) Both elbows up, (15) Crossing hands, (16) Index finger always up, (17) Right arm from the top, (18) Let arm from the top, (19) Reverse both hands, (20) Right reverse, (21) Left reverse and right crossed

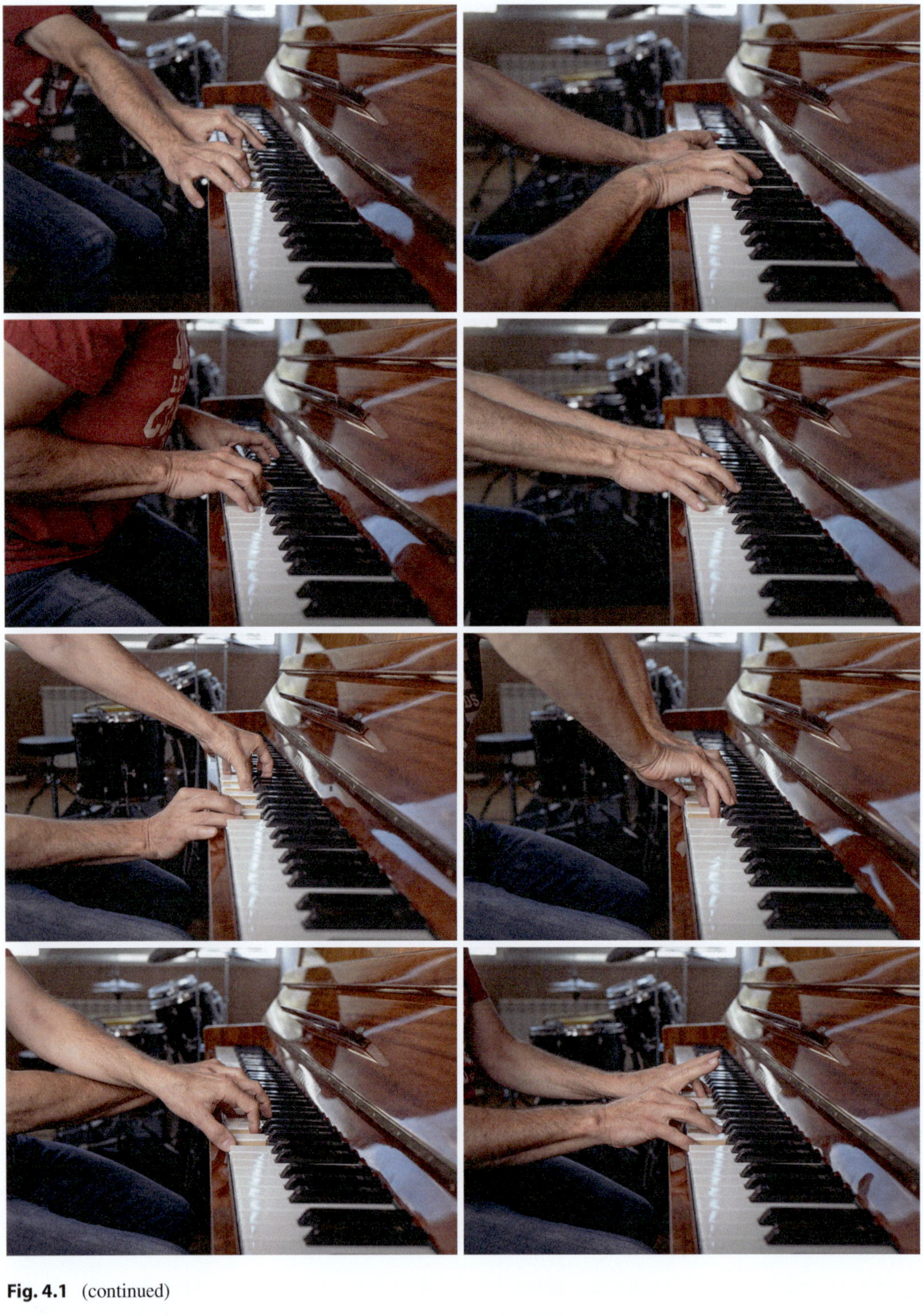

Fig. 4.1 (continued)

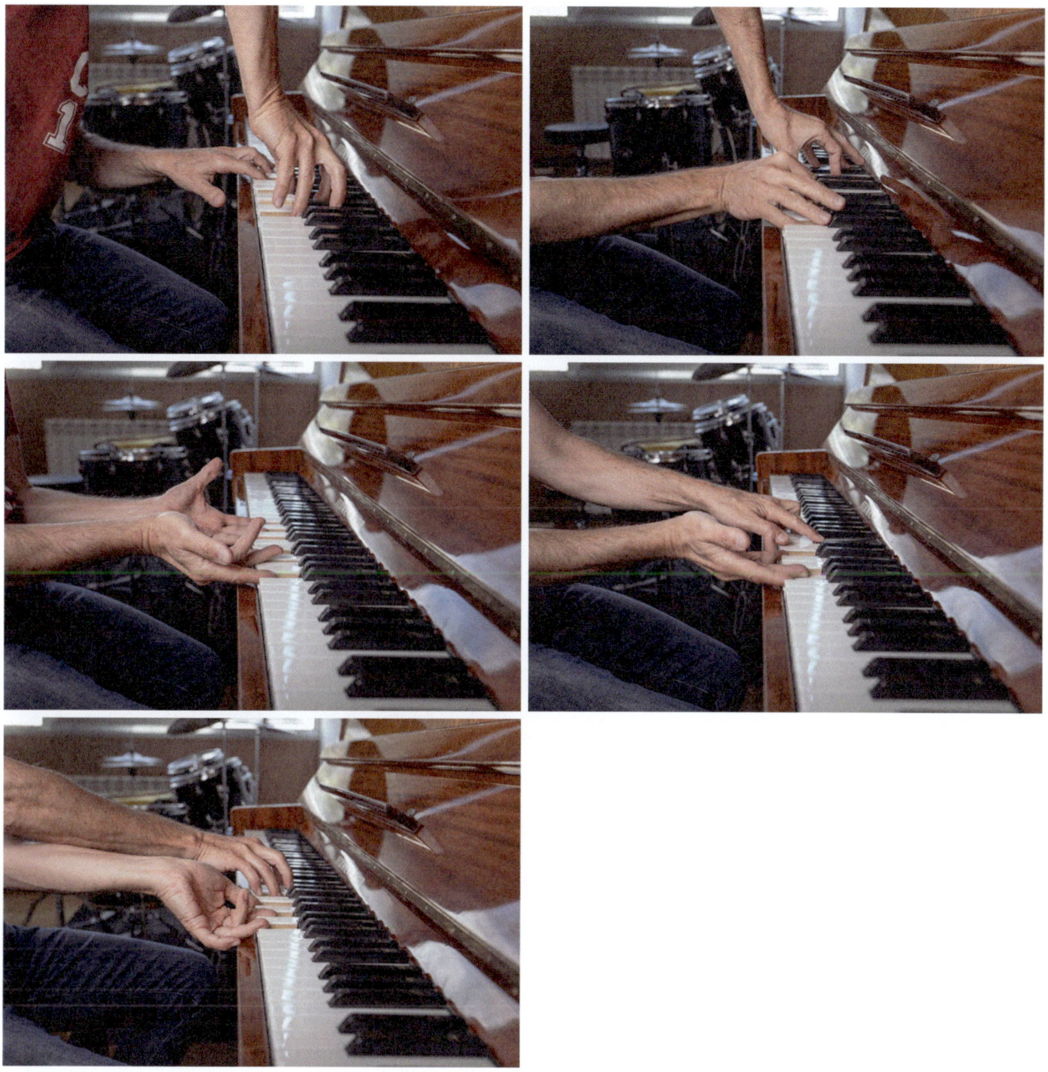

Fig. 4.1 (continued)

burn calories in a short time and improve cardiovascular fitness and endurance, it has also been demonstrated that it increases cognitive flexibility (Mekari et al. 2020). Coordinative exercises may include activities like juggling tennis balls or bouncing a table tennis ball on a racket, with the patterns constantly changing and gradually becoming more challenging. Additionally, exercises using an exercise ladder laid on the ground are incorporated, where the patient steps between the rungs, jumps, or moves from one step to the next in varied and increasingly challenging patterns.

The treatment for musician's dystonia is primarily based on SMR exercises. The patient will perform SMR, along with DL or ST activities. In the initial stages of treatment, we alternate between these approaches: one of the seven SMR exercises is combined with DL, the next exercise is paired with ST, and so on.

This approach is tailored to each patient. If a patient tends to have a high need for control, we might incorporate more ST exercises. If the dystonia manifests more in specific movements and we want to destabilize these patterns, we emphasize DL, depending on the treatment goals at each stage.

After a few weeks—this timeline varies depending on the patient and can range from the second week to two months—we introduce what we call "free playing." This means that, after completing the daily SMR exercises, the patient will play simple, progressive exercises on their instrument without splints, gradually increasing the difficulty. As the patient progresses, we incorporate technical exercises and, eventually, repertoire. Even during this free playing phase, the patient continues to alternate between DL and ST exercises. As the patient's condition improves and results become more stable, we allow the musician to incorporate some minutes of completely free playing (no SMR, no DL, no ST).

4.3 Factors Associated with Good Outcomes and a Case Study

Since incorporating differential learning (DL) into our protocol, we have seen a significant improvement in results. However, applying DL to musicians poses certain challenges. First, DL is a completely different approach compared to what most musicians typically use to correct their problems and errors. We ask them to destabilize the system and trust in the self-organization process. They are not supposed to guide the process. Additionally, we do not provide advice on postural or technical corrections as these corrections activate the declarative working memory and put unnecessary stress on the system. Therefore, the first challenge is helping them understand the value of this approach. The fact that there are few studies applying DL to musicians does not help much either. Evidence from sports, while relevant, often fails to fully convince them, although musicians generally acknowledge that they are indeed high-performance athletes.

Their personality and the way they have been trained play a significant role in whether they ultimately accept and succeed with DL. It is true that, in the case of musicians with dystonia—a condition that, in a large percentage of cases, prevents them from playing and makes it very difficult to find appropriate treatment—there is often a greater openness to approaches like DL. However, their personality remains a limiting factor.

4.3.1 Analysis of Treated Patients

To better understand the predictive aspect of a musician's personality and behavior in the successful acceptance and execution of DL, we reviewed the medical histories of 173 consecutive MD patients who had been treated with DL alone or in combination with SMR over the past 4 years at our center. Of these, 112 had completed their treatment by the time of the analysis and are included in the data.

For each patient, we identified periods of clear clinical improvement or, conversely, times when there was no clinical change or even regression to a previous condition. When such instances occurred, we investigated whether they coincided with notable changes in the patient's behavior, mindset, or approach to treatment.

We ultimately selected four characteristic cases that, in our opinion, clearly illustrate the most common trajectories of these patients. We identified the major characteristics of the two primary groups and outlined the key factors that we believe determined the outcomes (see Tables 4.5 and 4.6).

4.3.2 Demonstrative Cases

The individual characteristics of the four selected subjects are summarized in Table 4.7.

4.3.2.1 Case 1

A 34-year-old professional guitarist started experiencing right ring finger weakness while playing, which progressively worsened over 12 months. He initially tried to address the issue with technical exercises, but when the problem

Table 4.5 Factors facilitating the application and effectiveness of DL

Understanding and mental flexibility	Grasping the concept of DL and the specific objectives of each exercise
	Being mentally flexible, willing to accept other perspectives, and breaking away from existing beliefs
	Allowing oneself to experiment and break habitual work and behavioral patterns
Consistency and adaptability	Following the recommended guidelines
	Maintaining regularity and consistency in practice. Making clear that patience and patient do have the same origin
	Embracing diversity by making many changes and trying various approaches, including in daily activities (ADLs)
	Accepting that improvement may not follow fixed timelines and avoiding setting rigid goals (e.g., specific recovery deadlines or expected progress within a set time frame)
Body awareness and physical activities	Having the ability to perceive the body while also accepting the need to disregard some of this information when performing exercises
	Complementing treatment with additional activities such as physical exercise, relaxation, and stretching, instead of focusing exclusively on treatment
Motivation and feedback	Experiencing improvements, such as reduced pain or better coordination, serves as motivation
	Realizing that using DL can yield the same or better results with less effort, or improve technical skills in areas not explicitly worked on
	Understanding that DL is compatible with their development as musicians and with their learning process
	Knowing that another musician has successfully benefited from DL provides a reference point for encouragement

Table 4.6 Factors hindering the application and effectiveness of DL

Personality traits	Being too analytical and observant
	Being obsessive and controlling, needing to constantly monitor the affected area, and unable to let go of that control. Anxiety arises from not being able to control symptoms
	Having strong, clear ideas about how the affected area should behave (as a symptom for external control) and an inability to accept that conscious control or instruction is not the only way to determine motor response
Consistency and discipline	Irregular treatment routine
	Taking breaks, such as during vacations or days off
	Lack of variation in exercises
Distraction and overthinking	Distraction from treatment by continuously seeking information, alternative methods, or cures that worked for others. Engaging in social media forums about MD (impatience)
	Lack of focus or concentration.

(continued)

Table 4.6 (continued)

Emotional and cognitive aspects	Poor emotional management: apathy, demotivation, anxiety, frustration
	Hurry to recover, expecting immediate results
	Past experiences with dystonia treatments that did not work, projecting these failures onto current efforts
	Comparing oneself to the progress of other musicians
	Questioning the ongoing treatment
	Difficulty accepting worsening symptoms as a normal and desirable part of the destabilization process, aimed at encouraging the body to explore solutions
	Wanting to know the reason behind everything, overthinking rather than focusing on exercises
	Limiting beliefs, such as "classical practice is superior" or "this approach won't help my playing"
	Poor management of personal issues
	Being overly negative and skeptical
	High dependence on the external environment and opinions from others, including confrontation with the teacher's instructions
	Viewing classical learning as the only way to achieve musical results (because it was taught by an external teacher) and doubting that DL could help both dystonia and playing ability
	Lack of clear goals
	Being impatient
Lack of flexibility	Closed-mindedness
	Inconsistency or lack of persistence in treatment

Table 4.7 Demonstrative case summary

Case	Gender	Age	Instrument	Affected area	Protocol	Treatment duration *(months)*	Outcome	Follow-up after treatment *(months)*
1	Male	34	Classical guitar	Right hand	DL	19	Complete recovery	12
2	Male	26	Oboe	Cervical	DL	13	Complete recovery	18
3	Female	36	Violin	Right arm	DL + SMR	13	Complete recovery	20
4	Male	41	Violin	Left hand	DL + SMR	14	Partial improvement	0

escalated, he modified his playing style to avoid using the affected finger. Eventually, involuntary flexion of the ring and little fingers appeared, prompting him to seek medical help.

Diagnosis

Primary focal dystonia of the right hand, with a normal neurological exam outside of guitar playing.

Treatment and Outcome

A neurorehabilitation program was developed to accommodate his professional demands. He practiced 20–30 min daily using DL and ST. After initial improvement, he experienced setbacks, particularly when the tension in his hand increased. To address this, the exercises were intensified with more frequent variations. He also used techniques like focusing on breathing during difficult passages to manage symptoms in live performances. Over time, these adjustments led to significant improvements. After 19 months, he reported his hand function as completely normal and even better than before the dystonia. One year later, he remained symptom-free and continued using DL as part of his regular practice routine.

4.3.2.2 Case 2

A 26-year-old professional oboe player developed neck tension followed by involuntary head turning while playing. Over a few months, these symptoms began to affect his daily activities, and he was eventually unable to play the oboe. His condition worsened to the point that dystonia was triggered by simply sitting, causing frequent headaches and forcing him to spend much of the day in bed.

Diagnosis

Cervical dystonia, confirmed after normal neurological and imaging results.

Treatment and Outcome

Fifteen months after symptom onset, he began a rehabilitation program including physical therapy and 20–30 min of DL and ST exercises. He initially played the oboe only during rehabilitation sessions, gradually improving. After 3 months, he was tired of doing the exercises because of the great mental effort they required and the difficulty of constantly looking for new variations. He was advised that it is not always necessary to create new variations of ST as he can combine them or make them in a different (better random) order. He was also advised to look for and download new applications for the tablet with new games and challenges. A major breakthrough came when breathing variations were incorporated into his exercises, significantly reducing tension (Komori 2018). Although the mental effort required by the exercises caused fatigue, introducing new challenges and games helped maintain motivation. After 10 months, he could play for 30–45 min daily without significant symptoms. Further exercises involving external resistance and coordination challenges solidified his progress. By month 13, he was playing normally, and an 18-month follow-up confirmed no return of symptoms.

4.3.2.3 Case3

A 36-year-old violinist with a decade of experience in a national symphony orchestra switched from wrist to arm vibrato, which caused difficulties in high positions on the violin. She eventually reverted to wrist vibrato, but soon developed forearm tension and difficulties vibrating with multiple fingers. After a year off for maternity leave, she found herself completely unable to perform vibrato.

Diagnosis

Focal dystonia, diagnosed after a normal neurological examination, except when vibrato was attempted.

Treatment and Outcome

She began a neurorehabilitation protocol centered around SMR, DL, and ST. Being creative and resourceful, she constantly adapted her exercises, leading to significant improvement within 2 months. However, family stress slowed her progress temporarily. Once resolved, she regained momentum, working on specific techniques such as slow vibrato. After 10 months, she felt close to full recovery but plateaued. A month-long focus on exercises rather than performance brought her to near-complete recovery. By month 13, she returned to her orchestra position without any symptoms. A follow-up 20 months later confirmed her full recovery.

4.3.2.4 Case 4

A 41-year-old violinist developed involuntary flexion of his left ring finger after increasing his practice to improve technical skills. Despite attempting postural reeducation and botulinum toxin injections, he saw no improvement.

Diagnosis

Focal dystonia, confirmed by normal neurological findings outside of violin playing.

Treatment and Outcome

He began a neurorehabilitation program including SMR, ST, and variation exercises. From the outset, he struggled with the protocol, particularly with letting go of control over his finger movements. Although he experienced some improvement, he found it difficult to follow the prescribed exercises correctly. Over time, this led to only partial progress. Despite regular adjustments to the program and his attempts to vary his exercises, his need to control his finger movements remained a barrier. After 14 months, he decided to discontinue therapy due to the mental strain and inability to fully adhere to the protocol, despite some progress.

4.4 Differential Learning in Musicians with Other Pathologies

Since we incorporated DL as a tool to improve musicians' health, we have been experimenting and expanding its use to nearly all of our patients. Our primary goal at the Institute is to resolve the pathologies that come to us as effectively as possible—whether it is a trigger finger, a contracture, a radial neuritis, or anything else. We also use DL to prevent relapses and help patients return to their maximum performance as quickly as possible.

We apply DL as soon as the musician begins playing during their recovery. At the start, when they are playing for short periods, we try to ensure that all this playing time involves DL. This approach, aside from making the system more flexible again, brings other advantages. It prevents them from repeating the same movements too many times and thus overloading structures that are already strained due to the injury. It also helps avoid establishing compensatory patterns (or resolving existing ones) and keeps them from focusing too much on the musical outcome.

In the later stages, when individuals are more active or have returned to work, they often resist committing extensive time to DL. In such cases, we offer targeted guidance to ensure they at least disrupt their routine periodically, especially when symptoms resurface, or they encounter obstacles in their physical or technical progress. We also assist them in selecting the most critical technical exercises or sections of their repertoire where applying DL is most beneficial, based on their specific condition and the areas identified for improvement.

Once their time at our center ends and their pathology is resolved, a high proportion of musicians continue using DL. They do so either as a preventive measure or because they realize that it is helpful in their work as musicians. Those who are clearest about this are the ones who have students. They see that DL can help not only to prevent injuries in their students but also to resolve issues that traditional repetition-based learning methods fail to address, especially when students become blocked and stagnate. Some musicians apply DL themselves. The most common scenario is that they use it for specific problems, whether technical or otherwise, while some apply it more broadly to everything.

It is fascinating to listen to the YouTube conversation between Joseph Alessi (American trombonist, current principal trombone of the New York Philharmonic, professor at the Juilliard School, and one of the most recognized soloists today) and Danielle Morandini (Principal Trombone of the Teatro alla Scala in Milan). Both suffered from facial paralysis, which temporarily sidelined their careers. They were treated at our center and, among other strategies, incorporated DL into their recovery process. They found that DL helped them in many ways, but what surprised them most was how the simple introduction of fluctuations to the system led to improvements and resolved technical aspects without them working on these issues directly. For example, he reached very high notes that he had never played or practiced before (Alessi 2022).

The most challenging part is convincing musicians that DL can help them learn and consolidate their skills more effectively, with less risk of injury, compared to traditional learning. Moreover, the flexibility they gain makes them more resilient to performance drops under pressure. We still lack studies, similar to those conducted in sports, that demonstrate DL is not a waste of time from a technical and musical perspective, but is at least as effective, if not more so.

4.5 Conclusion

The application of DL in musicians' rehabilitation, particularly for those suffering from conditions like MD, has proven to be an effective approach to enhancing system flexibility and promoting recovery. Traditional methods often focus on perfecting specific techniques or maintaining consistency, which can inadvertently lead to increased rigidity and a higher risk of injury. In contrast, DL introduces intentional variability, encouraging the musician's neuromuscular system to adapt and self-organize, which is crucial for overcoming the maladaptive motor patterns that characterize MD.

Our experience and data demonstrate that DL significantly improves outcomes in musicians' rehabilitation by fostering adaptability and reducing the reliance on compensatory mechanisms. Musicians who adopt DL into their regular practice routines often find it beneficial for preventing future injuries and enhancing their technical abilities in ways that traditional methods may not.

Interestingly, the idea of introducing variability in practice is not entirely new. The renowned cellist Mstislav Rostropovich famously advised musicians to "Practice wrong!"—encouraging them to explore different, and perhaps musically "wrong," versions during practice (Demenga 2014). This approach aligns closely with the principles of DL, where the goal is to destabilize the system and allow for the emergence of new, more adaptable patterns of performance.

Furthermore, our analysis of factors associated with successful DL outcomes highlights the importance of mental flexibility, consistency in its practice, and avoiding, as much as possible, control. Musicians who embrace the concept of DL, allowing themselves to experiment and break habitual patterns and break away from existing beliefs, tend to achieve better results.

Moreover, the broader application of DL across various conditions affecting musicians has shown that it is a versatile tool, capable of addressing a range of physical challenges. Its ability to break down rigid patterns and introduce beneficial variability makes it a valuable component of modern musicians' health strategies.

In conclusion, the integration of DL into musicians' rehabilitation protocols represents a paradigm shift from traditional repetition-based learning to a more dynamic, adaptive approach that aligns with the complex and individualized nature of musical performance. This method not only aids in the recovery from specific conditions like focal dystonia but also contributes to the overall resilience and sustainability of a musician's career.

Questions

1. In what ways is the adaptability of a musician's motor system crucial for injury prevention and long-term performance?
2. How does focal dystonia illustrate the consequences of excessive rigidity in movement patterns?
3. What are the key differences between traditional rehabilitation approaches and differential learning when addressing musician-related injuries?
4. Why has conventional music education emphasized imitating fixed models, and what are the potential drawbacks of this approach?
5. How does the principle of self-organization in DL contrast with explicit technical correction in traditional pedagogy?
6. How do sensory motor retuning (SMR) and differential learning (DL) complement each other when rehabilitating injured musicians?
   A. SMR strengthens finger muscles, while DL focuses on rhythm and timing.
   B. SMR isolates healthy movement patterns; DL restores them through repetition.
   C. SMR alters perception and proprioception; DL introduces variability to enhance adaptability.
   D. SMR and DL are used sequentially: SMR before injury and DL after.
   E. SMR is cognitive therapy, while DL is purely physical.

7. Why may some musicians resist DL, and how can teachers ease its adoption?
   A. Musicians resist DL because it discourages creativity, which teachers must accept.
   B. Musicians see DL as disorganized; teachers can convince them with scientific evidence.
   C. Musicians find DL boring; teachers should use humor to make it engaging.
   D. Musicians find DL uncomfortable due to unpredictability; teachers should clarify its purpose and guide creativity.
   E. Musicians are too experienced for DL; teachers should only apply it to beginners.
8. How do instrument setup, posture, or practice routines affect neuromotor flexibility in musicians?
   A. They have minimal impact if musicians warm up properly.
   B. Uniform routines build consistency, which always enhances flexibility.
   C. Repetition of fixed setups fosters accuracy and reduces stress.
   D. Lack of variability in posture and routines reduces flexibility and adaptability.
   E. Only incorrect posture affects flexibility, not practice routines.
9. How can deliberate variability in practice enhance—rather than destabilize—performance consistency?
   A. It increases conscious control of movements during concerts.
   B. It confuses the motor system temporarily, which weakens automatisms.
   C. It forces the body to abandon bad habits through constant correction.
   D. It trains the performer to focus more on the final sound than the movement.
   E. It builds flexible automatisms that are more resilient to change.
10. What is a practical way to integrate DL into a musician's daily routine without hindering technical progress?
   A. Replace all scales with DL noise exercises and stop repertoire work entirely.
   B. Practice only random gestures for 2 months before returning to pieces.
   C. Begin each session with a 5-min block of systematic variations or practice a technique or part of a piece that is not improving as expected, to observe results. Then proceed to normal repertoire, gradually letting variability become an implicit habit.
   D. Avoid DL on concert days because it erases motor memory.
   E. Use DL only in physiotherapy clinics, never in the practice room.

References

Albrecht S, Janssen D, Quarz E, Newell KM, Schöllhorn WI (2014) Individuality of movements in music--finger and body movements during playing of the flute. Hum Mov Sci 35:131–144. https://doi.org/10.1016/j.humov.2014.03.010

Alessi J, Morandini D. Bell's Palsy/Ramsey Hunt syndrome – a cautionary tale (2022) https://youtu.be/yumhZ1KwjlQ?si=sIyJJzrmf_Vh_zo8

Almeida A, George D, Smith J, Wolfe J (2013) The clarinet: how blowing pressure, lip force, lip position and reed "hardness" affect pitch, sound level, and spectrum. J Acoust Soc Am 134(3):2247–2255. https://doi.org/10.1121/1.4816538

Andrews MH, Gorman AD, Crowther RH (2024) Functional movement variability to maintain delivery speed in cricket fast bowling. Eur J Sport Sci 24(4):415–421. https://doi.org/10.1002/ejsc.12045

Bartlett R, Wheat J, Robins M (2007) Is movement variability important for sports biomechanists? Sports Biomech 6(2):224–243. https://doi.org/10.1080/14763140701322994

Bara-Jimenez W, Catalan MJ, Hallett M, Gerloff C (1998) Abnormal somatosensory homunculus in dystonia of the hand. Abstract Annals of Neurology 44(5):828–31 https://doi.org/10.1002/ana.v44:5; https://doi.org/10.1002/ana.410440520

Bauer HU, Schöllhorn WI (1997) Self-organizing maps for the analysis of complex movement patterns. Neural Process Lett 5:193–199. https://doi.org/10.1023/A:1009643721719
Baugh LA, Marotta JJ (2009) When What's Left Is Right: Visuomotor Transformations in an Aged Population. PLoS ONE 4(5): e5484. https://doi.org/10.1371/journal.pone.0005484
Beckers F, Verheyden B, Aubert AE (2006) Aging and nonlinear heart rate control in a healthy population. Am J Physiol Heart Circ Physiol 290(6):H2560–H2570. https://doi.org/10.1152/AJPHEART.00903.2005
Bella SD, Palmer C (2011) Rate effects on timing, key velocity, and finger kinematics in piano performance. PLoS One 6(6):e20518. https://doi.org/10.1371/journal.pone.0020518
Berardelli A, Rothwell JC, Hallett M, Thompson PD, Manfredi M, Marsden CD (1998) The pathophysiology of primary dystonia Brain 121(Pt 7):1195–12. https://doi.org/10.1093/brain/121.7.1195. PMID: 9679773.
Bernstein NA (1935) The problem of the interrelation of co-ordination and localization. Arch Biol Sci 38:1–34. (in Russian). Translated into English in Bernstein NA (1967) The coordination and regulation of movements. Pergamon Press, Oxford. p 196
Bertsch M (1997) Variabilities in trumpet sounds. A lot of variables and aspects makes trumpets sounding different. An attempt to systematize. In: Myers A (ed) Proceedings of the international symposium of musical acoustics, vol II, pp 401–406
Betzel RF, Satterthwaite TD, Gold JI, Bassett DS (2017) Positive affect, surprise, and fatigue are correlates of network flexibility. Sci Rep 7(1):520. https://doi.org/10.1038/s41598-017-00425-z
Butković A, Vukojević N, Carević S (2021) Music performance anxiety and perfectionism in Croatian musicians. Psychol Music 50(1):100–110. https://doi.org/10.1177/0305735620978692
Butefisch CM, Boroojerdi B, Chen R, Battaglia F, Hallett M (2005) Taskdependent intracortical inhibition is impaired in focal hand dystonia. Abstract Movement Disorders 20(5):545–51. https://doi.org/10.1002/mds.v20:5; https://doi.org/10.1002/mds.20367
Buttkus F, Weidenmüller M, Schneider S, Jabusch H-C, Nitsche MA, Paulus W, Altenmüller E (2010) Failure of cathodal direct current stimulation to improve fine motor control in musician's dystonia. Abstract Movement Disorders 25(3):389–94 https://doi.org/10.1002/mds.v25:3; https://doi.org/10.1002/mds.22938
Byl NN, McKenzie A (2000) Treatment effectiveness for patients with a history of repetitive hand use and focal hand dystonia. Journal of Hand Therapy 13(4):289–301 https://doi.org/10.1016/S0894-1130(00)80021-6
Cleveland SE (1959) Personality dynamics in torticollis. J Nerv Ment Dis 129:150–161. https://doi.org/10.1097/00005053-195908000-00004
Côté JN (2014) Adaptations to neck/shoulder fatigue and injuries. In: Levin MF (ed) Progress in motor control: advances in experimental medicine and biology. Springer, New York, pp 205–222. https://doi.org/10.1007/978-1-4939-1338-1_13
Demenga T (2014) The art of distraction is more effective than repetitive practice. The Strad. https://www.thestrad.com/the-art-of-distraction-ismore-effective-than-repetitive-practice/5344.article
Demos AP, Lisboa T, Chaffin R (2016) Flexibility of expressive timing in repeated musical performances. Front Psychol 4(7):1490. https://doi.org/10.3389/fpsyg.2016.01490
Fedorowich L, Emery K, Gervasi B, Côté JN, Feil M, Oberfeld T (2013) Gender differences in neck/shoulder muscular patterns in response to repetitive motion induced fatigue. J Electromyogr Kinesiol 23(5):1183–1189. https://doi.org/10.1016/j.jelekin.2013.06.005
Elbert T, Candia V, Altenmüller E, Rau H, Sterr A, Rockstroh B, Pantev C and Taub E (1998) Alteration of digital representations in somatosensory cortex in focal hand dystonia. NeuroReport 9(16):3571–5. https://doi.org/10.1097/00001756-199811160-00006
Ferrari JR, Mautz WT (1997) Predicting perfectionism: applying tests of rigidity. J Clin Psychol 53(1):1–6. https://doi.org/10.1002/(sici)1097-4679(199701)53:1<1::aid-jclp1>3.0.co;2-y
Furuya S, Altenmüller E (2013) Flexibility of movement organization in piano performance. Front Hum Neurosci 16(7):173. https://doi.org/10.3389/fnhum.2013.00173
Furuya S, Tanibuchi R, Nishioka H, Kimoto Y, Hirano M, Oku T (2023) Passive somatosensory training enhances piano skill in adolescent and adult pianists: a preliminary study. Ann N Y Acad Sci 1519(1):167–172. https://doi.org/10.1111/nyas.14939
Gibson HB (1972) Writer's cramp: a behavioural approach. Behav Res Ther 10(4):371–380. https://doi.org/10.1016/0005-7967(72)90060-5
Haken H (1983) Synergetics: An Introduction: Nonequilibrium Phase Transitions and Self-Organization in Physics, Chemistry and Biology. Springer, Berlin.
Henz D, Schöllhorn WI (2018) Temporal courses in EEG theta and alpha activity in the dynamic health qigong techniques Wu Qin xi and Liu Zi Jue. Front Psychol 8:2291. https://doi.org/10.3389/fpsyg.2017.02291
Herholz SC, Zatorre RJ (2012) Musical training as a framework for brain plasticity: behavior, function, and structure. Neuron 76(3):486–502. https://doi.org/10.1016/j.neuron.2012.10.011
Hodges PW (2011) Pain and motor control: From the laboratory to rehabilitation. J Electromyogr Kinesiol 21(2)220–8 https://doi.org/10.1016/j.jelekin.2011.01.002
Horisawa S, Goto S, Taira T, Ochiai T, Nakajima T (2013) Long-term improvement of musician's dystonia after stereotactic ventro-oral thalamotomy. Ann Neurol 74(2):648. https://doi.org/10.1002/ana.23877
Ioannou CI, Altenmüller E (2014) Psychological characteristics in musician's dystonia: a new diagnostic clas-

sification. Neuropsychologia 61:80–88. https://doi.org/10.1016/j.neuropsychologia.2014.06.011

Ioannou CI, Furuya S, Altenmüller E (2016) The impact of stress on motor performance in skilled musicians suffering from focal dystonia: physiological and psychological characteristics. Neuropsychologia 85:226–236. https://doi.org/10.1016/j.neuropsychologia.2016.03.029

Jabusch HC, Altenmüller E (2006) Focal dystonia in musicians: from phenomenology to therapy. Adv Cogn Psychol 2(2):207–220. https://doi.org/10.2478/V10053-008-0056-6

Kast V, Leukel C (2016) Motor experts care about consistency and are reluctant to change motor outcome. PLoS One 11(8):e0161798. https://doi.org/10.1371/journal.pone.0161798

Komori T (2018) The relaxation effect of prolonged expiratory breathing. Ment Illn 10(1):7669. https://doi.org/10.4081/mi.2018.7669

Kotani S, Furuya S (2018) State anxiety disorganizes finger movements during musical performance. J Neurophysiol 120(2):439–451. https://doi.org/10.1152/jn.00813.2017

Latash ML, Scholz JP, Schöner G (2007) Toward a New Theory of Motor Synergies. Motor Control 11(3):276–308 https://doi.org/10.1123/mcj.11.3.276

Lashley KS (1933) Integrative function of the cerebral cortex. Physiol Rev 13(1):1–42. https://doi.org/10.1152/physrev.1933.13.1.1

Lohmann K, Schmidt A, Schillert A, Winkler S, Albanese A, Baas F, Bentivoglio AR, Borngräber F, Brüggemann N, Defazio G, Del Sorbo F, Deuschl G, Edwards MJ, Gasser T, Gómez-Garre P, Graf J, Groen JL, Grünewald A, Hagenah J, Hemmelmann C, Jabusch H-C, Kaji R, Kasten M, Kawakami H, Kostic VS, Liguori M, Mir P, Münchau A, Ricchiuti F, Schreiber S, Siegesmund K, Svetel M, Tijssen MAJ, Valente EM, Westenberger A, Zeuner KE, Zittel S, Altenmüller E, Ziegler A, Klein C (2014) Genome-wide association study in musician's dystonia: A risk variant at the arylsulfatase G locus? ABSTRACT Movement Disorders 29(7):921–7 https://doi.org/10.1002/mds.v29.7; https://doi.org/10.1002/mds.25791

Madeleine P, Mathiassen SE, Arendt-Nielsen L (2008) Changes in the degree of motor variability associated with experimental and chronic neck-shoulder pain during a standardised repetitive arm movement. Exp Brain Res 185(4):689–698. https://doi.org/10.1007/s00221-007-1199-2

Manor B, Costa MD, Hu K, Newton E, Starobinets O, Kang HG et al (2010) Physiological complexity and system adaptability: evidence from postural control dynamics of older adults. J Appl Physiol 109(6):1786–1791. https://doi.org/10.1152/japplphysiol.00390.2010

Mekari S, Neyedli HF, Fraser S, O'Brien MW, Martins R, Evans K, Earle M, Aucoin R, Chiekwe J, Hollohan Q, Kimmerly DS, Dupuy O (2020) High-intensity interval training improves cognitive flexibility in older adults. Brain Sci 10(11):796. https://doi.org/10.3390/brainsci10110796

McKenzie AL, Nagarajan SS, Roberts TP, Merzenich MM, Byl NN (2003). Somatosensory representation of the digits and clinical performance in patients with focal hand dystonia. Am J Phys Med Rehabil 82(10):737–49. https://doi.org/10.1097/01.PHM.0000087458.32122.14. PMID: 14508403.

McKenzie AL, Goldman S, Barrango C, Shrime M, Wong T, Byl N (2009) Differences in Physical Characteristics and Response to Rehabilitation for Patients with Hand Dystonia: Musicians' Cramp. Compared to Writers' Cramp. Journal of Hand Therapy 22(2):172–82 https://doi.org/10.1016/j.jht.2008.12.006

Moura N, Vidal M, Aguilera AM, Vilas-Boas JP, Serra S, Leman M (2023) Knee flexion of saxophone players anticipates tonal context of music. npj Sci Learn 8(1):1–7. https://doi.org/10.1038/s41539-023-00172-z

Paulig J, Jabusch HC, Großbach M, Boullet L, Altenmüller E (2014) Sensory trick phenomenon improves motor control in pianists with dystonia: prognostic value of glove-effect. Front Psychol 5:1012. https://doi.org/10.3389/fpsyg.2014.01012

Pfordresher PQ, Chow K (2019) A cost of musical training? Sensorimotor flexibility in musical sequence learning. Psychon Bull Rev 26(3):967–973. https://doi.org/10.3758/s13423-018-1535-5

Phillips E, Portus M, Davids K, Renshaw I (2012) Performance accuracy and functional variability in elite and developing fast bowlers. J Sci Med Sport 15(2):182–188. https://doi.org/10.1016/j.jsams.2011.07.006

Pujol JJ, Roset-Llobet D, Rosinés-Cubells J, Deus B, Narberhaus J, Valls-Solé A, Capdevila A, Pascual-Leone (2000) Brain Cortical Activation during Guitar-Induced Hand Dystonia Studied by Functional MRI NeuroImage 12(3):257–67 https://doi.org/10.1006/nimg.2000.0615

Quartarone A, Siebner HR, Rothwell JC (2006) Task-specific hand dystonia: can too much plasticity be bad for you? Trends in Neurosciences 29(4):192–9 https://doi.org/10.1016/j.tins.2006.02.007

Ranganathan R, Newell KM (2010) Emergent flexibility in motor learning. Exp Brain Res 202(4):755–764. https://doi.org/10.1007/s00221-010-2177-7

Repšaitė V, Vainoras A, Berškienė K, Baltaduonienė D, Daunoravičienė A, Sendžikaitė E (2015) The effect of differential training-based occupational therapy on hand and arm function in patients after stroke: results of the pilot study. Neurol Neurochir Pol 49(3):150–155. https://doi.org/10.1016/j.pjnns.2015.06.001

Rosenkranz K, Butler K, Williamon A, Rothwell JC (2009) Regaining Motor Control in Musician's Dystonia by Restoring Sensorimotor Organization. The Journal of Neuroscience 29(46):14627–14636 https://doi.org/10.1523/JNEUROSCI.2094-09.2009

Ridding MC, Sheean G, Rothwell JC, Inzelberg R, Kujirai T (1995) Changes in the balance between motor cortical excitation and inhibition in focal, task specific dystonia. J Neurol Neurosurg Psychiatry. 59(5):493–8. https://doi.org/10.1136/jnnp.59.5.493. PMID: 8530933; PMCID: PMC1073711.

Rosset-Llobet J, Fàbregas-Molas S (2013) La dystonie du musician. Manuel pratique à l'usage des musiciens et de leurs thérapeutes. Montauvan: Alexitère editions
Rosset-Llobet J, Fàbregas-Molas S (2018) Rehabilitation and plasticity of task-specific focal hand dystonia. In: Dressler D, Altenmüller E, Krauss J (eds) Treatment of dystonia. Cambridge University Press, Cambridge, pp 256–260. https://doi.org/10.1017/9781316459324.052
Rosset-Llobet J, Candia V, Fàbregas S, Ray W, Pascual-Leone A (2007) Secondary motor disturbances in 101 patients with musician's dystonia. J Neurol Neurosurg Psychiatry 78(9):949–953. https://doi.org/10.1136/jnnp.2006.107953
Rosset-Llobet J, Garcia-Elias M, Montero J, Valls-Solé J, Pascual-Leone A (2009) Linburg's syndrome, can it cause focal dystonia? Mov Disord 24(11):1704–1706. https://doi.org/10.1002/mds.22592
Rosset-Llobet J, Pascual-Leone A, Fàbregas-Molas S, Role of female reproductive hormones in musicians' dystonia (2012) Med Probl Perform Art 27(3):156–158. https://doi.org/10.21091/mppa.2012.3027
Sadnicka A, Rosset-Llobet J (2019) A motor control model of task-specific dystonia and its rehabilitation. Prog Brain Res 249:269–283. https://doi.org/10.1016/bs.pbr.2019.04.011
Schöllhorn WI (2000) Applications of systems dynamic principles to technique and strength training. Acta Academiae Olympiquae Estoniae 7:67–85
Schöllhorn WI (2005) Differenzielles Lehren und Lernen von Bewegung – Durch veränderte Annahmen zu neuen Konsequenzen [Differential teaching and learning of movement – through changed assumptions to new consequences]. In: Gabler H, Göhner U, Schiebl F (eds) Zur Vernetzung von Forschung und Lehre in Biomechanik, Sportmotorik und Trainingswissenschaft. Czwalina, pp 125–135
Schöllhorn WI, Nigg BM, Stefanyshyn DJ, Liu W (2002) Identification of individual walking patterns using time discrete and time continuous data sets. Gait Posture 15(2):180–186. https://doi.org/10.1016/s0966-6362(01)00193-x
Schöllhorn WI, Mayer-Kress G, Newell KM, Michelbrink M (2009) Time scales of adaptive behavior and motor learning in the presence of stochastic perturbations. Hum Mov Sci 28(3):319–333. https://doi.org/10.1016/j.humov.2008.10.005
Schöllhorn WI, Beckmann H, Davids K (2010) Exploiting system fluctuations: differential training in physical prevention and rehabilitation programs for health and exercise. Medicina 46(6):365–373. https://doi.org/10.3390/medicina46060052
Schöllhorn WI, Rizzi N, Slapšinskaitė-Dackevičienė A, Leite N (2022) Always pay attention to which model of motor learning you are using. Int J Environ Res Public Health 19(2):711. https://doi.org/10.3390/ijerph19020711
Schuele S, Jabusch H, Lederman R, Altenmüller E (2005) Botulinum toxin injections in the treatment of musician's dystonia. Neurology 64(2):341–343. https://doi.org/10.1212/01.WNL.0000149768.36634.92
Seifert L, Komar J, Araújo D, Davids K (2016) Neurobiological degeneracy: a key property for functional adaptations of perception and action to constraints. Neurosci Biobehav Rev 69:159–165. https://doi.org/10.1016/j.neubiorev.2016.08.006
Sheehy MP, Marsden CD (1982) Writers' cramp-a focal dystonia. Brain 105(Pt 3):461–480. https://doi.org/10.1093/brain/105.3.461
Shine JM, Koyejo O, Poldrack RA (2016) Temporal metastates are associated with differential patterns of time-resolved connectivity, network topology, and attention. Proc Natl Acad Sci USA 113(35):9888–9891. https://doi.org/10.1073/pnas.1604898113
Stergiou N, Decker LM (2011) Human movement variability, nonlinear dynamics, and pathology: is there a connection? Hum Mov Sci 30(5):869–888. https://doi.org/10.1016/j.humov.2011.06.002
Tamura Y, Ueki Y, Lin P, Vorbach S, Mima T, Kakigi R, Hallett M (2009) Disordered plasticity in the primary somatosensory cortex in focal hand dystonia. Brain 132(3):749–55 https://doi.org/10.1093/brain/awn348
Thorpe CT, Chaudhry S, Lei II, Varone A, Riley GP, Birch HL, Clegg PD, Screen HR (2015) Tendon overload results in alterations in cell shape and increased markers of inflammation and matrix degradation. Scand J Med Sci Sports 25(4):e381–91. https://doi.org/10.1111/sms.12333. Epub 2014 Dec 30. PMID: 25639911
Tubiana R, Chamagne P (1983) Occupational "cramps" of the upper limb. Ann Chir Main 2(2):134–142. https://doi.org/10.1016/S0753-9053(83)80049-5
Turner C, Visentin P, Oye D, Rathwell S, Shan G (2022) An examination of trunk and right-hand coordination in piano performance: a case comparison of three pianists. Front Psychol 13:838554. https://doi.org/10.3389/fpsyg.2022.838554
Uehara K, Yasuhara M, Koguchi J, Oku T, Shiotani S, Morise M, Furuya S (2023) Brain network flexibility as a predictor of skilled musical performance. Cereb Cortex 33(20):10492–10503. https://doi.org/10.1101/2023.04.26.538360
van Emmerik REA and van Wegen EEH (2000) On variability and stability in human movement. J Appl Biomech 16(4):394–406. https://doi.org/10.1123/jab.16.4.394
Van Emmerik RE, Hamill J, McDermott WJ (2005) Variability and coordinative function in human gait. Quest 57(1):102–123. https://doi.org/10.1080/00336297.2005.10491845
Van Vugt FT, Treutler K, Altenmüller E, Jabusch HC (2013) The influence of chronotype on making music: circadian fluctuations in pianists' fine motor skills. Front Hum Neurosci 7:347. https://doi.org/10.3389/fnhum.2013.00347

Velut L, Vergez C, Gilbert J, Sanchez P (2015) Simultaneous and in vivo measurements of control parameters used in trumpet performance. In: Proceedings of the third Vienna talk on music acoustics. University of Music and Performing Arts Viena, p 3

Williamon A, Aufegger L, Wasley D, Looney D, Mandic DP (2013) Complexity of physiological responses decreases in high-stress musical performance. J R Soc Interface 10(89):20130719. https://doi.org/10.1098/rsif.2013.0719

Wilson C, Perkin OJ, McGuigan MP, Stokes KA (2016) The effect of age on technique variability and outcome variability during a leg press. PLoS One 11(10):e0163764. https://doi.org/10.1371/journal.pone.0163764

5 Differential Learning in the Rehabilitation of Patients After a Stroke

Viktorija Kaktienė

Abbreviations

BMI	Body mass index
BP	Blood pressure
DALYs	Disability-adjusted life years
DM	Diabetes mellitus
DL	Differential learning
ESO	European Stroke Organisation
fMRI	Functional magnetic resonance imaging
FPG	Fasting plasma glucose
LDL	Low-density lipoprotein
LMIC	Low- and middle-income countries
MMSE	Mini-Mental State Examination
MRI	Magnetic resonance imaging
PET	Positron emission tomography
SBP	Systolic blood pressure

5.1 The Burden of Stroke: Risk Factors, Demographic Challenges, and Global Trends

Stroke remains one of the leading causes of disability and mortality worldwide, ranking among the top cardiovascular diseases (GBD 2019 Stroke Collaborators 2021; Roth et al. 2020). It is a highly prevalent condition, causing severe impairments and long-lasting consequences for survivors (Udvardi et al. 2023). As a major global health issue (Feigin et al. 2014; Krishnamurthi et al. 2013; Mendis 2013), the significance of stroke is expected to grow in the future due to ongoing demographic shifts, including population aging and health transitions in developing countries (Roth et al. 2015).

Currently, stroke is the second leading contributor to disease burden in Europe (Feigin et al. 2022). Projections suggest that stroke incidence

V. Kaktienė (✉)
Sports Medicine Clinic, Lithuanian University of Health Sciences, Kaunas, Lithuania
e-mail: viktorija.kaktiene@lsmuni.lt; viktorija.kaktiene@gmail.com

W. I. Schöllhorn, A. Slapšinskaitė-Dackevičienė (eds.), *Differential Learning in Physiotherapy*,
https://doi.org/10.1007/978-3-031-98787-8_5

will increase by 34% in the coming decades, with the number of ischemic strokes in individuals over 80 anticipated to triple between 2010 and 2060. Additionally, a 27% increase in the number of stroke survivors is expected, leading to a corresponding rise in health and non-healthcare expenditures related to stroke (Lucas-Noll et al. 2023). Stroke remains the third leading cause of death and disability globally (Feigin et al. 2022) and the primary cause of adult disability in Europe (Wafa et al. 2020).

Regional differences in Europe show that age-standardized stroke incidence has decreased due to improved prevention and treatment strategies. However, the absolute number of cases remains high because of the aging population, with approximately 1.1 million new cases reported annually. Forecasts for Europe from 2017 to 2047 predict a 17% decrease in stroke mortality but a 27% increase in stroke prevalence (Wafa et al. 2020). These trends highlight the growing demand for stroke rehabilitation services and underscore the pressing need for innovative strategies to address this global health crisis effectively.

Being a heterogeneous disease, stroke has contrasting consequences on human physiology, depending on whether the stroke is subarachnoid hemorrhage, ischemic stroke, or intraparenchymal hemorrhage, each varying in pathophysiology (Lekander et al. 2017). Epidemiologic studies can help identify the risk factors that lead to stroke. Marking the risk factors for certain precarious diseases helps deal with the morbidity.

Unmodifiable Risk Factors

1. **Age**
   Stroke incidences increase with age between 45 and 85 years and almost double with each passing decade. The risk of having a stroke is highest among 55–65 years. In a study of stroke prevalence in the United Kingdom, it was revealed that at the age of 40, there are 10 deaths/100,000 population, whereas there are 100 deaths/100,000 population at the age of 75. The stroke rate is doubled in both genders after 55 for each passing decade. Age is declared as an independent, unmodifiable risk factor for experiencing intracranial atherosclerosis (ICAD), and its prevalence increases with each passing decade (23% for the age group of 50–60 years, 43% for 60–70 years, 65% for 70–80 years, and 80% for the population > 80 years) (Elkind and Sacco 1998).
2. **Ethnicity**
   Results of a stroke study to determine ethnicity as a risk factor showed that Black people are at 2.1 times greater risk of subarachnoid hemorrhage and 1.4 times greater risk of intracerebral hemorrhage than white people (Broderick et al. 1992). The ratio of affected population with intracranial stenosis is higher in Hispanic and African Americans than in white Americans. A comparative autopsy supports this data study (aorta and coronary arteries) for ICAD between African and white Americans (O'Donnell et al. 2010). Similarly, stroke incidence among Asian populations is much higher than in those of North European descent.
3. **Gender**
   Gender differences in stroke incidence vary across different regions, with some studies reporting higher rates in men, others in women, and some finding no significant gender differences. The National Stroke Epidemiology Survey found no statistically significant gender-based differences in overall stroke incidence or age-adjusted incidence. In a review of 18 studies from various countries (including the United States, Japan, Russia, Italy, and Finland), researchers concluded that the incidence of stroke in women was 1.24 times higher than in men (range: 1.09–1.42) (Vyas et al. 2021). Recent Canadian data reveals that, over the course of their lives, women face a higher risk of ischemic stroke and transient ischemic attack (TIA) compared to men (Chen et al. 2018; Sun et al. 2019). The estimated global lifetime risk of stroke from the age of 25 onward is 24.7% (23.3–26.0) for men and 25.1% (23.7–26.5)

for women, though geographic variations exist (Katan and Luft 2018). Approximately 55,000 more fatal strokes occur annually in women than in men (Gokhale et al. 2015). Throughout adulthood, strokes account for a larger proportion of deaths in women compared to men. However, due to differences in reproductive health, the prevalence and impact of stroke risk factors in women diverge from those in men. Conditions such as high blood pressure (BP), atrial fibrillation, diabetes, abdominal obesity, migraine with aura, emotional stress, and depression are more prevalent among women and contribute more significantly to their stroke risk.

4. **Genetics**
   Epidemiological studies indicate that genetic factors play a significant role in stroke risk (Markus 2012). Several single-gene disorders can lead to both ischemic and hemorrhagic strokes, often resulting in specific subtypes of stroke. The most common of these is cerebral autosomal dominant arteriopathy with subcortical infarcts and leukoencephalopathy (CADASIL), a monogenic cause of cerebral small vessel disease (SVD). While these monogenic causes are crucial for individual patients, they are rare and contribute minimally to the overall population-level stroke risk (Markus 2010).
5. **Heredity/Family Stroke History**
   Heredity is one of the well-studied risk factors. Previous studies have divulged that genetic factors play an important role in developing premature ICAD-atherosclerosis in the body's vascular system via proliferation of the smooth muscle, angiogenesis impairment, and endothelial injury (Khan et al. 2009).
6. **Social Status**
   Social status is a significant risk factor for stroke, particularly in the United States. Low social status, including lower education levels, reduced income, and limited social support, is associated with a higher risk of stroke. Studies indicate that individuals with lower social status are more likely to experience stroke and tend to have poorer health outcomes following it (Avendano et al. 2006).

Modifiable Risk Factors

1. **Alcohol Consumption**
   Studies on stroke have shown a curvilinear relationship between ischemic stroke and alcohol consumption, with low alcohol intake providing a protective effect and excessive consumption increasing the risk (Miah et al. 2012). Women consuming three drinks per day were found to be at higher risk than men (White et al. 2005). Heavy alcohol consumption (more than 14 drinks per week for men and more than 7 drinks per week for women) may increase the risk of any type of stroke, particularly small artery occlusion in ischemic stroke.
2. **Diabetes Mellitus**
   Diabetic patients are more prone to atherogenic risk factors, such as hypertension, irregular blood lipids, and obesity, leading to a higher susceptibility toward atherosclerosis (Chambless et al. 2000). Diabetes mellitus (DM) has been confirmed as an independent risk factor for ischemic stroke (Lackland et al. 2014). Studies have shown that the population suffering from DM has twice the risk of experiencing thromboembolic stroke, and glucose-intolerant people have double the risk of brain infarction compared to nondiabetic individuals (White et al. 2013).
3. **High Blood Pressure**
   According to the 2018 guidelines from the European Society of Cardiology (ESC) and the European Society of Hypertension (ESH) for managing arterial hypertension, high blood pressure (hypertension) is defined as a systolic blood pressure (SBP) of 140 mmHg or higher or a diastolic blood pressure (DBP) of 90 mmHg or higher. The guidelines also emphasize that blood pressure readings consistently above 130/80 mmHg, even under ambulatory monitoring conditions, should be regarded as indicative of hypertension. This threshold is consistent with the criteria used

for diagnosing hypertension in various clinical environments, including ambulatory blood pressure (BP) monitoring. Ambulatory BP monitoring provides a thorough evaluation of blood pressure fluctuations throughout the day and night, offering a more precise assessment compared to traditional office-based measurements. Hypertension is diagnosed based on ambulatory BP monitoring when the 24-hour average is ≥130/80 mmHg, the daytime average is ≥135/85 mmHg, and the nighttime average is ≥120/70 mmHg. These thresholds align with those used for office-based measurements of ≥140/90 mmHg, underscoring the significance of consistently elevated blood pressure readings for the diagnosis of hypertension (Williams et al. 2018). High blood pressure is a significant precursor for ischemic and intracranial hemorrhage. Blood pressure > 140/90 mmHg has been reported in 77% of the population during their first stroke attack. Diabetic stroke patients with blood pressure < 120/85 have 50% less lifetime risk than those with hypertension (Choudhury et al. 2015).

4. **Hyperlipidemia**
   Hyperlipidemia is directly associated with coronary heart disease but has uncertain effects on stroke (Rincon et al. 2009). High cholesterol, especially low-density lipoprotein (LDL), and low high-density lipoprotein (HDL) levels have been associated with an increased risk of stroke. Dyslipidemia, particularly high cholesterol, is directly linked with intracranial stenosis (Jetten et al. 2010).
5. **Obesity**
   Abdominal obesity is an independent risk factor for stroke in all ethnic groups. Obesity is a major contributor to hypertension, type II diabetes, and coronary heart disease, all of which increase stroke risk. Emphasis on weight reduction and obesity prevention is crucial in stroke prevention and rehabilitation programs (Elijovich et al. 2009; Towfighi et al. 2010).
6. **Sleep Apnea and Drug Use**
   Obstructive sleep apnea has been identified as an independent risk factor for stroke, significantly increasing the risk of stroke (Yaggi et al. 2005). The prevalence of sleep apnea in stroke patients exceeds 60%, compared to 4% in the general population (Young et al. 1993). Drug use, particularly stimulants such as cocaine and amphetamines, increases stroke risk by acutely elevating blood pressure and leading to vessel constriction (Westover et al. 2007).
7. **Smoking**
   Smoking doubles the risk of stroke. Studies like the Nurses' Health and Framingham studies have shown that quitting smoking significantly reduces the risk of stroke within 2–4 years. This risk reduction trend was observed across moderate and heavy smokers of all age groups (Miah et al. 2012). Both modifiable and unmodifiable risk factors contribute significantly to the incidence of stroke, leading to substantial long-term healthcare needs. The economic costs of poststroke care are enormous (GBD 2016 Stroke Collaborators 2019). As of now, approximately 34% of the global total healthcare expenditure is spent on stroke. The average healthcare cost of stroke per person, including inpatient care, rehabilitation, and follow-up care, is estimated at USD 140,048 in the United States (Katan and Luft 2018). The most recent Global Burden of Disease (GBD) 2019 stroke burden estimates (GBD 2019 Stroke Collaborators 2021) showed that stroke remains the second leading cause of death and the third leading cause of death and disability combined (as expressed by disability-adjusted life years (DALYs)) lost in the world. The estimated global cost of stroke is over USD891 billion (1.12% of the global GDP) (Owolabi et al. 2022).

In recent decades, the burden of stroke among people under the age of 65 has increased significantly. There is an alarming shift in the overall stroke burden to younger age groups, particularly in low- and middle-income countries. The worldwide incidence of stroke in the 20–64-year age group has increased by 25%. Among men, the incidence is notably high in the age range of 55–64 years (Katan and Luft 2018). This increase is attributed to the epidemic rise in cardiovascular risk factors among young adults in regions such as Russia, China, and India (Gorelick 2019).

Asia, home to more than 60% of the world's population, has the highest incidence rate of stroke, followed by Eastern Europe, with the lowest incidence observed in central Latin America. Mortality caused by stroke is higher in Asia compared to Western Europe, America, or Australasia and similar to Eastern Europe (Venketasubramanian et al. 2017).

From 1990 to 2019, the burden (in terms of the absolute number of cases) increased substantially (70.0% increase in incident strokes, 43.0% deaths from stroke, 102.0% prevalent strokes, and 143.0% DALYs lost), with the bulk of the global stroke burden (86.0% of deaths and 89.0% of DALYs) residing in lower-income and lower-middle-income countries (LMIC). There were large geographical differences in age-standardized stroke incidence (sixfold), mortality (15-fold), prevalence (fourfold), and DALYs (20-fold) rates, with the highest rates in LMIC (particularly in Eastern Europe, Asia, and sub-Saharan Africa) (GBD 2019 Stroke Collaborators 2021).

Although the absolute number of DALYs due to stroke in males (77.0 million) exceeded that in females (66.0 million) at the global level in 2019, the point estimates of incident and prevalent strokes were higher in females (6.4 million incident strokes and 56.4 million prevalent strokes) than in males (5.8 million incident strokes and 45.0 million prevalent strokes), and there were no noticeable sex differences in the number of stroke-related deaths (Tables 5.1 and 5.2). Although age-standardized incidence rates did not differ significantly between males and

Table 5.1 External variations

Used tools	
Conventional occupational therapy	Occupational therapy based on DL
Tree with clips of the same color and resistance to strengthen hand muscles, improve coordination and accuracy of movements, and enhance fine motor skills and hand–eye coordination	*Tree with clips of different colors* and varying resistance to strengthen hand muscles, improve coordination and accuracy of movement, enhance fine motor skills and hand–eye coordination, and develop cognitive functions
Tree with rings of the same texture and color to improve movement coordination and accuracy, increase the range of motion, and develop hand–eye coordination	*Tree with rings of different shapes and colors* to improve movement coordination and accuracy, increase the range of motion, and enhance hand–eye coordination and cognitive functions
Occupational therapy hoop with rings of the same texture and color to increase the range of motion and improve fine motor skills	*Occupational therapy hoop with rings of different textures and colors* to increase the range of motion and improve fine motor skills
A pipe system with rings of uniform texture and color, designed to increase the range of motion and improve wrist function	*A pipe system with rings of varying textures and colors, designed* to increase the range of motion and improve wrist function
Pins of the same size and color to improve fine motor skills, movement accuracy, and hand–eye coordination	*Multicolored pins* to improve fine motor skills, movement accuracy, and cognitive functions
Blocks of the same size, shape, and color to improve fine motor skills, movement coordination and accuracy, hand–eye coordination, and cognitive functions	*Blocks of different sizes, shapes, and colors* to improve fine motor skills, movement coordination and accuracy, hand–eye coordination, and cognitive functions
Letters of the same size and color to improve fine motor skills, cognitive functions, and hand–eye coordination	*Letters of different sizes, shapes, and colors* to improve fine motor skills, hand–eye coordination, and cognitive functions
Therapeutic putty to increase finger and hand muscle strength	*Therapeutic putty of different colors (strengths)* to increase finger and hand muscle strength
	Wall with variously arranged letters and numbers of different sizes and colors to improve coordination, balance, hand–eye coordination, and cognitive functions

Table 5.2 Internal variations

Variation in the frequency and kind of problem	Variations during the sessions are introduced by the occupational therapist Variations during the sessions are introduced by the individual (ask the patients to state a task for themselves and complete it)
Variation in the body posture (static)	*Sitting* (straight, sideways, leaning to the left, leaning to the right, etc.) *Standing* (straight, on the right foot, on the left foot, turned to the left, turned to the right, etc.) *Squatting* (straight, sideways, with one leg bent and the other extended on the floor, etc.) *Kneeling* (on both knees, turned to the right, turned to the left, bending forward, kneeling on the right knee, kneeling on the left knee, etc.) *Involving the unaffected upper limb*. While performing tasks with the affected upper limb, the subjects are asked to perform additional tasks with the unaffected arm (e.g., pronation and supination of the arm; holding it extended to the side; punching, bending and extending; lifting up and lowering; placing behind the head and then lifting up; placing behind the head and then lowering; placing the arm on the table; flexion and extension of the fingers; pronation and supination of the hand; etc.)
Variation in the movement execution (dynamic)	*Variations when changing the speed of performance*. As the subject is performing the tasks, the occupational therapist may ask them to perform the tasks at a different speed—e.g., to begin slowly and then accelerate or decelerate or to perform slowly, fast, more slowly, etc. *Variations in different environments*. The tasks are performed in the occupational therapy room, at the table, at the windowsill, by the wall, in the lobby, in the ward, etc.
Variation in the stimulation of different senses	*Variation in music*. Music of various styles is used during exercise performance *Active involvement of the individual* in exercise performance and their well-grounded motivation

females, age-standardized death rates were greater in males than in females (96.4 per 100,000 vs. 73.5 per 100,000), as were DALYs rates (2024.3 per 100,000 vs. 1531.3per 100,000). The lifetime risk of stroke has also increased over the last 20 years by 50% and is now one in four people (GBD 2016 Lifetime Risk of Stroke Collaborators et al. 2018).

From 1990 to 2019, the total number of stroke-related DALYs due to risk factors increased from 91.5 million to 125.0 million, with a decrease in the high-income countries (from 16.4 million to 13.1 million in 2019) and an increase in the LMIC (from 75.1 million in 1990 to 111.0 million in 2019), with the largest (almost fourfold) increase in the age-standardized stroke-related DALYs globally due to high body mass index (BMI). The five leading risk factors for stroke were high systolic blood pressure (SBP; contributing to 55.5% of total stroke DALYs), high BMI (24.3%), high fasting plasma glucose (FPG; 20.2%), ambient particulate matter pollution (20.1%), and smoking (17.6%). Metabolic risks (high SBP, high BMI, high FPG, high LDL cholesterol, and kidney dysfunction) accounted for 70.3% of stroke-related DALYs (70.3% in females and 70.1% in males), dietary risks (diet high in sodium and red meat and low in fruits, vegetables, whole grains, and alcohol consumption) for 30.0% (27.5% in females and 32.1% in males), behavioral risks (smoking and dietary risks) for 46.6% (37.0% in females and 54.6% in males), and environmental risks (air pollution cluster, low ambient temperature, high ambient temperature, and lead exposure) for 37.3% (36.0% in females and 38.4% in males). From 1990 to 2019, there was a significant reduction in the contribution of behavioral, dietary, and environmental risks (5.4%, 7.9%, and 8.2%, respectively) but a significant increase in the contribution of metabolic risks (8.4%), especially due to the increase in high BMI (52.7%) and high FPG (39.3%) (Feigin et al. 2022).

5.1.1 Upper Limb Impairments Caused by Stroke: Challenges and Opportunities for Recovery

Stroke is a leading cause of permanent disability (Diener and Hankey 2020), with the majority of patients experiencing upper limb impairments (Langhorne et al. 2009; Pollock et al. 2014). Approximately 80% of individuals with stroke experience hemiparesis of the upper extremity (van Delden et al. 2009; Haaland et al. 2012; Langhorne et al. 2011; Lawrence et al. 2001; Taube et al. 2015), leading to chronic impairments such as muscle weakness, muscle contracture, abnormal muscle tone, edema, pain, limited range of motion of the joints, and movement control disorders (Bleyenheuft and Gordon 2014; Norouzi-Gheidari et al. 2021). The initial severity of motor impairment often predicts the chances of recovery (Coupar et al. 2012), with patients suffering from mild paresis having a reasonable likelihood of full recovery (Kwakkel et al. 2003). However, those with severe upper limb paresis are less likely to regain full function. Indeed, in 30–50% of stroke survivors, the affected arm remains severely impaired even 6 months after stroke, leading to significant challenges in performing daily activities and often requiring assistance from family members or caregivers (Veerbeek et al. 2011). A major health goal for these patients is to recover their motor function and regain independence (Levin and Demers 2021). Upper extremity motor impairment after stroke significantly impedes the performance of daily activities and affects patients' quality of life (Campbell and Khatri 2020; Crichton et al. 2016; GBD 2016 Lifetime Risk of Stroke Collaborators et al. 2018; Johnson et al. 2016; Krishnamurthi et al. 2013; Langhorne et al. 2009; Langhorne et al. 2011; Mayo et al. 2002), underscoring the critical need for effective rehabilitation strategies to address these impairments.

Upper limb dysfunction following a stroke is not a singular phenomenon but rather a complex syndrome characterized by a combination of symptoms, including loss of strength and dexterity, increased movement variability, heightened resting muscle tone, and the development of abnormal synergies (Krakauer and Thomas Carmichael 2017). One common abnormality is the flexor synergy, where an attempt to move the affected arm results in the shoulder rising, the elbow contracting, and the palm turning upward. This dysfunction is thought to result from a loss of precise regulation in the timing between flexor and extensor muscles.

Recovery of upper limb function can be achieved either by regaining the ability to perform movements that were entirely lost (Kitago et al. 2015) or by improving the accuracy and/or speed of movements that have been preserved (Kitago et al. 2013; Park et al. 2016). However, the dynamic nature of impairments—whereby they may change as motor recovery progresses—complicates the treatment process, necessitating a flexible and versatile therapeutic approach. Recovery of hand function after stroke represents the hardest target for clinicians (Baldan et al. 2021). Proper treatment mediation for functional activity is essential to restore upper limb function and regain independence (Chien et al. 2020). Improving upper limb function in patients after a stroke enables them to perform daily tasks independently; such task performance can improve motor control in these patients.

Given the rising burden of stroke, there is an urgent need for innovative tools and strategies, such as differential training, that can effectively facilitate the restoration of motor function in this patient population (Angerhöfer et al. 2021). The development and implementation of such treatments are critical to improving patient outcomes, as traditional approaches may not be sufficient to address the complex and evolving nature of upper limb impairments after stroke. Therefore, the urgency for effective treatments (Lin et al. 2021) that can adapt to the dynamic recovery process and address multiple impairments simultaneously cannot be overstated.

5.1.2 The Importance of Early Rehabilitation After Stroke: The Path to Independence and Functional Recovery

Annually, of the 12.2 million people worldwide who suffer a stroke, 5 million require urgent rehabilitation (Feigin et al. 2022). Once stroke damage is established, there is currently no available treatment to restore lost functions. To optimize recovery, extensive and early rehabilitation is essential (Motolese et al. 2022). Early rehabilitation significantly improves functional recovery, with patients who receive early intervention achieving greater independence and reduced long-term care needs (Coleman et al. 2017). Early, coordinated, and multidisciplinary rehabilitation plays a major part in motor recovery after stroke (Malik et al. 2022). According to Chen et al. (2016), early and active rehabilitation supported by a team of specialists, helps reduce the number of complications and shortens the duration of physical recovery (Rodgers and Price 2017). Rehabilitation must be proactive, person-centered, and goal-oriented (Langhorne et al. 2020). Research indicates that neurological and functional recovery in individuals who have experienced a stroke is most likely to occur within the first 3 months from the onset of the illness (Kwakkel and Kollen 2013). Both human and nonhuman animal studies demonstrate that most recovery from impairment takes place during this period, driven by spontaneous reorganization as well as increased responsiveness to enriched environments and training (Zeiler and Krakauer 2013). Other studies suggest that rehabilitation should begin on the first day after the stroke. It should be timely, appropriate, and comprehensive to maximize individual functions and achieve the highest possible level of independence—physically, psychologically, socially, and financially (Langhorne et al. 2020). The primary objective of stroke rehabilitation is to reduce neurological impairments and restore independence in patients' daily activities (Tarri et al. 2018).

In conclusion, the global burden of stroke continues to rise, with growing disparities in incidence, mortality, and disability between high-income countries and low- and middle-income countries (LMICs). The increasing prevalence of risk factors, such as high blood pressure, obesity, and diabetes, has contributed to a sharp rise in stroke-related disability-adjusted life years (DALYs), especially among younger populations. As demographic shifts and aging populations lead to a higher incidence of stroke, the economic costs of care are projected to increase, placing immense pressure on healthcare systems worldwide.

In light of this, rehabilitation remains a critical component of stroke recovery, helping survivors regain independence and improve their quality of life. However, as stroke recovery varies greatly among individuals, there is an urgent need for continued research into more effective rehabilitation methods. By advancing innovative approaches—such as personalized therapies and differential learning techniques—rehabilitation can be significantly enhanced. Addressing modifiable risk factors and expanding access to effective stroke care and rehabilitation will be essential in reducing the global stroke burden and improving outcomes for survivors across the world.

5.2 Pathway to Recovery: Modern Strategies and Innovations in Stroke Rehabilitation

Rehabilitation after a stroke should be based on simple, repetitive, and unidirectional or, better still, complex and multidirectional movements in all spatial planes, such as circular or spiral movements. It should also incorporate a feedback system, as this seems to bring about earlier and better motor and functional outcomes (Masiero and Carraro 2008).

The literature identifies several key principles of rehabilitation that influence the treatment of individuals after a stroke. One of these principles is that the central nervous system of adults is plastic and adaptive (Dobkin and Dorsch 2013). Neuroplasticity has been variously attributed to redundancy (parallel distributed pathways), changes in synaptic strength, axonal sprouting with the formation of new synapses, assumption of function by contralateral homologous cortex, and substitution of uncrossed pathways (Green 2003). Neuroplasticity is believed to be the basis for both learning in the intact brain and relearning in the damaged brain that occur through physical rehabilitation (Kleim and Jones 2008). Stroke recovery therapies promote favorable neuroplasticity, both during spontaneous recovery and the chronic phase. Practice of activities in sufficient quantity and quality is the key to learning and plasticity. Research studies emphasize key therapeutic variables, such as dose, intensity, and timing (Richards and Cramer 2021). Neuroscience research has made significant advances in understanding experience-dependent neuroplasticity, and these findings are beginning to be integrated with research on the degenerative and regenerative effects of brain damage (Kleim and Jones 2008).

There are three stages of recovery after a stroke: the acute stage (lasting up to 2 weeks), the subacute stage (lasting approximately 6 months after the onset), and the chronic stage (lasting 1 year after stroke and, sometimes, for the remainder of the patient's life) (Kelly-Hayes et al. 2003).

Current Canadian Stroke Best Practices and American Heart Association guidelines state that inpatient stroke rehabilitation should provide task-specific therapy (defined as physiotherapy, occupational therapy, and speech and language therapy) for at least 3 hours per day, 5 days per week (Winstein et al. 2016; Teasell et al. 2020). Evidence supports that more therapy results in improved outcomes (Wang et al. 2013). Unfortunately, many institutions struggle to provide this rehabilitation intensity. A 2018 Canadian study found that inpatients in stroke rehabilitation participated in only 8.5 hours per week of therapy, which is much below the guideline recommendation of 15 hours per week (Barrett et al. 2018). Outside of therapy, stroke rehabilitation inpatients spend most of their days in a sedentary manner (Barrett et al. 2018; Putman et al. 2016; Sjöholm et al. 2014). Numerous barriers prevent meeting current stroke rehabilitation guidelines, including insufficient staff; timing mismatches with other patient activities, such as investigations for stroke workup (CTs, echocardiograms, and Holter monitors); and a rise in the number of patients requiring stroke rehabilitation (Bayley et al. 2012; Foley et al. 2012).

The European Stroke Organisation (ESO) has released a European Stroke Action Plan (ESAP) (Norrving et al. 2018) and defined 30 targets and 72 research priorities within seven domains to improve stroke services. One of these domains is stroke rehabilitation for improving management, outcome, and quality of life after stroke by 2030 (Norrving et al. 2018). Rehabilitation was defined following the WHO as "a set of measures that assist individuals, who experience or are likely to experience disability, to achieve and maintain optimal functioning in interaction with their environments" (Anon 2011).

One of the important tasks of rehabilitation is the regular assessment of the patient's condition and the selection of appropriate rehabilitation measures. The use of alternative rehabilitation methods is becoming more common, given that standard poststroke rehabilitation is not always effective enough in improving the patient's functional condition (van de Ven et al. 2017). Scientific research (Shapi'i et al. 2015) confirms that with conventional rehabilitation methods, many stroke survivors still have residual functional disabilities that impair their ability to perform daily activities. This can be attributed to insufficient therapy dosage, the repetitive and boring nature of exercises, low patient engagement and motivation, and the lack of objective feedback necessary to achieve significant functional improvement. This is further supported by a study that states that input as a repetitive train of identical sensory stimulation is not effective. The input should be variable. When identical input is repeated, it loses its informational value, and the system will quickly adapt to it. Neural networks are shaped by both input and variation (Mulder and Hochstenbach 2001).

Rehabilitation is said to be a holistic process that should begin as early as possible for individuals after experiencing a stroke, aiming for their active engagement in activities. Engagement and active participation in activities are generally the primary goals of rehabilitation, and these aspects are crucial for improving individuals' quality of life and simultaneously reducing economic costs (Andrenelli et al. 2015). Therefore, it is essential to individualize rehabilitation interventions as early as possible, according to each individual's needs and determining factors (Rodgers and Price 2017). As stated in the recommendations, all patients with stroke should receive rehabilitation therapy as early as possible once they are medically stable and able to participate in active rehabilitation [Evidence Level A] (Teasell et al. 2020).

5.3 Neuroplasticity Unleashed: Pathways to Recovery and Innovation in Stroke Rehabilitation

Traditional approaches to stroke rehabilitation have predominantly centered on facilitating functional recovery through compensatory strategies to alleviate the consequences of impairments rather than addressing their underlying causes (Grefkes and Fink 2020). However, a growing realization within the scientific and medical communities has underscored the extraordinary transformative potential embedded within neuroplasticity. This recognition has prompted a paradigm shift in stroke rehabilitation, emphasizing the harnessing of neuroplasticity to facilitate functional recovery and promote substantial and enduring improvements in long-term outcomes for stroke survivors (Aderinto et al. 2023).

Neurological injuries, such as strokes, can lead to significant loss of motor function. A stroke often results in neuronal death and permanent dysfunction, causing substantial damage to the motor cortex. This damage impairs motor control and can lead to decreased autonomy and a diminished quality of life. Fortunately, neuroplasticity offers the potential for partial recovery of the lost functionality over time. This plasticity enables the brain to reorganize itself by forming new connections among residual neurons, which can help compensate for those that have been lost (Zeiler and Krakauer 2013). Despite the promise of neuroplasticity, the recovery process is often slow and incomplete, even with the most effective conventional rehabilitation therapies (Ting et al. 2021).

Recent advancements in our understanding of activity-dependent plasticity have led to the development of neuromodulation interventions, designed to harness neuroplasticity more effectively. This approach aims to achieve faster and more complete recovery by capitalizing on the brain's ability to adapt and reorganize. Notably, there is a critical period of enhanced plasticity during the 1–3 months following an ischemic stroke, where both spontaneous and intervention-mediated recovery are maximized. During this window, the brain's capacity for reorganization is at its peak, making it an optimal time for implementing therapeutic strategies to facilitate motor recovery (Zeiler and Krakauer 2013).

Stroke induces a plastic state in the brain. This period of enhanced plasticity leads to the sprouting of new axons, the formation of new synapses, and the remapping of sensorimotor functions and is associated with motor recovery. This is a remarkable process in the adult brain, which is normally constrained in its levels of neuroplasticity and connectional change. Recent evidence indicates that these changes are driven by molecular systems that underlie learning and memory, such as changes in cellular excitability during memory formation (Joy and Thomas Carmichael 2021).

Following a stroke, the brain demonstrates remarkable restorative abilities through neuroplasticity. It enables the generation of new neurons, the establishment of fresh neural pathways, and the modification of cellular structures in response to environmental changes. Neuroplasticity encompasses various mechanisms, including interhemispheric lateralization, new connections by association between cortical regions within the injured area, and the reorganization of cortical representational maps (Alia et al. 2017). Studies conducted on animal models provide compelling evidence that the most significant advancements in recovery occur within a limited time frame of heightened neuroplasticity following a stroke. Notably, altered neural activity and connectivity, both in function and structure, have been observed in the perilesional and remote regions and the contralateral hemisphere (Su and Wendong 2020). These changes are believed to underlie the mechanisms responsible for spontaneous recovery. One notable change attributed to neuroplasticity is the modulation of local cortical structure and function, where the affected regions of the brain undergo adaptive modifications to compensate for the lost function (Pekna et al. 2012). Additionally, neuroplasticity can lead to the modulation of brain regions distant from the injury site, indicating a network-wide reorganization to support functional recovery (Pekna et al. 2012). Furthermore, a significant alteration occurs in the interaction between the ipsilesional and contralesional hemispheres as the brain adapts and redistributes functions across these regions (Fekonja et al. 2022). Another aspect of neuroplasticity is the remapping of somatotrophic representation, involving the reorganization of sensory and motor maps within the brain to accommodate changes in the body (Kolasinski et al. 2016).

Exploring neuroplasticity mechanisms in stroke survivors has heavily relied on noninvasive functional neuroimaging techniques, including positron emission tomography (PET) and functional magnetic resonance imaging (fMRI). PET enables the analysis of local perfusion and glucose metabolism changes, while fMRI detects variations in blood flow and oxygenation (Frizzell et al. 2022). During movements of the affected hand, increased brain activity has been observed in both the unaffected and affected hemispheres (Astrakas et al. 2021). Recruiting additional brain regions in the unaffected hemisphere has been associated with better motor recovery. Longitudinal studies have demonstrated that changes in brain activity over time are closely linked to functional recovery. Initially, motor activity decreases shortly after a stroke, gradually increasing until it reaches levels comparable to those in healthy individuals (Crone and Elzinga 2015; Rehme et al. 2011).

Furthermore, fMRI connectivity studies have provided valuable insights into the functional connections between different brain areas in stroke patients. Reduced functional connectivity between the lesioned and unaffected hemispheres has been observed (Carter et al. 2010). However, improved functional recovery in later stages correlates with establishing functional connections between specific brain regions following a stroke. Analyses of effective connections have demonstrated that the unaffected hemisphere can either facilitate or suppress activity in the lesioned hemisphere, depending on the severity of motor impairment (Bajaj et al. 2016).

5.4 Differential Learning: A Novel Approach to Stroke Rehabilitation

In this section, the author will discuss the role of occupational therapy in improving upper limb function in individuals who have experienced a stroke, focusing on both conventional methods and those incorporating differential learning. To the best of our knowledge, we were the first to apply DL to the rehabilitation of neurological patients (Repšaitė 2015). Neurological injuries, such as strokes, often result in neuronal death and permanent dysfunction in the motor cortex. This damage disrupts essential motor functions, making it challenging for individuals to regain movement and coordination in the affected areas of the body. In the literature (Kitago et al. 2013; Levin et al. 2009; Raghavan et al. 2010), it is noted that motor deficits following a stroke can improve through two distinct mechanisms: true recovery and compensation. While it is common to refer to poststroke improvements in performance as recovery, it is crucial to differentiate between true recovery and compensatory mechanisms. True recovery involves the restoration of pre-stroke movement patterns (i.e., a reduction in impairment), whereas compensation refers to the use of alternative movements or strategies to complete a motor task (i.e., engaging different muscle groups, joints, or effectors).

Effective stroke rehabilitation is built on several key principles, with one of the most important being the plasticity and adaptability of the adult central nervous system. For the best recovery outcomes, rehabilitation should focus on tasks that are not only specific and meaningful to the patient but also challenging and motivating. Neuroplasticity offers hope for partial recovery, as the brain can reorganize itself by forming new connections among surviving neurons. The brain's intrinsic ability to adapt provides a valuable foundation for the development of innovative strategies that enhance recovery and restore lost functions (Aderinto et al. 2023). However, the perfect approach to asking the patient to decide how to perform the task in rehabilitation is still being actively researched, as no single method has yet proven to be universally optimal.

One such method that holds promise in facilitating this process is DL. By introducing variability and promoting movement in diverse conditions, differential learning creates the challenges needed to stimulate the brain's plasticity, making it a powerful tool for stroke rehabilitation. The search for the most effective rehabilitation strategies continues, but DL offers a compelling approach to unlocking the brain's potential for recovery.

Early and intensive rehabilitation is crucial in improving functional recovery after stroke, as it significantly enhances the quality of life for patients, supports their independence, and reduces the need for hospitalization and long-term care. Studies indicate that timely rehabilitation is associated with better recovery outcomes and lower healthcare costs (Bernhardt et al. 2017). These findings highlight that the earlier the rehabilitation begins, the more favorable the recovery prospects and the lesser the long-term financial burden on the healthcare system.

Economic analyses further confirm that early rehabilitation can reduce disability levels and improve the quality of life for stroke patients, while delays in rehabilitation increase long-term healthcare expenses (Langhorne 2007). The economic burden of stroke care is substantial, accounting for approximately 1.7% of total healthcare expenditures (Feigin et al. 2017), underscoring the need for effective strategies that can minimize these costs.

This is where DL comes into play. While traditional rehabilitation methods and their early application contribute to immediate improvements, they often focus primarily on compensatory strategies rather than addressing the underlying mechanisms of motor recovery (Grefkes and Fink 2020). This approach, while beneficial in the short term, may not lead to long-lasting improvements in recovery. DL, by fostering motor variability and encouraging the brain to adapt in diverse, dynamic conditions, can provide the challenges necessary for stimulating long-term brain plasticity and promoting sustainable recovery (Schöllhorn et al. 2010). Therefore, while early rehabilitation lays the foundation for functional improvements, integrating DL into the rehabilitation process offers a promising approach for achieving superior and more lasting recovery outcomes.

The DL method, which promotes the development of motor variability, has been studied in sports, where research has shown (Schöllhorn et al. 2010) that this method can enhance adaptation by providing natural individual movement variability. This allows athletes to achieve similar or even better results than traditional practice. Given that stroke rehabilitation also requires the development of motor and sensory skills, the application of DL principles may be beneficial for improving patients' adaptation to the demands of daily activities.

Furthermore, DL application in the training process can promote more effective motor skill learning by ensuring greater variability and personalized adaptation (Schöllhorn et al. 2010). This is especially relevant in stroke rehabilitation, where individual patient needs and responses can vary significantly. Thus, the DL method can become an essential part of rehabilitation, complementing traditional methods and being adapted to each patient individually.

5.4.1 Protocol of a Study on Differential Learning

In designing the activity and study protocol, we drew inspiration from sports research, where the differential learning method has been widely used and shown to deliver impressive results. Because of some skepticism of the clinic responsible at that time, the protocol consisted of three sessions per week of traditional occupational therapy and two sessions per week of occupational therapy based on DL. The duration of each session was 45 min. In occupational therapy sessions, stroke survivors engage in targeted activities to regain control and strength. They work on improving balance, increasing the range of motion in the affected upper limb, and building hand and finger strength. Exercises also focus on refining movement coordination, boosting execution accuracy, restoring wrist function, and enhancing fine motor skills. Cognitive skills are developed alongside physical abilities, supporting a well-rounded recovery process. A variety of occupational therapy tools support the development of these functions, including therapy hoops, pipe systems, ring trees, clothespins, pegs, blocks, shape puzzles, therapy putty, and alphabet exercises. Each tool is thoughtfully chosen to target specific motor and cognitive skills essential for recovery. Although the tools used in occupational therapy sessions are typically standardized, incorporating differential learning techniques introduces variations in size, color, and texture to boost engagement and adaptability (see Table 5.1 for detailed descriptions of each tool).

5.4.2 Evidence-Based Benefits of the Differential Learning Method for Individuals After Stroke

Our study set out to explore the impact of differential learning on the functional movements and independence of individuals who have experienced a stroke, grounded in the principle of functional unity. We wanted to understand how this innovative approach could potentially enhance recovery and restore daily functioning. As we began, it was essential to carefully define the criteria for selecting participants, ensuring that we included individuals at varying stages of recovery, all with different needs and goals, while also ensuring their ability to comprehend the provided information and be moderately dependent so that they can complete the task across all functional levels of the body. These selection criteria were established through a pilot study.

Inclusion Criteria

1. Mini-Mental State Examination (MMSE): ≥ 11 points
2. Barthel index: 50–65 points

Exclusion Criteria

1. Mini-Mental State Examination (MMSE): < 11 points
2. Barthel index: < 50–65 points
3. Motor aphasia
4. Sensory aphasia
5. Sensorimotor aphasia
6. Recurrent cerebral infarction

With this diverse group in mind, we then crafted a methodology that combined traditional occupational therapy with differential learning–based techniques. This allowed us to compare the two approaches and assess the effectiveness of each. Throughout the research, we focused on creating an environment that was both challenging and supportive, ensuring that every participant had the opportunity to engage in movements that would improve their functional independence. By integrating differential learning, we aimed to offer a fresh, evidence-backed approach that could significantly impact their recovery journey.

The methods of the study were the following: information abstracted from medical records, arm function measurements obtained by applying the Wolf motor function test (Wolf et al. 2009), and measurements of hand grip strength using a dynamometer.

Prior to the study, patients were randomized into two groups—conventional therapy and the studied group—based on their medical documents (MMSE and the Barthel index) and their registration in the registry of the Second Department of Physical Medicine and Rehabilitation.

For the conventional therapy group, the training program consisted of five sessions per week (conducted daily, except on weekends), each lasting 45 minutes, and was adapted to individual, regular occupational therapy based on task repetition. The occupational therapy procedures aimed to improve the range of motion in the affected arm; increase the strength of the hand and fingers; enhance movement coordination and accuracy, wrist function, and fine motor skills; and develop cognitive abilities. To support these goals, the following occupational therapy equipment was utilized: a range of motion arc; a zigzag type supinator and pronator (PVC pipe); a tree with rings of the same color and texture; pins of the same color and resistance force; pegs and blocks of the same size and color; figures of the same size, shape, and color; exercise putty of the same color; and letters of the same size and color.

Conventional therapy group subjects performed the exercises with their affected arm and continuously repeated the same movements. All tasks for training the affected upper limb, as well as daily activity tasks, were performed without changing the environment, the speed of exercising, or the initial body position (i.e., all exercises were performed in the sitting position).

For the DL group, the training program objectives were the same as for the conventional therapy group (see above). In contrast, the program consisted of three sessions per week of regular occupational therapy and two sessions per week of occupational therapy based on the differential training technique (conducted daily, except on weekends), each lasting 45 min.

In the DL group, occupational therapy procedures targeted the same goals as the conventional therapy group: improving coordination, balance, range of motion in the affected upper limb, hand and finger strength, wrist function, fine motor skills, and cognitive abilities. The same occupational therapy equipment was used; however, the items varied in size, color, and texture, aligning with the principles of differential learning to introduce variation.

All the tasks for the training of the affected upper limb were performed by applying the DL approach—i.e., the tasks were performed in different contexts and on different functional levels of the body, every time, changing the conditions of the problems, with not more than three repetitions, and actively involving the subjects in exercise performance.

The application of occupational therapy based on DL was based on the variations presented in Table 5.2.

Our findings on the upper limb function of all individuals revealed significant improvements following the applied interventions. The subjects who received occupational therapy combined with differential training performed a greater proportion of tasks aimed at improving the upper limb function more effectively (Repšaitė et al. 2015). These results can be explained by the fact that the same tasks were performed in constantly different situations, at different functional body levels, and with active patient involvement in task execution. This is supported by the literature, which states that improvements in movement performance through DL are superior to traditional training based on exercise repetition and correction. In addition, DL can help improve performance execution even after the learning period (Frank et al. 2008).

Our research also revealed that the hand muscle strength in both hands increased in subjects after undergoing DL-based occupational therapy, whereas no significant changes were observed after traditional occupational therapy alone (Repšaitė et al. 2013). These results can be attributed to the fact that DL included exercises that engaged the muscles surrounding the wrist and hand, utilizing tools of varying sizes and shapes, changes in initial body positions, and active subject participation in the activity.

5.4.3 Variations of Differential Learning

In conventional occupational therapy sessions, most tasks are typically done while seated at a table. However, in occupational therapy that uses differential learning, tasks are performed in various body positions—standing, squatting, kneeling, or sitting. This approach keeps the environment, support base, and task conditions constantly changing so that patients avoid performing the same action in the same way each time. Every session encourages active engagement, where patients must adapt to new challenges and conditions, making the learning process more dynamic and effective.

Occupational therapy based on differential learning was conducted using the following variations (a detailed description of the variations is provided in Table 5.2):

It is important to note that during occupational therapy sessions based on DL, each task is repeated not more than two or three times before a variation is introduced (Carr and Shepherd 2010; Schöllhorn et al. 2009), either suggested by the occupational therapist or by asking the patient to decide how to perform the task next (Fallahpour et al. 2011). The therapist does not and does not have to correct the tasks, allowing the patient to make mistakes, thus introducing noise and performing "incorrect" actions and learning not to judge the deviations from expectations. Why two or three repetitions? Carr and Shepherd (2010) suggest that high brain activity persists during the first three repetitions of a task, as the brain's automation program kicks in afterward. Differential learning refers to these variations in their original sense. However, since in conventional occupational therapy, variation is typically understood in a naïve manner, similar to Schmidt's variability of practice theory (Schmidt 1975), as performing the same task differently each time (by changing the speed of execution, body position, and functional body level; involving the healthy upper limb; etc.), even if it is done correctly, it is important to explain to the patient that, in this case, it is closer to a mistake rather than a variation.

Approximately every two or three repetitions, either the therapist or the patient introduces a variation. The degree of variation needed will vary for each patient, aiming to create enough fluctuation to challenge the system without causing excessive discomfort. The goal is to provide a challenge that destabilizes the patient just enough to promote progress, without overwhelming them.

Various literature sources indicate that the most common and oldest theory for learning specific movements is the repetition theory, which states that target movements are copied and repeated to achieve mastery. This approach suggests that learners improve their skills simply by repeating them (Schöllhorn et al. 2010). According to Feys et al. (2004), the recovery of hand function in individuals who have experienced a stroke can be effectively facilitated through occupational therapy based on movement repetition, which actively involves the individual's hand in the exercises. In contrast, Frank et al. (2008) highlight that improvements in movement execution using differential learning (DL) surpass those achieved through traditional repetition-based training. Unlike repetition-focused methods, DL incorporates variability, presenting the patient with new challenges that require adaptation to different conditions. This approach stimulates neuroplasticity and fosters long-term motor learning. Consequently, while repetition proves beneficial for specific aspects of recovery, DL provides additional advantages by enhancing adaptability and ensuring better retention of movements beyond the training period.

It is also essential to emphasize the importance of trunk function training in the rehabilitation of individuals who have experienced a stroke. The role of trunk stability in performing functional movements with all extremities is highly significant. Ryerson et al. (2008) state that good trunk stability is essential for balance and the use of limbs when performing daily functional activities and higher-level tasks. The findings of the study conducted by Michaelsen et al. (2006) confirm that performing tasks with a stable trunk improves upper limb function more effectively than performing tasks with an unstable trunk (Kitago et al. 2013; Michaelsen et al. 2006). This can be successfully achieved through training based on differential learning, i.e., performing the same tasks in various environments (e.g., at a table in the occupational therapy room, near a window sill, in a corridor, or by a countertop), at different functional body levels (e.g., sitting, standing, squatting, or kneeling), and actively involving the patient in task execution.

You may confidently integrate the DL method into occupational and physical therapy sessions for stroke survivors. This approach is not only affordable but also highly effective, offering a

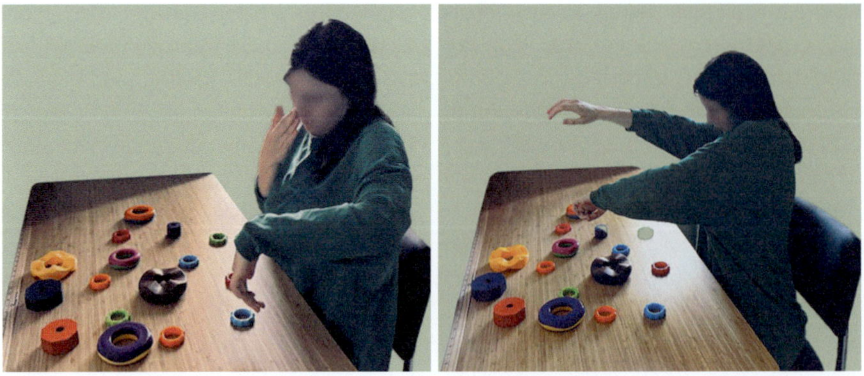

Fig. 5.1 *Variations of sitting* straight *at the table:* using the affected upper limb to reach *differently colored and shaped figures, involving the unaffected upper limb*

dynamic way to enhance recovery by continuously adapting to each patient's needs and progress. You may apply the session protocol mentioned above as a guide, refer to the variations presented in Table 5.2, and be creative—develop your own variations and combine them, but most importantly, do not instruct the patient to repeat the same task more than three times. While some patients may initially find this challenging or even unacceptable, they eventually seek more diverse variations, as it enriches the task, making it seem less monotonous, always different, and ultimately provides them with significant, evidence-based benefits (Figs. 5.1, 5.2, 5.3, 5.4, 5.5, 5.6, and 5.7).

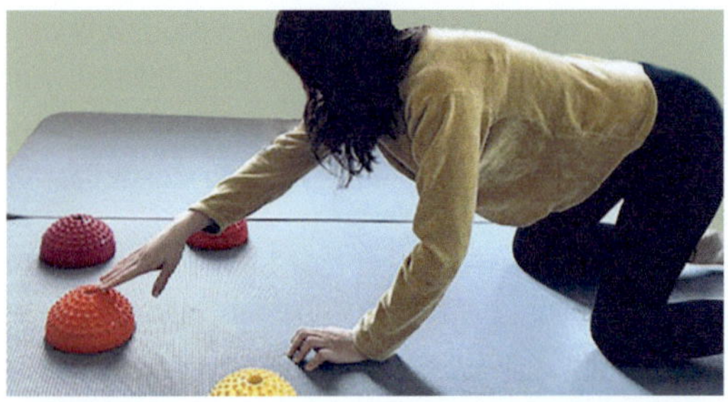

Fig. 5.2 *Variation of kneeling* on both knees: using the unaffected upper limb to reach for figures of different colors while utilizing the affected upper limb for support

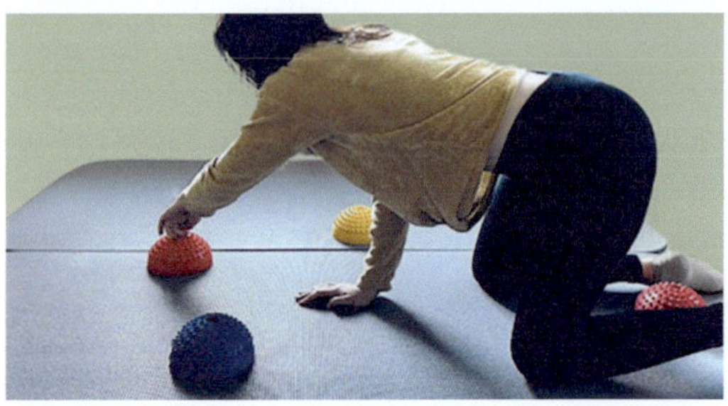

Fig. 5.3 *Variation of kneeling* on both knees: using the affected upper limb to reach for figures of different colors

5.4.4 The Impact of Olfactory Perception on Cognitive Function in Stroke Rehabilitation

In this chapter, I will explore the intriguing relationship between olfactory perception and cognitive function, particularly in individuals who have suffered an ischemic stroke. Over recent years, scientific research has increasingly focused on cognitive function impairments, revealing a significant link between olfactory disorders and various pathologies. Despite these advancements, there remains a gap in studies specifically assessing how olfactory dysfunctions impact cognitive abilities in stroke survivors.

To address this gap, we were the first to conduct a study that directly investigates olfactory perception disorders in individuals who have experienced ischemic stroke. Our research not only aimed to identify the presence of these disorders but also sought to evaluate the effectiveness of correcting olfactory dysfunctions through occupational therapy. This pioneering study opens up new possibilities for rehabilitation, suggesting that addressing olfactory impairments may play a vital role in enhancing cognitive recovery and overall quality of life for stroke survivors.

The criteria for participant selection were:

Inclusion Criteria

1. Mini-Mental State Examination (MMSE) score of ≥11 points (for individuals with mild or moderate cognitive impairment)
2. First-time ischemic stroke survivors
3. No diagnosed aphasia
4. Stable somatic condition, with sufficient vision and hearing to assess cognitive functions and apply therapeutic interventions
5. Individuals familiar with the purpose and course of the study and who provided written consent to participate in the research

Exclusion Criteria

1. Recurrent ischemic stroke
2. MMSE score < 11 points (for individuals with severe cognitive impairment)

The Following Assessment Tools Were Used in the Study

1. Mini-Mental State Examination (MMSE) to assess cognitive functions
2. Scandinavian Odor Identification Test (SOIT) to assess olfactory perception disorders, consisting of 16 different scents

Again, all participants who met the selection criteria were randomly assigned to two groups:

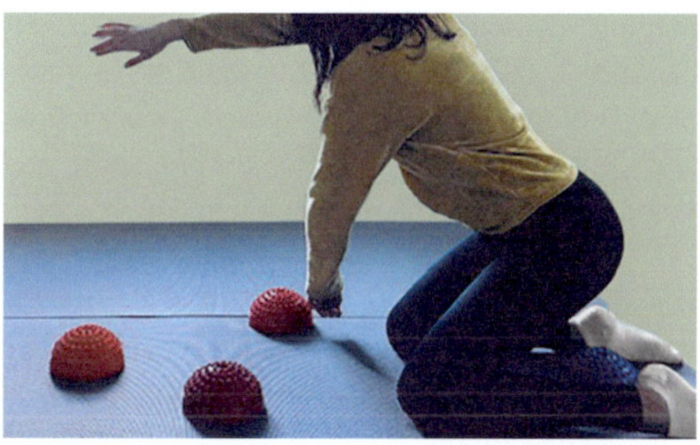

Fig. 5.4 *Variation of kneeling* on both knees: using the affected upper limb to reach for figures of different colors, involving the unaffected upper limb in the variation performance

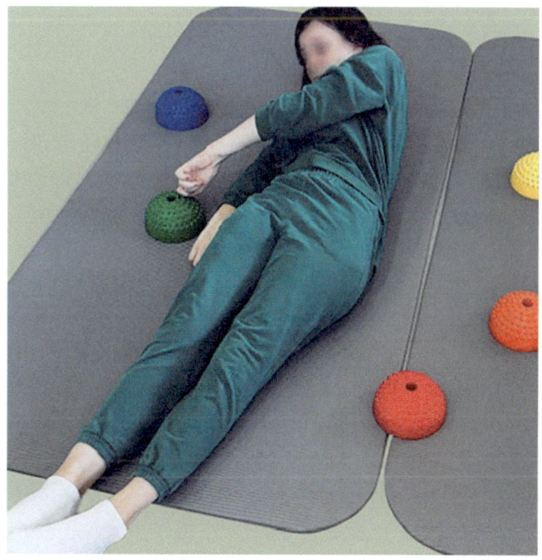

Fig. 5.6 *Variation of lying on the back:* using the affected upper limb to reach for figures of different colors

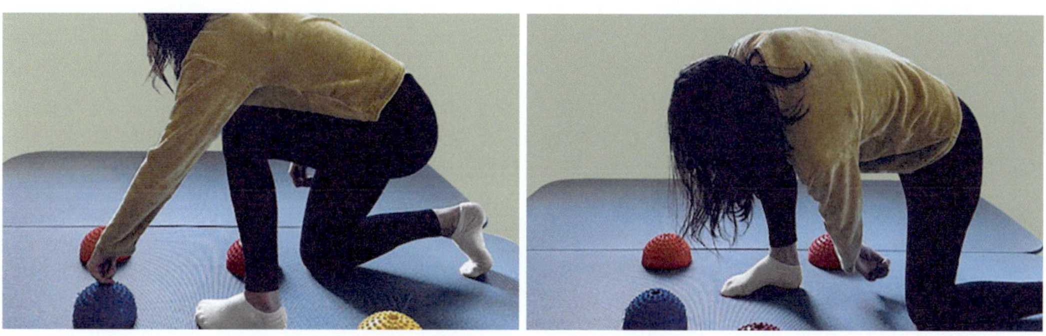

Fig. 5.5 *Variations of kneeling* on one knee: using the affected upper limb to reach for figures of different colors

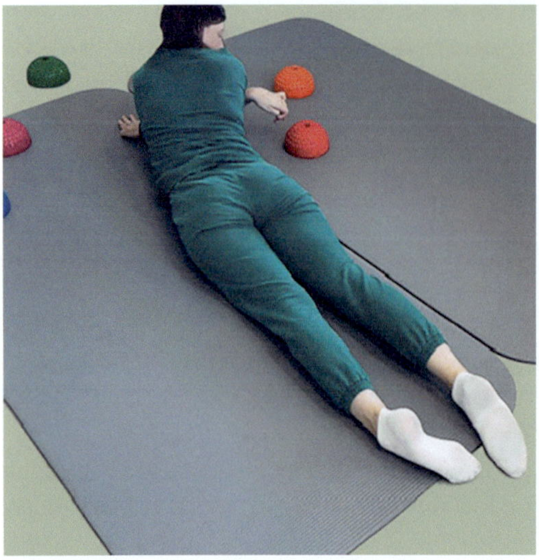

Fig. 5.7 *Variation of lying on the stomach:* using the affected upper limb to reach for figures of different colors

group I (intervention group) and group II (intervention group). All participants were assessed at the beginning and at the end of the study. Cognitive functions were trained for all individuals who had an ischemic stroke according to a personalized and adapted occupational therapy program.

Each participant in group I underwent 15 occupational therapy sessions, each lasting 30 min, conducted five times a week. Various occupational therapy tools were used for cognitive function training, such as different objects, letters, numbers, and pictures. Tasks involved recognizing different forms and colors. No tasks related to the training of olfactory perception were included.

Each participant in group II also underwent 15 occupational therapy sessions, each lasting 30 min, conducted five times a week. However, their sessions included tasks that trained olfactory perception with various scents, a kind of transferring DL to other sensory systems. The occupational therapy protocol for this group involved three sessions per week dedicated to cognitive tasks related to scent perception and two sessions per week dedicated to cognitive tasks unrelated to scents, using the same tools as in group I. The tasks related to scent perception included recognizing scents from pictures used in the test, finding scent bottle pictures according to names, reading texts about scents and identifying them, and memory tasks involving cards with scent-related names and pictures.

Upon completing the study, we found significant improvement in the cognitive functions, scent recognition, and identification in all participants who had suffered an ischemic stroke. Those who engaged in scent-related cognitive tasks alongside occupational therapy demonstrated significantly improved differentiation of grapefruit and juniper berry scents compared to those who received standard occupational therapy. Interestingly, participants who underwent occupational therapy combined with scent perception tasks showed significant associations between cognitive function scores (attention, language, abstraction, orientation, and long-term recall) and the perception of lavender, grapefruit, tea tree, mint, and anise scents. In contrast, those who only received conventional occupational therapy demonstrated significant associations between visual–spatial abilities/executive function, naming, attention, language, abstraction, and the perception of cinnamon, mint, resin, and vinegar scents (Strimaitytė et al. 2019).

5.5 Summary

This chapter highlights the transformative potential of differential learning (DL) in stroke rehabilitation, emphasizing its role in fostering neuroplasticity and promoting functional recovery. Traditional rehabilitation methods, while effective, often rely on repetitive task execution, which may limit adaptability and engagement. In contrast, DL introduces variability and challenges, enabling patients to develop motor and cognitive skills dynamically. By adapting tasks to the patient's needs and varying conditions, DL leverages the brain's plasticity to achieve superior outcomes compared to conventional approaches.

Our research demonstrated significant improvements in upper limb function, hand muscle strength, and overall recovery among stroke survivors who engaged in DL-based occupational therapy. This method's success lies in its capacity to stimulate neural networks, enhance retention of learned skills, and encourage active patient participation, ultimately contributing to long-term functional independence. Furthermore, extending DL principles to sensory systems, such as olfactory perception, revealed promising results in cognitive function enhancement, opening new avenues for innovative rehabilitation techniques.

The findings underscore the value of integrating DL into clinical practice, providing a compelling, evidence-based approach to address the complexities of stroke recovery. By adopting DL, healthcare professionals can enrich rehabilitation programs, improve patient outcomes, and reduce the economic burden of long-term care. This chapter serves as an invitation to explore and implement DL in stroke rehabilitation, offering a pathway to more effective, personalized, and engaging recovery strategies.

Practical Reflection Questions

1. How does differential learning (DL) differ from traditional occupational therapy methods in stroke rehabilitation?
   A. DL encourages patients to perform tasks only according to specific fixed patterns, without changing the conditions.
   B. DL focuses on performing tasks under varying conditions, promoting brain plasticity and movement variability.
   C. Traditional occupational therapy typically involves tasks performed in a specific environment to reduce variability.
   D. DL uses only a particular physiological posture, preventing the patient from adapting their movement in different conditions.
2. Why is it important to introduce variations in tasks during differential learning–based occupational therapy?
   A. Variations help maintain patient interest and motivation, as the tasks become more engaging.
   B. Variations help the brain adapt and reorganize, promoting better retention of motor skills and long-term functional improvements.
   C. Variations reduce therapy time, as patients achieve their goals more quickly.
   D. Variations are only necessary to ensure that patients perform tasks in different positions.
3. What is the reasoning behind limiting task repetitions to only two or three times in DL-based occupational therapy?
   A. Repeating the same movement pattern multiple times can enhance muscle memory and motor skills without requiring adaptation.
   B. Repeating tasks too often is necessary for patients to fully master a skill, and limiting repetitions would hinder progress.
   C. Limiting repetitions encourages brain adaptation and plasticity, preventing patients from becoming too comfortable with a single movement, thus promoting better functional recovery.
   D. Task repetitions should be limited to ensure that patients experience sufficient rest to avoid fatigue and optimize recovery time.
4. How does differential learning promote long-term brain plasticity in stroke rehabilitation?
   A. Introducing task variations forces the brain to adapt and reorganize, leading to better retention of motor skills and more sustainable functional improvements.
   B. Differential learning promotes brain plasticity by using only repetitive tasks.
   C. The brain is unable to adapt to different task variations, so no significant long-term plastic changes occur.
   D. Long-term changes in brain structure occur only when tasks are performed in exactly the same way every time.
5. What is the significance of performing tasks at varying body positions in differential learning–based occupational therapy?
   A. It helps improve strength in a single, fixed position.
   B. It allows the therapist to evaluate the patient's ability to maintain a static posture.
   C. It encourages the patient to focus exclusively on one movement pattern.
   D. It challenges the body and the brain in different ways, enhancing motor learning and promoting functional adaptability.

6. What role does trunk stability play in stroke rehabilitation, and how can DL help in this regard?
   A. Trunk stability is important only for restoring balance, but it does not affect limb function.
   B. Trunk stability helps only with walking, but it is not necessary for other daily movements.
   C. Trunk stability is crucial as it provides the foundation for proper limb movement and balance in functional activities, and DL can assist by encouraging tasks in various body positions.
   D. Trunk stability is not important in rehabilitation, as the focus is solely on the upper limbs.
7. How does the use of differential learning in stroke rehabilitation impact healthcare costs?
   A. Differential learning can reduce healthcare costs by promoting faster and more sustainable recovery, reducing the duration of hospital stay and long-term care requirements.
   B. Differential learning may increase healthcare costs as the rehabilitation process takes longer.
   C. Differential learning has no impact on healthcare costs.
   D. Differential learning requires greater investment in rehabilitation technologies, thus increasing costs.

References

Aderinto N, AbdulBasit MO, Olatunji G, Adejumo T (2023) Exploring the transformative influence of neuroplasticity on stroke rehabilitation: a narrative review of current evidence. Ann Med Surg 85(9):4425–4432. https://doi.org/10.1097/MS9.0000000000001137

Alia C, Spalletti C, Lai S, Panarese A, Lamola G, Bertolucci F, Vallone F, Di Garbo A, Chisari C, Micera S, Caleo M (2017) Neuroplastic changes following brain ischemia and their contribution to stroke recovery: novel approaches in Neurorehabilitation. Front Cell Neurosci 11. https://doi.org/10.3389/fncel.2017.00076

Andrenelli E, Ippoliti E, Coccia M, Millevolte M, Cicconi B, Latini L, Lagalla G, Provinciali L, Ceravolo MG, Capecci M (2015) Features and predictors of activity limitations and participation restriction 2 years after intensive rehabilitation following first-ever stroke. Eur J Phys Rehabil Med 51(5):575–585

Angerhöfer C, Colucci A, Vermehren M, Hömberg V, Soekadar SR (2021) Post-stroke rehabilitation of severe upper limb paresis in Germany – toward long-term treatment with brain-computer interfaces. Front Neurol 12:772199. https://doi.org/10.3389/fneur.2021.772199

Anon (2011) World report on disability 2011

Astrakas LG, Li S, Ottensmeyer MP, Pusatere C, Moskowitz MA, Aria Tzika A (2021) Peak activation shifts in the sensorimotor cortex of chronic stroke patients following robot-assisted rehabilitation therapy. Open Neuroimag J 14:8–15. https://doi.org/10.2174/1874440002114010008

Avendano M, Kawachi I, Van Lenthe F, Boshuizen HC, Mackenbach JP, Van den Bos GAM, Fay ME, Berkman LF (2006) Socioeconomic status and stroke incidence in the US elderly: the role of risk factors in the EPESE study. Stroke 37(6):1368–1373. https://doi.org/10.1161/01.STR.0000221702.75002.66

Bajaj S, Housley SN, David W et al (2016) Dominance of the unaffected hemisphere motor network and its role in the behavior of chronic stroke survivors. Front Hum Neurosci 10:650. https://doi.org/10.3389/fnhum.2016.00650

Baldan F, Turolla A, Rimini D, Pregnolato G, Maistrello L, Agostini M, Jakob I (2021) Robot-assisted rehabilitation of hand function after stroke: development of prediction models for reference to therapy. J Electromyogr Kinesiol 57:102534. https://doi.org/10.1016/j.jelekin.2021.102534

Barrett M, Snow JC, Kirkland MC, Kelly LP, Gehue M, Downer MB, McCarthy J, Ploughman M (2018) Excessive sedentary time during in-patient stroke rehabilitation. Top Stroke Rehabil 25(5):366–374. https://doi.org/10.1080/10749357.2018.1458461

Bayley MT, Hurdowar A, Richards CL, Korner-Bitensky N, Wood-Dauphinee S, Eng JJ, McKay-Lyons M, Harrison E, Teasell R, Harrison M, Graham ID (2012) Barriers to implementation of stroke rehabilitation evidence: findings from a multi-site pilot project. Disabil Rehabil 34(19):1633–1638. https://doi.org/10.3109/09638288.2012.656790

Bernhardt J, Godecke E, Johnson L, Langhorne P (2017) Early rehabilitation after stroke. Curr Opin Neurol 30(1):48–54. https://doi.org/10.1097/WCO.0000000000000404

Bleyenheuft Y, Gordon AM (2014) Precision grip in congenital and acquired hemiparesis: similarities in impairments and implications for Neurorehabilitation. Front Hum Neurosci 8:459. https://doi.org/10.3389/fnhum.2014.00459

Broderick JP, Brott T, Tomsick T, Huster G, Miller R (1992) The risk of subarachnoid and intracerebral hemorrhages in blacks as compared with whites. N Engl J Med 326(11):733–736. https://doi.org/10.1056/NEJM199203123261103

Campbell BCV, Khatri P (2020) Stroke. Lancet (London, England) 396(10244):129–142. https://doi.org/10.1016/S0140-6736(20)31179-X

Carr JH, Shepherd RB (2010) Neurological rehabilitation, 2nd edn

Carter AR, Astafiev SV, Lang CE, Connor LT, Rengachary J, Strube MJ, Pope DLW, Shulman GL, Corbetta M (2010) Resting interhemispheric functional magnetic resonance imaging connectivity predicts performance after stroke. Ann Neurol 67(3):365–375. https://doi.org/10.1002/ana.21905

Chambless LE, Folsom AR, Clegg LX, Richey Sharrett A, Eyal Shahar F, Nieto J, Rosamond WD, Evans G (2000) Carotid Wall thickness is predictive of incident clinical stroke: the atherosclerosis risk in communities (ARIC) study. Am J Epidemiol 151(5):478–487

Chen L, Fang J, Ma R, Xudong G, Chen L, Li J, Shouyu X (2016) Additional effects of acupuncture on early comprehensive rehabilitation in patients with mild to moderate acute ischemic stroke: a multicenter randomized controlled trial. BMC Complement Altern Med 16:226. https://doi.org/10.1186/s12906-016-1193-y

Chen Z, Iona A, Parish S, Yiping Chen Y, Guo FB, Yang L, Bian Z, Holmes MV, Lewington S, Lacey B, Gao R, Liu F, Zhang Z, Chen J, Walters RG, Collins R, Clarke R, Peto R, Li L, Biobank CK, collaborative group (2018) Adiposity and risk of Ischaemic and Haemorrhagic stroke in 0·5 million Chinese men and women: a prospective cohort study. Lancet Glob Health 6(6):e630–e640. https://doi.org/10.1016/S2214-109X(18)30216-X

Chien W-T, Chong Y-Y, Tse M-K, Chien C-W, Cheng H-Y (2020) Robot-assisted therapy for upper-limb rehabilitation in subacute stroke patients: a systematic review and meta-analysis. Brain and Behavior 10(8):e01742. https://doi.org/10.1002/brb3.1742

Choudhury MJH, Chowdhury MTI, Nayeem A, Jahan WA (2015) Modifiable and non-modifiable risk factors of stroke: a review update. J Natl Inst Neurosci Bangladesh 1(1):22–26. https://doi.org/10.3329/jninb.v1i1.22944

Coleman ER, Moudgal R, Lang K, Hyacinth HI, Awosika OO, Kissela BM, Feng W (2017) Early rehabilitation after stroke: a narrative review. Curr Atheroscler Rep 19(12):59. https://doi.org/10.1007/s11883-017-0686-6

Coupar F, Pollock A, Rowe P, Weir C, Langhorne P (2012) Predictors of upper limb recovery after stroke: a systematic review and meta-analysis. Clin Rehabil 26(4):291–313. https://doi.org/10.1177/0269215511420305

Crichton SL, Bray BD, McKevitt C, Rudd AG, Wolfe CDA (2016) Patient outcomes up to 15 years after stroke: survival, disability, quality of life, cognition and mental health. J Neurol Neurosurg Psychiatry 87(10):1091–1098. https://doi.org/10.1136/jnnp-2016-313361

Crone EA, Elzinga BM (2015) Changing brains: how longitudinal functional magnetic resonance imaging studies can inform us about cognitive and social-affective growth trajectories. WIREs Cogn Sci 6(1):53–63

Diener H-C, Hankey GJ (2020) Primary and secondary prevention of ischemic stroke and cerebral hemorrhage: JACC focus seminar. J Am Coll Cardiol 75(15):1804–1818. https://doi.org/10.1016/j.jacc.2019.12.072

Dobkin BH, Dorsch A (2013) New evidence for therapies in stroke rehabilitation. Curr Atheroscler Rep 15(6):331. https://doi.org/10.1007/s11883-013-0331-y

Elijovich L, Andrew Josephson S, Fung GL, Smith WS (2009) Intermittent atrial fibrillation may account for a large proportion of otherwise cryptogenic stroke: a study of 30-day cardiac event monitors. J Stroke Cerebrovasc Dis 18(3):185–189. https://doi.org/10.1016/j.jstrokecerebrovasdis.2008.09.005

Elkind MS, Sacco RL (1998) Stroke risk factors and stroke prevention. Semin Neurol 18(4):429–440. https://doi.org/10.1055/s-2008-1040896

Fallahpour M, Tham K, Joghataei MT, Jonsson H (2011) Perceived participation and autonomy: aspects of functioning and contextual factors predicting participation after stroke. J Rehabil Med 43(5):388–397. https://doi.org/10.2340/16501977-0789

Feigin VL et al (2014) Global and regional burden of stroke during 1990-2010: findings from the global burden of disease study 2010. Lancet (London, England) 383(9913):245–254. https://doi.org/10.1016/s0140-6736(13)61953-4

Feigin VL, Norrving B, Mensah GA (2017) Global burden of stroke. Circ Res 120(3):439–448. https://doi.org/10.1161/CIRCRESAHA.116.308413

Feigin VL, Brainin M, Norrving B, Martins S, Sacco RL, Hacke W, Fisher M, Pandian J, Lindsay P (2022) World stroke organization (WSO): global stroke fact sheet 2022. Int J Stroke 17(1):18–29. https://doi.org/10.1177/17474930211065917

Fekonja LS, Wang Z, Cacciola A, Timo Roine D, Aydogan B, Mewes D, Vellmer S, Vajkoczy P, Picht T (2022) Network analysis shows decreased Ipsilesional structural connectivity in glioma patients. Commun Biol 5(1):258. https://doi.org/10.1038/s42003-022-03190-6

Feys H, De Weerdt W, Verbeke G, Steck GC, Capiau C, Kiekens C, Dejaeger E, Van Hoydonck G, Vermeersch G, Cras P (2004) Early and repetitive stimulation of the arm can substantially improve the long-term outcome after stroke: a 5-year follow-up study of a randomized trial. Stroke 35(4):924–929. https://doi.org/10.1161/01.STR.0000121645.44752.f7

Foley N, Andrew McClure J, Meyer M, Salter K, Bureau Y, Teasell R (2012) Inpatient rehabilitation following stroke: amount of therapy received and associations with functional recovery. Disabil Rehabil 34(25):2132–2138. https://doi.org/10.3109/09638288.2012.676145

Frank TD, Michelbrink M, Beckmann H, Schöllhorn WI (2008) A quantitative dynamical systems approach to differential learning: self-organization principle and order parameter equations. Biol Cybern 98(1):19–31. https://doi.org/10.1007/s00422-007-0193-x

Frizzell TO, Phull E, Khan M, Song X, Grajauskas LA, Gawryluk J, D'Arcy RCN (2022) Imaging functional neuroplasticity in human White matter tracts. Brain Struct Funct 227(1):381–392. https://doi.org/10.1007/s00429-021-02407-4

GBD 2016 Lifetime Risk of Stroke Collaborators et al (2018) Global, regional, and country-specific lifetime risks of stroke, 1990 and 2016. N Engl J Med 379(25):2429–2437. https://doi.org/10.1056/NEJMoa1804492

GBD 2016 Stroke Collaborators (2019) Global, regional, and National Burden of stroke, 1990-2016: a systematic analysis for the global burden of disease study 2016. Lancet Neurol 18(5):439–458. https://doi.org/10.1016/S1474-4422(19)30034-1

GBD 2019 Stroke Collaborators (2021) Global, regional, and National Burden of stroke and its risk factors, 1990-2019: a systematic analysis for the global burden of disease study 2019. Lancet Neurol 20(10):795–820. https://doi.org/10.1016/S1474-4422(21)00252-0

Gokhale S, Caplan LR, James ML (2015) Sex differences in incidence, pathophysiology, and outcome of primary intracerebral hemorrhage. Stroke 46(3):886–892. https://doi.org/10.1161/STROKEAHA.114.007682

Gorelick PB (2019) The global burden of stroke: persistent and disabling. Lancet Neurol 18(5):417–418. https://doi.org/10.1016/S1474-4422(19)30030-4

Green JB (2003) Brain reorganization after stroke. Top Stroke Rehabil 10(3):1–20. https://doi.org/10.1310/H65X-23HW-QL1G-KTNQ

Grefkes C, Fink GR (2020) Recovery from stroke: current concepts and future perspectives. Neurol Res Pract 2:17. https://doi.org/10.1186/s42466-020-00060-6

Haaland KY, Mutha PK, Rinehart JK, Daniels M, Cushnyr B, Adair JC (2012) Relationship between arm usage and instrumental activities of daily living after unilateral stroke. Arch Phys Med Rehabil 93(11):1957–1962. https://doi.org/10.1016/j.apmr.2012.05.011

Jetten J, Haslam C, Pugliese C, Tonks J, Alexander Haslam S (2010) Declining autobiographical memory and the loss of identity: effects on Well-being. J Clin Exp Neuropsychol 32(4):408–416. https://doi.org/10.1080/13803390903140603

Johnson W, Onuma O, Owolabi M, Sachdev S (2016) Stroke: a global response is needed. Bull World Health Organ 94(9):634–634A. https://doi.org/10.2471/BLT.16.181636

Joy MT, Thomas Carmichael S (2021) Encouraging an excitable brain state: mechanisms of brain repair in stroke. Nat Rev Neurosci 22(1):38–53. https://doi.org/10.1038/s41583-020-00396-7

Katan M, Luft A (2018) Global burden of stroke. Semin Neurol 38(2):208–211. https://doi.org/10.1055/s-0038-1649503

Kelly-Hayes M, Beiser A, Kase CS, Scaramucci A, D'Agostino RB, Wolf PA (2003) The influence of gender and age on disability following ischemic stroke: the Framingham study. J Stroke Cerebrovasc Dis 12(3):119–126. https://doi.org/10.1016/S1052-3057(03)00042-9

Khan NI, Naz L, Mushtaq S, Rukh L, Ali S, Hussain Z (2009) Ischemic stroke: prevalence of modifiable risk factors in male and female patients in Pakistan. Pak J Pharm Sci 22(1):62–67

Kitago T, Liang J, Huang VS, Hayes S, Simon P, Tenteromano L, Lazar RM, Marshall RS, Mazzoni P, Lennihan L, Krakauer JW (2013) Improvement after constraint-induced movement therapy: recovery of normal motor control or task-specific compensation? Neurorehabil Neural Repair 27(2):99–109. https://doi.org/10.1177/1545968312452631

Kitago T, Goldsmith J, Harran M, Kane L, Berard J, Huang S, Ryan SL, Mazzoni P, Krakauer JW, Huang VS (2015) Robotic therapy for chronic stroke: general recovery of impairment or improved task-specific skill? J Neurophysiol 114(3):1885–1894. https://doi.org/10.1152/jn.00336.2015

Kleim JA, Jones TA (2008) Principles of experience-dependent neural plasticity: implications for rehabilitation after brain damage. J Speech Lang Hear Res 51(1):S225–S239. https://doi.org/10.1044/1092-4388(2008/018)

Kolasinski J, Makin TR, Logan JP, Jbabdi S, Clare S, Stagg CJ, Johansen-Berg H (2016) Perceptually relevant remapping of human Somatotopy in 24 hours. elife 5. https://doi.org/10.7554/eLife.17280

Krakauer JW, Thomas Carmichael S (2017) Broken movement: the neurobiology of motor recovery after stroke, 1st edn. MIT Press (Massachusetts Institute of Technology Press), Cambridge

Krishnamurthi RV et al (2013) Global and regional burden of first-ever Ischaemic and Haemorrhagic stroke during 1990-2010: findings from the global burden of disease study 2010. Lancet Glob Health 1(5):e259–e281. https://doi.org/10.1016/S2214-109X(13)70089-5

Kwakkel G, Kollen BJ (2013) Predicting activities after stroke: what is clinically relevant? Int J Stroke 8(1):25–32. https://doi.org/10.1111/j.1747-4949.2012.00967.x

Kwakkel G, Kollen BJ, van der Grond J, Prevo AJH (2003) Probability of regaining dexterity in the flaccid upper limb: impact of severity of paresis and time since onset in acute stroke. Stroke 34(9):2181–2186. https://doi.org/10.1161/01.STR.0000087172.16305.CD

Lackland DT, Roccella EJ, Deutsch AF, Fornage M, George MG, Howard G, Kissela BM, Kittner SJ, Lichtman JH, Lisabeth LD, Schwamm LH, Smith EE, Towfighi A (2014) Factors influencing the decline in stroke mortality a statement from the American Heart Association/American Stroke Association. Stroke 45(1):315–353

Langhorne P (2007) Early supported discharge after stroke. J Rehabil Med 39(2):103–108. https://doi.org/10.2340/16501977-0042

Langhorne P, Coupar F, Pollock A (2009) Motor recovery after stroke: a systematic review. Lancet Neurol 8(8):741–754. https://doi.org/10.1016/S1474-4422(09)70150-4

Langhorne P, Bernhardt J, Kwakkel G (2011) Stroke rehabilitation. Lancet (London, England) 377(9778):1693–1702. https://doi.org/10.1016/S0140-6736(11)60325-5

Langhorne P, Ramachandra S, Stroke Unit Trialists' Collaboration (2020) Organised inpatient (stroke unit) care for stroke: network meta-analysis. Cochrane Database Syst Rev 4(4):CD000197. https://doi.org/10.1002/14651858.CD000197.pub4

Lawrence ES, Coshall C, Dundas R, Stewart J, Rudd AG, Howard R, Wolfe CD (2001) Estimates of the prevalence of acute stroke impairments and disability in a multiethnic population. Stroke 32(6):1279–1284. https://doi.org/10.1161/01.str.32.6.1279

Lekander I, Willers C, von Euler M, Lilja M, Sunnerhagen KS, Pessah-Rasmussen H, Borgström F (2017) Relationship between functional disability and costs one and two years post stroke. PLoS One 12(4):e0174861. https://doi.org/10.1371/journal.pone.0174861

Levin MF, Demers M (2021) Motor learning in neurological rehabilitation. Disabil Rehabil 43(24):3445–3453. https://doi.org/10.1080/09638288.2020.1752317

Levin MF, Kleim JA, Wolf SL (2009) What do Motor 'recovery' and 'compensation' mean in patients following stroke? Neurorehabil Neural Repair 23(4):313–319. https://doi.org/10.1177/1545968308328727

Lin DJ, Erler KS, Snider SB, Bonkhoff AK, DiCarlo JA, Lam N, Ranford J, Parlman K, Cohen A, Freeburn J, Finklestein SP, Schwamm LH, Hochberg LR, Cramer SC (2021) Cognitive demands influence upper extremity motor performance during recovery from acute stroke. Neurology 96(21):e2576–e2586. https://doi.org/10.1212/WNL.0000000000011992

Lucas-Noll J, Clua-Espuny JL, Lleixà-Fortuño M, Gavaldà-Espelta E, Queralt-Tomas L, Panisello-Tafalla A, Carles-Lavila M (2023) The costs associated with stroke care continuum: a systematic review. Heal Econ Rev 13(1):32. https://doi.org/10.1186/s13561-023-00439-6

Malik AN, Tariq H, Afridi A, Rathore FA (2022) Technological advancements in stroke rehabilitation. J Pak Med Assoc. 72(8):1672–1674

Markus HS (2010) Unravelling the genetics of Ischaemic stroke. PLoS Med 7(3):e1000225. https://doi.org/10.1371/journal.pmed.1000225

Markus HS (2012) Stroke genetics: prospects for personalized medicine. BMC Med 10:113. https://doi.org/10.1186/1741-7015-10-113

Masiero S, Carraro E (2008) Upper limb movements and cerebral plasticity in post-stroke rehabilitation. Aging Clin Exp Res 20(2):103–108. https://doi.org/10.1007/BF03324755

Mayo NE, Wood-Dauphinee S, Côté R, Durcan L, Carlton J (2002) Activity, participation, and quality of life 6 months Poststroke. Arch Phys Med Rehabil 83(8):1035–1042. https://doi.org/10.1053/apmr.2002.33984

Mendis S (2013) Stroke disability and rehabilitation of stroke: World Health Organization perspective. Int J Stroke 8(1):3–4. https://doi.org/10.1111/j.1747-4949.2012.00969.x

Miah MNA, Azhar MA, Rahman A, Halder D, Akteruzzaman M, Kundu NC (2012) Risk factors of stroke in young and old age group-a comparative study. J Med 13(2):138–142

Michaelsen SM, Dannenbaum R, Levin MF (2006) Task-specific training with trunk restraint on arm recovery in stroke: randomized control trial. Stroke 37(1):186–192. https://doi.org/10.1161/01.STR.0000196940.20446.c9

Motolese F, Capone F, Di Lazzaro V (2022) Chapter 21: new tools for shaping plasticity to enhance recovery after stroke. In: Quartarone A, Ghilardi MF, Boller F (eds) Handbook of clinical neurology, vol 184, 1st edn. Elsevier, Amsterdam, pp 299–315

Mulder T, Hochstenbach J (2001) Adaptability and flexibility of the human motor system: implications for neurological rehabilitation. Neural Plast 8(1–2):131–140. https://doi.org/10.1155/NP.2001.131

Norouzi-Gheidari N, Archambault PS, Monte-Silva K, Kairy D, Sveistrup H, Trivino M, Levin MF, Milot M-H (2021) Feasibility and preliminary efficacy of a combined virtual reality, robotics and electrical stimulation intervention in upper extremity stroke rehabilitation. J Neuroeng Rehabil 18(61). https://doi.org/10.1186/s12984-021-00851-1

Norrving B, Barrick J, Davalos A, Dichgans M, Cordonnier C, Guekht A, Kutluk K, Mikulik R, Wardlaw J, Richard E, Nabavi D, Molina C, Bath PM, Sunnerhagen KS, Rudd A, Drummond A, Planas A, Caso V (2018) Action plan for stroke in Europe 2018-2030. Eur Stroke J 3(4):309–336. https://doi.org/10.1177/2396987318808719

O'Donnell MJ, Xavier D, Liu L, Zhang H, Chin SL, Rao-Melacini P, Rangarajan S, Islam S, Pais P, McQueen MJ, Mondo C, Damasceno A, Lopez-Jaramillo P, Hankey GJ, Dans AL, Yusoff K, Truelsen T, Diener H-C, Sacco RL, Ryglewicz D, Czlonkowska A, Weimar C, Wang X, Yusuf S (2010) Risk factors for Ischaemic and intracerebral Haemorrhagic stroke in 22 countries (the INTERSTROKE study): a case-control study. Lancet (London, England) 376(9735):112–123. https://doi.org/10.1016/S0140-6736(10)60834-3

Owolabi MO et al (2022) Primary stroke prevention worldwide: translating evidence into action. Lancet Public Health 7(1):e74–e85. https://doi.org/10.1016/S2468-2667(21)00230-9

Park H, Kim S, Winstein CJ, Gordon J, Schweighofer N (2016) Short-duration and intensive training improves long-term reaching performance in individuals with chronic stroke. Neurorehabil Neural Repair 30(6):551–561. https://doi.org/10.1177/1545968315606990

Pekna M, Pekny M, Nilsson M (2012) Modulation of neural plasticity as a basis for stroke rehabilitation. Stroke 43(10):2819–2828. https://doi.org/10.1161/STROKEAHA.112.654228

Pollock A, Farmer SE, Brady MC, Langhorne P, Mead GE, Mehrholz J, van Wijck F (2014) Interventions for improving upper limb function after stroke. Cochrane

Database Syst Rev 2014(11):CD010820. https://doi.org/10.1002/14651858.CD010820.pub2

Putman K, de Wit L, Schupp W, Ilse B, Berman P, Connell L, Dejaeger E, de Mieyer A-M, de Weerdt W, Feys H, Walter J, Lincoln N, Louckx F, Anneleen M, Birgit S, Smith B, Leys M (2016) Use of time by physiotherapists and occupational therapists in a stroke rehabilitation unit: a comparison between four European rehabilitation Centres. Disabil Rehabil 28(22):1417–1424

Raghavan P, Santello M, Gordon AM, Krakauer JW (2010) Compensatory motor control after stroke: an alternative joint strategy ForObject-dependent shaping of hand posture. J Neurophysiol 103:3034–3043. https://doi.org/10.1152/jn.00936.2009

Rehme AK, Fink GR, Von Cramon DY, Grefkes C (2011) The role of the contralesional motor cortex for motor recovery in the early days after stroke assessed with longitudinal FMRI. Cereb Cortex 21(4):756–768. https://doi.org/10.1093/cercor/bhq140

Repšaitė V (2015) The effect of differential training on functional training movements and independence in patients with stroke. Doctoral dissertation, Institute of Sport, Lithuanian University of Health Sciences

Repšaitė V, Baltaduonienė D, Vainoras A (2013) Asmenų, Persirgusių Galvos Smegenų Infarktu, Savarankiškumo Ir Plaštakos Raumenų Jėgos Pokyčiai Taikant Įprastą Ir Diferencinio Mokymo Metodika Paremtą Ergoterapiją. Sveikatos Mokslai 23(4):90–93. https://doi.org/10.5200/sm-hs.2013.097

Repšaitė V, Vainoras A, Berškienė K, Baltaduonienė D, Daunoravičienė A, Sendžikaitė E (2015) The effect of differential training-based occupational therapy on hand and arm function in patients after stroke: results of the pilot study. Neurol Neurochir Pol 49(3):150–155. https://doi.org/10.1016/j.pjnns.2015.04.001

Richards LG, Cramer SC (2021) Advances in stroke: therapies targeting stroke recovery. Stroke 52(1):348–350. https://doi.org/10.1161/STROKEAHA.120.033231

Rincon F, Sacco RL, Kranwinkel G, Qiu X, Paik MC, Boden-Albala B, Elkind MSV (2009) Incidence and risk factors of intracranial atherosclerotic stroke: the northern Manhattan stroke study. Cerebrovasc Dis (Basel, Switzerland) 28(1):65–71. https://doi.org/10.1159/000219299

Rodgers H, Price C (2017) Stroke unit care, inpatient rehabilitation and early supported discharge. Clin Med (Lond) 17(2):173–177. https://doi.org/10.7861/clinmedicine.17-2-173

Roth GA, Forouzanfar MH, Moran AE, Barber R, Nguyen G, Feigin VL, Naghavi M, Mensah GA, Murray CJL (2015) Demographic and epidemiologic drivers of global cardiovascular mortality. N Engl J Med 372(14):1333–1341. https://doi.org/10.1056/NEJMoa1406656

Roth GA et al (2020) Global burden of cardiovascular diseases and risk factors, 1990-2019: update from the GBD 2019 study. J Am Coll Cardiol 76(25):2982–3021. https://doi.org/10.1016/j.jacc.2020.11.010

Ryerson S, Byl NN, Brown DA, Wong RA, Hidler JM (2008) Altered trunk position sense and its relation to balance functions in people post-stroke. J Neurol Phys Ther 32(1):14–20. https://doi.org/10.1097/NPT.0b013e3181660f0c

Schmidt RA (1975) A schema theory of discrete motor skill learning. Psychol Rev 82(4):225–260

Schöllhorn WI, Mayer-Kress G, Newell KM, Michelbrink M (2009) Time scales of adaptive behavior and motor learning in the presence of stochastic perturbations. Hum Mov Sci 28(3):319–333. https://doi.org/10.1016/j.humov.2008.10.005

Schöllhorn WI, Beckmann H, Davids K (2010) Exploiting system fluctuations. Differential training in physical prevention and rehabilitation programs for health and exercise. Medicina (Kaunas) 46(6):365–373

Shapi'i A, Mat Zin NA, Elaklouk AM (2015) A game system for cognitive rehabilitation. Biomed Res Int 493562. https://doi.org/10.1155/2015/493562

Sjöholm A, Skarin M, Churilov L, Nilsson M, Bernhardt J, Lindén T (2014) Sedentary behaviour and physical activity of people with stroke in rehabilitation hospitals. Stroke Res Treat 2014:591897. https://doi.org/10.1155/2014/591897

Strimaitytė E, Kaktienė V, Baltaduonienė D (2019) Asmenų, patyrusių galvos smegenų insultą, kvapų suvokimo sutrikimai ir jų korekcija, taikant ergoterapiją. Health Sci 29(6):68–71. https://doi.org/10.35988/sm-hs.2019.102

Su F, Wendong X (2020) Enhancing brain plasticity to promote stroke recovery. Front Neurol 11:554089. https://doi.org/10.3389/fneur.2020.554089

Sun L, Clarke R, Bennett D, Guo Y et al (2019) Causal associations of blood lipids with risk of ischemic stroke and intracerebral hemorrhage in Chinese adults. Nat Med 25(4):569–574. https://doi.org/10.1038/s41591-019-0366-x

Tarri M, Brihmat N, Gasq D, Lepage B, Loubinoux I, De Boissezon X, Marque P, Castel-Lacanal E (2018) Five-day course of paired associative stimulation fails to improve motor function in stroke patients. Ann Phys Rehabil Med 61(2):78–84. https://doi.org/10.1016/j.rehab.2017.11.002

Taube W, Mouthon M, Leukel C, Hoogewoud H-M, Annoni J-M, Keller M (2015) Brain activity during observation and motor imagery of different balance tasks: an FMRI study. Cortex 64:102–114. https://doi.org/10.1016/j.cortex.2014.09.022

Teasell R, Salbach NM, Foley N, Mountain A, Cameron JI, de Jong A, Acerra NE, Bastasi D, Carter SL, Fung J, Halabi M-L, Iruthayarajah J, Harris J, Kim E, Noland A, Pooyania S, Rochette A, Stack BD, Symcox E, Timpson D, Varghese S, Verrilli S, Gubitz G, Casaubon LK, Dowlatshahi D, Patrice Lindsay M (2020) Canadian stroke best practice recommendations: rehabilitation, recovery, and community participation following stroke. Part one: rehabilitation and recovery following stroke; 6th edition update 2019. Int J Stroke 15(7):763–788. https://doi.org/10.1177/1747493019897843

Ting WK-C, Fadul FA-R, Fecteau S, Ethier C (2021) Neurostimulation for stroke rehabilitation. Front Neurosci 15:649459. https://doi.org/10.3389/fnins.2021.649459

Towfighi A, Zheng L, Ovbiagele B (2010) Weight of the obesity epidemic: rising stroke rates among middle-aged women in the United States. Stroke 41(7):1371–1375. https://doi.org/10.1161/STROKEAHA.109.577510

Udvardi V, Szabó G, Fazekas G (2023) The effects of mindfulness-based interventions in post-stroke rehabilitation. Ideggyogy Sz 76(1–2):11–17. https://doi.org/10.18071/isz.76.0011

van de Ven RM, Buitenweg JIV, Schmand B, Veltman DJ, Aaronson JA, Nijboer TCW, Kruiper-Doesborgh SJC, van Bennekom CAM, Sascha MC, Rasquin KR et al (2017) Brain training improves recovery after stroke but waiting list improves equally: a multicenter randomized controlled trial of a computer-based cognitive flexibility training. PLoS One 12(3):e0172993. https://doi.org/10.1371/journal.pone.0172993

van Delden A, Lex EQ, Lieke C, Peper E, Harlaar J, Daffertshofer A, Zijp NI, Nienhuys K, Koppe P, Kwakkel G, Beek PJ (2009) Comparing unilateral and bilateral upper limb training: the ULTRA-stroke program design. BMC Neurol 9:57. https://doi.org/10.1186/1471-2377-9-57

Veerbeek JM, Kwakkel G, van Wegen EEH, Ket JCF, Heymans MW (2011) Early prediction of outcome of activities of daily living after stroke: a systematic review. Stroke 42(5):1482–1488. https://doi.org/10.1161/STROKEAHA.110.604090

Venketasubramanian N, Yoon BW, Pandian J, Navarro JC (2017) Stroke epidemiology in south, east, and South-East Asia: a review. J Stroke 19(3):286–294. https://doi.org/10.5853/jos.2017.00234

Vyas MV, Silver FL, Austin PC, Yu AYX, Pequeno P, Fang J, Laupacis A, Kapral MK (2021) Stroke incidence by sex across the lifespan. Stroke 52(2):447–451. https://doi.org/10.1161/STROKEAHA.120.032898

Wafa HA, Wolfe CDA, Emmett E, Roth GA, Johnson CO, Wang Y (2020) Burden of stroke in Europe: thirty-year projections of incidence, prevalence, deaths, and disability-adjusted life years. Stroke 51(8):2418–2427. https://doi.org/10.1161/STROKEAHA.120.029606

Wang H, Camicia M, Terdiman J, Mannava MK, Sidney S, Elizabeth Sandel M (2013) Daily treatment time and functional gains of stroke patients during inpatient rehabilitation. PM & R 5(2):122–128. https://doi.org/10.1016/j.pmrj.2012.08.013

Westover AN, McBride S, Haley RW (2007) Stroke in young adults who abuse amphetamines or cocaine: a population-based study of hospitalized patients. Arch Gen Psychiatry 64(4):495–502. https://doi.org/10.1001/archpsyc.64.4.495

White H, Boden-Albala B, Wang C, Elkind MSV, Rundek T, Wright CB, Sacco RL (2005) Ischemic stroke subtype incidence among whites, blacks, and hispanics: the northern Manhattan study. Circulation 111(10):1327–1331. https://doi.org/10.1161/01.CIR.0000157736.19739.D0

White CL, Pergola PE, Szychowski JM, Talbert R, Cervantes-Arriaga A, Clark HD, Del Brutto OH, Godoy IE, Hill MD, Pelegrí A, Sussman CR, Taylor AA, Valdivia J, Anderson DC, Conwit R, Benavente OR (2013) Blood pressure after recent stroke: baseline findings from the secondary prevention of small subcortical strokes trial. Am J Hypertens 26(9):1114–1122. https://doi.org/10.1093/ajh/hpt076

Williams B et al (2018) 2018 ESC/ESH guidelines for the management of arterial hypertension. Eur Heart J 39(33):3021–3104. https://doi.org/10.1093/eurheartj/ehy339

Winstein CJ, Stein J, Arena R, Bates B, Cherney LR, Cramer SC et al (2016) Guidelines for adult stroke rehabilitation and recovery: a guideline for healthcare professionals from the American Heart Association/American Stroke Association. Stroke 47(6):e98–e169. https://doi.org/10.1161/STR.0000000000000098

Wolf TJ, Baum C, Conner LT (2009) Changing face of stroke: implications for occupational therapy practice. Am J Occup Ther 63(5):621–625. https://doi.org/10.5014/ajot.63.5.621

Yaggi HK, Concato J, Kernan WN, Lichtman JH, Brass LM, Mohsenin V (2005) Obstructive sleep apnea as a risk factor for stroke and death. N Engl J Med 353(19):2034–2041. https://doi.org/10.1056/NEJMoa043104

Young T, Palta M, Dempsey J, Skatrud J, Weber S, Badr S (1993) The occurrence of sleep-disordered breathing among middle-aged adults. N Engl J Med 328(17):1230–1235. https://doi.org/10.1056/NEJM199304293281704

Zeiler SR, Krakauer JW (2013) The interaction between training and plasticity in the poststroke brain. Curr Opin Neurol 26(6):609–616. https://doi.org/10.1097/WCO.0000000000000025

Differential Learning Approaches in Anterior Cruciate Ligament Rehabilitation: Enhancing Recovery

6

Alli Gokeler, Jo Verschueren, and Bruno Tassignon

6.1 Introduction

Anterior cruciate ligament (ACL) injuries are a significant concern in the sports medicine community, affecting athletes across various sports. The incidence of ACL injuries varies by age, sex, and type and level of sports. Female athletes have a higher incidence of ACL injuries compared to male athletes. In a systematic review, the injury rate for girls was 0.084 per 1000 athlete-exposures (AEs) versus 0.060 for boys, resulting in a relative risk (RR) of 1.40 for females (Bram et al. 2021). The highest relative risk for ACL injuries in females was observed in basketball (RR 4.14) and soccer incident rate (IR 0.166) (Bram et al. 2021). For males, football had the highest number of injuries, but the overall injury rate per exposure was lower than that of females (Gornitzky et al. 2016). Non-contact ACL injuries accounted for 55% of all ACL injuries in team ball sports, with a higher incidence in competition settings (Chia et al. 2022). Girls' soccer had the highest injury rate (IR 0.148) among high school sports (Gornitzky et al. 2016). Among adolescent athletes, ACL injuries are increasingly common. The risk is particularly high in sports like soccer and basketball, with girls facing a nearly 10% risk of sustaining an ACL injury throughout their high school career (Bram et al. 2021).

6.1.1 Anatomy, Biomechanics and Sensory Function of the ACL

Anatomically, the ACL is an intra-articular but extrasynovial ligament located within the knee joint. It originates from the posteromedial aspect of the lateral femoral condyle and inserts into the anterior intercondylar area of the tibia. The ACL consists of two functional bundles: the anteromedial (AM) bundle, which provides stability during knee flexion, and the posterolateral (PL) bundle, which contributes to rotational stability and is more taut in knee extension (Zantop et al. 2006). Biomechanically, the ACL plays a critical role by resisting anterior tibial translation, preventing the tibia from sliding forward relative to the femur, and controlling rotational stability

A. Gokeler (✉)
Exercise Science and Neuroscience unit, Department Exercise & Health, Faculty of Science, Paderborn University, Paderborn, Germany

Faculty of Health, Amsterdam University of Applied Sciences, Amsterdam, the Netherlands
e-mail: alli.gokeler@uni-paderborn.de

J. Verschueren
Human Physiology and Sports Physiotherapy Research Group, Vrije Universiteit Brussel, Brussels, Belgium

B. Tassignon
Rehabilitation Sciences, Capacity group Rehabilitation Sciences & Physiotherapy, Research Group Rehabilitation Research Center, University Hasselt, Hasselt, Belgium

W. I. Schöllhorn, A. Slapšinskaitė-Dackevičienė (eds.), *Differential Learning in Physiotherapy*,
https://doi.org/10.1007/978-3-031-98787-8_6

during pivoting or cutting movements. During activities such as jumping, landing, and sudden changes in direction, the ACL experiences significant stress. The ACL is composed of dense connective tissue with a rich supply of mechanoreceptors, contributing to proprioception, and receives its blood supply primarily from the middle genicular artery (Fu et al. 1999). Mechanoreceptors within the ligament provide feedback to the brain about the position and movement of the knee, which helps in coordinating muscle activity and ensuring joint stability (Hogervorst and Brand 1998).

6.1.2 Intrinsic and Extrinsic Risk Factors

Multiple intrinsic risk factors have been linked to increased ACL injury risk. For example, the increased incidence of ACL injuries in females is attributed to anatomical differences such as wider pelvises, increased quadriceps (Q) angles, and steeper tibial slopes, all of which predispose females to greater knee valgus during dynamic activities (Saber et al. 2024).

Hormonal fluctuations have been implicated in ACL laxity, potentially modifying injury risk, although data remain limited and further research is necessary to elucidate these relationships (Mancino et al. 2023). These findings underscore the multifactorial nature of ACL injury risk, highlighting the importance of considering a range of intrinsic factors in both research and the development of targeted prevention strategies. Extrinsic risk factors are external to the individual and involve environmental, equipment, and activity-related aspects. Important extrinsic factors include certain surfaces, such as artificial floors, which may increase the risk of ACL injuries compared to natural grass (Pasanen et al. 2008). Shoes that have high friction coefficients with the playing surface can increase the risk (Dowling et al. 2010).

6.1.3 Mechanism of ACL Injury and Consequences

The ACL can be injured through both contact and noncontact mechanisms. Non-contact injuries are more common and often occur during activities that involve sudden stops, changes in direction, or landing from a jump. Most commonly, there is a combination of a rotated trunk away from the injured side, an abducted hip, slight knee flexion, and a flat foot position, all contributing to the dynamics of valgus collapse (Della Villa et al. 2020).

The consequences of ACL injury are notoriously impactful. First, it poses a large personal burden due to the large number of days of absence from sports. In the Australian High Performance Sports System, a median return-to-sport (RTS) time of 369 days was reported following ACL injuries (Rigg et al. 2023). Second, after undergoing ACLR, only 53% of football players return to competition within 3 years (Sandon et al. 2025).

Third, ACL injuries result in a significant financial burden to society due to the operation and subsequent rehabilitation (Ross et al. 2023). Fourth, athletes after ACLR injury have an increased risk of sustaining second ACL injuries. Of those athletes under 25 years of age, 25% suffer a second ACL injury within 24 months after RTS (Wiggins et al. 2016). Finally, the prevalence of early osteoarthritis is 36% 10 years after ACLR (Webster and Hewett 2022).

6.1.4 Outcomes After ACL Reconstruction

6.1.4.1 Biomechanics

After ACLR, patients often exhibit altered biomechanics, such as unloading the reconstructed limb and shifting from knee to hip and ankle strategies to dissipate load from the injured knee (Johnston et al. 2018). Additionally, between limbs, there is often a shift from the reconstructed limb to the uninjured limb, further exacerbating the risk of injury to the uninjured knee (Gokeler et al. 2022a, b). These biomechanical changes can be subtle but have significant implications for the long-term health and function of the knee joint. For instance, altered gait patterns and asymmetrical loading can increase the wear and tear on the joint surfaces, leading to degenerative changes over time (Gokeler et al. 2013).

Understanding these biomechanical factors is crucial for developing targeted rehabilitation strategies that address not only strength and mobility but also the quality of movement patterns to reduce the risk of further injury and degeneration.

Neurophysiological Changes

Beyond biomechanical factors, neurophysiological changes after ACL injury and reconstruction play a critical role in rehabilitation and the risk of re-injury. After ACLR, alterations in the central nervous system's processing of sensory information can lead to changes in motor control. This can manifest as delayed muscle activation patterns, reduced proprioception, and an increased reliance on visual cues for balance and movement control (Piskin et al. 2022). These changes include sensory motor reweighting demonstrated by increased visual reliance and higher cognitive activity for motor planning and execution (Piskin et al. 2022; Tortoli et al. 2024). These adaptations can affect an athlete's ability to perform complex movements and respond to dynamic environments, critical aspects of sports participation. The brain's role in coordinating movement and ensuring joint stability is paramount. Addressing these neurophysiological changes through rehabilitation is essential for restoring optimal function and reducing the risk of further injury.

General Principles of Rehabilitation After ACLR

To achieve the often desired goal by the patient—that is, RTS—optimizing all preceding phases of rehabilitation is paramount. The necessity of effective early-stage rehabilitation serves as the foundation for successful recovery (Buckthorpe et al. 2023). The early phase of rehabilitation after ACLR generally occurs immediately after surgery and is typically defined as the first 4–6 weeks following the procedure. This phase focuses on overcoming the effects of surgery and preparing the patient for entry into mid-stage rehabilitation. This phase is crucial for addressing dysfunctions that can impede knee function and hinder progression to subsequent rehabilitation stages.

Six key factors need to be considered during early-phase rehabilitation (Buckthorpe et al. 2023):

1. Pain and Swelling: Post-surgery, patients often experience significant pain and swelling, which can lead to a catabolic environment in the joint, adversely affecting recovery. The authors recommend utilizing various treatment modalities such as cryotherapy, compression, and elevation to manage these symptoms. Active range of motion (ROM) exercises should also be incorporated early to promote venous return and reduce swelling. Frequent medical consultations are suggested to monitor the patient's progress and address any complications that may arise, such as excessive swelling or signs of infection.
2. Knee Joint ROM: Achieving full knee extension and flexion is vital for successful rehabilitation. The authors emphasize that loss of knee extension by 2–4 weeks post-ACLR significantly increases the risk of complications such as cyclops lesions or arthrofibrosis. Therefore, early intervention through passive and active ROM exercises is necessary to prevent these issues and facilitate optimal knee biomechanics.
3. Arthrogenic Muscle Inhibition (AMI) and Muscle Strength: The rehabilitation process must focus on restoring muscle strength, particularly in the quadriceps, which is often inhibited post-surgery. The authors point out that residual strength deficits can hinder functional progression and lead to complications such as altered biomechanics and knee pain. They recommend early rehabilitation strategies aimed at overcoming AMI, such as neuromuscular electrical stimulation and blood flow restriction training, to enhance muscle activation and strength during this critical phase.
4. Movement Quality and Neuromuscular Control: There is a need to address movement quality early in rehabilitation, as poor movement mechanics can increase the risk of re-injury and affect long-term outcomes. Incorporating gait retraining and balance

exercises is warranted in the rehabilitation program. This approach should focus on restoring proper limb control and optimal kinematics during various functional tasks, emphasizing the importance of integrating both biomechanical and neuromechanical factors into early rehabilitation efforts.
5. Psycho-social-Cultural and Environmental Factors: The psychological aspect of rehabilitation is often overlooked but is crucial for the athlete's recovery. The authors highlight the emotional challenges that athletes face post-injury, including feelings of loss, frustration, and anxiety. Engaging with sports psychologists or providing emotional support through counseling can aid in managing these feelings and promoting a more positive rehabilitation experience. Understanding the socio-cultural context of the athlete's environment is also essential, as it influences their recovery journey.
6. Physical Fitness Preservation: Maintaining overall physical fitness during early rehabilitation is vital, especially for athletes who need to return to high-performance levels. The authors emphasize that while the primary focus should be on knee joint recovery, incorporating cardiovascular conditioning and strength training for adjacent joints is also essential. This multifaceted approach can help prevent deconditioning and promote a quicker return to sport.

There is a need for clear communication between the patient and the rehabilitation team to ensure that the patient understands their recovery process and feels supported throughout their journey. Moreover, clinicians should acknowledge the importance of structured planning and programming in rehabilitation. Rehabilitation should be approached as a continuum, with clear criteria for progression from early- to mid-stage rehabilitation based on measurable outcomes, such as pain levels, swelling, and strength. By establishing these criteria, rehabilitation professionals can more effectively monitor patient progress and make timely adjustments to the rehabilitation program as needed.

Optimizing early-stage rehabilitation post-ACLR is essential for improving patient outcomes and reducing the risk of re-injury. The authors provide a comprehensive overview of the key dimensions to consider during this phase, emphasizing the need for a holistic, individualized approach that integrates physical, psychological, and social factors. By focusing on these areas and implementing evidence-based strategies, rehabilitation professionals can better support athletes in their recovery and enhance their chances of a successful return to sport. After achieving the desired goals, the patient can progress to the mid-stage rehabilitation following ACLR, which is a critical period aimed at addressing various functional deficits to ensure optimal recovery and prepare the athlete for late-stage rehabilitation and return to sport. The primary goals of mid-stage rehabilitation can be categorized into three main areas: muscle strength, movement quality, and fitness reconditioning (Buckthorpe and Della Villa 2020).

1. First, a primary focus of mid-stage rehabilitation is the restoration of muscle strength, particularly in the knee extensors and flexors. Post-injury and surgery, patients often experience significant deficits in quadriceps muscle volume, neural activation, and overall strength. Research indicates that achieving knee extensor strength within 20% of the contralateral limb is essential to support functional recovery and prevent compensatory movement patterns that may lead to further injury (Failla et al. 2016). It is noted that many patients struggle to restore quadriceps strength adequately, with studies showing that over half of the patients have deficits greater than 10% compared to their uninjured limb at the time of return to sport. Therefore, targeted strength training becomes paramount, utilizing both isolated and closed kinetic chain exercises tailored to address these deficits while managing arthrogenic muscle inhibition that often accompanies ACL injuries.
2. Second, improving movement quality is crucial during the mid-stage rehabilitation process. Altered movement patterns, such as poor

joint control and balance, can increase the risk of both ipsilateral and contralateral injuries, as well as the development of osteoarthritis. Rehabilitation strategies should focus on retraining basic motor patterns, ensuring that the athlete can perform movements with optimal biomechanics. This involves incorporating exercises that enhance proprioception and joint stability, as well as addressing any muscle imbalances that may contribute to suboptimal movement mechanics.

3. The third primary goal is fitness reconditioning. It is essential to maintain and enhance the athlete's overall physical fitness during the rehabilitation process to prepare them for the demands of their sport. Evidence shows that athletes often experience declines in cardiovascular fitness after ACLR, which can be detrimental to their performance upon return (Gokeler et al. 2022a, b). Therefore, mid-stage rehabilitation should include structured cardiovascular conditioning, strength training for both the upper and lower body, as well as specific sessions focused on body composition and muscle morphology. This holistic approach not only emphasizes the recovery of knee function but also aims to improve overall athletic performance, potentially surpassing pre-injury levels.

The integration of these three goals—muscle strength, movement quality, and fitness reconditioning—requires careful program planning and periodization. Clinicians must adapt the rehabilitation strategies to the individual athlete's needs, taking into account their specific sport, previous injury history, and current functional status. Monitoring progress through screening tests is vital to ensure the athlete is meeting the necessary criteria for transitioning into the late-stage rehabilitation and return to sport.

In the stage of rehabilitation and RTS training after ACLR, clinicians should be cognizant of these key issues (Buckthorpe 2019; Gokeler et al. 2022a, b):

1. Explosive Neuromuscular Performance Deficits
   Many RTS protocols emphasize maximal muscle strength but neglect explosive force generation, or rate of force development (RFD), which is crucial for dynamic joint stability and athletic performance. Even with restored muscle strength, RFD deficits persist, increasing re-injury risk. Specific high-load and explosive strength training, including ballistic and plyometric exercises, should be incorporated to address these gaps.
2. Movement Quality and Retraining
   Poor movement mechanics contribute to re-injury risk. ACL injuries alter neuromuscular control, leading to movement asymmetries and improper biomechanics. Standard rehabilitation often fails to fully restore movement quality. A systematic movement retraining program addressing neuromuscular, biomechanical, and neurocognitive factors is necessary. This includes progressive movement coaching, biofeedback techniques, and scenario-based reactive training to mimic game situations.
3. Impact of Fatigue on Performance and Injury Risk
   Fatigue exacerbates neuromuscular deficits and alters biomechanics, increasing ACL re-injury risk. Acute fatigue affects decision-making and muscle control, while cumulative fatigue from training and match play can lead to overuse injuries. Rehabilitation should include training under fatigue conditions, progressive load management, and monitoring of acute-to-chronic workload ratios (ACWR) to ensure athletes develop tolerance to game-related demands.
4. Sport-Specific Retraining and Conditioning
   Returning to sport requires more than strength and movement training; it necessitates sport-specific skill retraining. On-field rehabilitation should bridge the gap between controlled rehabilitation settings and the chaotic nature of competitive sport. This includes reconditioning for high-intensity actions like sprinting, deceleration, and directional changes, ensuring athletes restore sport-specific fitness levels.
5. Progressive Loading for RTS

An often-overlooked aspect of ACL rehabilitation is ensuring that athletes achieve sufficient training volume before returning to full competition. Load management strategies should be in place to gradually increase training intensity and duration, avoiding spikes in workload that elevate injury risk. A structured RTS program should include progressive exposure to match-play conditions.

6. Comprehensive RTS Testing
   Traditional RTS testing is inadequate in predicting re-injury risk. A more holistic approach is needed, incorporating:
   - Muscle strength assessment (isokinetic testing)
   - RFD evaluation
   - Movement quality analysis under reactive and fatigued conditions
   - Sport-specific conditioning tests
   - Load management monitoring
   - Psychological readiness assessment

   Despite meeting RTS criteria, this has not been shown to reduce re-injury risk, nor does it guarantee complete performance. More advanced testing methods and individualized return-to-play protocols are required.

6.2 Rehabilitation Practices from a Motor Learning Perspective

Rehabilitation after ACLR is pivotal in determining the long-term success of the surgery and the athlete's return to sport. Clinical practice guidelines that include criteria for rehabilitation practices often focus on restoring strength and range of motion but may not adequately address the neurophysiological changes that occur after injury (Andrade et al. 2019). Blocked practice and instructions with an internal focus of attention are commonly used (Gokeler et al. 2023). Blocked practice in motor learning refers to a training approach where a single skill is repeatedly practiced in a consistent setting before moving on to learn another skill. Blocked practice is believed to enhance the initial acquisition of skills by allowing learners to focus intensely on mastering one task at a time. Traditionally, sentiments (there is a perfect technique/movement) and versatile training (not striving for a perfect technique) are diametrically opposed to each other. The common view regarding the goals of rehabilitation after ACLR is that the athlete (re) learns ideal motor skills (Risberg and Holm 2009). Any deviation and perceived error from the model that perfect movement ecxist, is corrected. However, movement variability always occurs when the same action is repeated, and even the elite athlete cannot reproduce identical movement patterns (Bartlett et al. 2007). Movement variability has been viewed as an unwanted source of error that should be eliminated or reduced. However, the functional role of movement variability is essential to expert performance in many sports.

6.2.1 Instructions with an Internal Focus of Attention

Instructions that promote an internal focus of attention direct the patient's awareness toward their own bodily movements and sensations. An internal focus can lead to overanalysis of body movements, which may result in a decrease in the fluidity and naturalness of movements, counteracting the goals of rehabilitation (Wulf and Lewthwaite 2016). Research has indicated that an internal focus of attention is not universally beneficial and can actually impair performance in tasks that are more automatic or involve multitasking, where an external focus might be more appropriate (Wulf and Prinz 2001).

Yet novel motor learning principles, such as differential learning, are not widely implemented. The theory of dynamical systems is the foundation of differential learning in that athletes can use a self-organized learning process by performing a variety of movement patterns (Schöllhorn 2000). Hence, the movement patterns themselves are purposefully varied during practice when using differential learning for movement skills. Athletes develop a customized motor solution that works best for them, given the physical limitations of their bodies and the environmental context. This is the result of the process of experimentation with various movement patterns, target goals, and alternative methods of performing a task (rather than only practicing the supposedly "correct" movement form). These principles could offer new avenues for rehabilitation, emphasizing the adaptation to variability and enhancing the reintegration of the injured limb into complex movement patterns. Traditional rehabilitation methods have typically focused on linear causality and structured exercises aimed at gradually restoring strength and mobility. However, emerging literature suggests that integrating differential learning into ACL rehabilitation might provide additional benefits, potentially enhancing the recovery process and possibly reducing the risk of re-injury (Tassignon et al. 2021).

6.3 Exploring the Potential of Differential Learning for ACL Rehabilitation

A study involving beginner male soccer players demonstrated that training with differential learning (DL) significantly improved kinematic and kinetic factors associated with noncontact ACL injuries compared to classical model and average-oriented approaches. The DL group showed greater changes in knee valgus and other critical biomechanical measures, suggesting that increased variability during training helps lower injury risk (Mohammadi Orangi et al. 2021). Another randomized controlled trial compared differential learning with self-controlled feedback and external focus of attention. It found that differential learning effectively reduced kinetic and kinematic risk factors for ACL injuries among athletes, indicating its potential as a beneficial training strategy (Ghanati et al. 2022). This approach focuses on variability and self-discovery, which are crucial for effective motor skill acquisition (Gokeler et al. 2023). By participating in a wide range of movements, individuals recovering from ACL injuries could potentially develop a more versatile motor repertoire, which may make them better prepared to handle various physical demands. This could be particularly beneficial for athletes who need to perform in different conditions.

In the upcoming section, a series of examples showcasing the application of DL principles in clinical practice will be presented, along with the underlying rationale. These examples serve as valuable tools for clinicians working with athletes after ACLR, offering innovative strategies to enhance rehabilitation and optimize performance outcomes. By integrating DL principles into daily care routines, clinicians can empower athletes to improve postural stability, movement control, and adaptability through personalized training approaches. The diversified exercises and targeted interventions based on DL not only address physical limitations but also stimulate cognitive engagement and skill acquisition. Through the adoption of these practices, clinicians can facilitate a comprehensive and dynamic rehabilitation process that goes beyond traditional methods, fostering resilience, creativity, and optimal functional recovery for athletes recovering from ACLR. Embracing the principles of DL in clinical care not only enriches the rehabilitation experience but also cultivates a supportive environment for athletes to thrive and excel in their athletic endeavors.

6.3.1 Postural Stability

Recent studies have highlighted postural stability deficits after ACLR (Lehmann et al. 2021). In the aftermath of ACLR, a deficiency in postural control in the affected leg can impede an athlete's capacity to effectively manage the movement of the body's center of mass over the base of support during dynamic sports activities. This underscores the critical significance of tailored RTS rehabilitation programs, as postural stability is a trait that can be improved and enhanced through targeted interventions. The increased variability and unpredictability in differential learning exercises challenge the neuromuscular system to adapt and develop more robust control strategies (Gholami et al. 2023).

6.3.2 Gait

A systematic review by Gokeler et al. found that altered gait patterns can persist for up to 5 years after ACLR (Gokeler et al. 2013). These persistent gait abnormalities may contribute to the early onset of osteoarthritis. Of particular interest, subjects with ACL deficiency exhibited significantly less variable walking patterns compared to healthy controls (Moraiti et al. 2010). A study by Frank et al. (2008) showed that a form of differential learning, characterized by noisy training sessions with varied exercises, leads to greater performance improvements compared to traditional learning methods. This improvement persists even during post-training periods, suggesting that differential learning fosters long-term retention of motor skills (Frank et al. 2008). These findings collectively indicate that differential learning can effectively enhance walking abilities by promoting individualized learning patterns and improving motor skills through varied and context-rich training environments.

In the early stages of rehabilitation following an ACL injury, gait training exercises are often implemented to address various aspects of motor control and balance. These exercises include walking straight, walking on a line, walking on two lines, and walking with internally or externally rotated feet, both symmetrically and asymmetrically. These activities are designed to challenge the leg muscles by requiring them to compensate for the small shear forces generated during movement. Additionally, exercises such as walking backward, walking with different arm movements, and performing movements on the heels or toes can further engage the lower extremity muscles. Variations such as pronation and supination of the foot can also be incorporated to promote coordination and muscular adaptation. Initially, slight changes in direction are introduced, with an increase in the angle of change as the patient progresses. To ensure proper technique and prevent overexertion, the speed of walking is limited by performing these exercises within a constrained 3x3 meter area. This structured approach allows for gradual progression, enhancing neuromuscular control and facilitating recovery of normal gait mechanics.

Here is an example of how differential learning could be applied to gait training:

- Varied Foot Placement: During gait training, instruct the individual to walk with varied foot placements. For example, have them alternate between taking wider steps, narrower steps, and steps of different lengths. This variability encourages the brain to adapt and find the most efficient movement patterns for different foot placements.
- Dynamic Surfaces: Conduct gait training on various surfaces (e.g., grass, sand, uneven terrain) to challenge the individual's proprioception and balance. This approach forces the individual to adjust their gait mechanics dynamically based on surface feedback.
- Obstacle Navigation: Introduce obstacles of varying heights and distances that the individual must navigate around while walking. This can include cones, small steps, or even uneven ground. The need to adapt their gait to avoid obstacles promotes variability in movement and enhances overall motor learning.
- Changing Speed and Rhythm: Encourage the individual to change their walking speed and rhythm frequently. For instance, they could walk slowly for a period, then speed up for a few seconds, and then walk backward or sideways. This variability helps to develop a more adaptable gait pattern.
- Incorporating Multitasking: During gait training, introduce dual-task scenarios where the individual must perform a cognitive task (like counting backward) while walking. This can enhance focus and adaptability, as the individual learns to manage their gait while attending to an additional task.

By implementing these varied practices, differential learning may help individuals develop a more robust and adaptable gait, which is crucial for rehabilitation post-ACLR.

6.3.3 Running

A systematic review indicated that individuals post-ACL reconstruction (ACLR) exhibit significant deficits in knee flexion motion and internal knee extension moment during the stance phase of running (Pairot-de-Fontenay et al. 2019). These deficits persist from 3 months to 5 years after surgery, suggesting that these biomechanical alterations do not resolve over time (Pairot-de-Fontenay et al. 2019). Research from the JUMP-ACL study demonstrated that both the injured and uninjured legs show altered biomechanics after ACL injury and reconstruction. Specifically, the ACLR-injured leg displayed increased hip adduction and knee valgus, while the uninjured leg also showed changes, indicating a compensatory mechanism that could increase the risk of future injuries (Goerger et al. 2015). It has been shown that running biomechanics in the surgical limb do not return to pre-injury levels within 1 year post-ACL-R (Knurr et al. 2021). The surgical limb consistently showed significant deficits compared to pre-injury measurements, while the nonsurgical limb remained stable (Knurr et al. 2021). Although more research is needed, the findings illustrate the potential of adding principles of DL to our current rehabilitation programs.

A similar approach described above for gait training can be followed. In addition, running up and down stairs, as well as performing a slalom pattern while navigating stairs, offers valuable insights into the dynamic movements of the human body. When running upstairs, the body relies on a powerful upward thrust, with the legs engaging primarily in extension at the hip and knee joints, while the arms assist by swinging opposite to the legs for balance and momentum. The arms, moving in a natural left-right alternation, help to stabilize the torso and generate forward motion. On the other hand, running downstairs involves a different set of movements: the body shifts to a controlled descent, where the quadriceps play a critical role in managing the impact forces, and the arms continue to swing but with more emphasis on deceleration and counterbalancing the body's downward motion. In a slalom pattern, when running up and down stairs while alternating direction, the arms perform more exaggerated cross-body movements to help steer the body through tight turns. This requires greater coordination and more dynamic arm motions, as each direction change demands quick shifts in torso alignment. These various activities highlight the distinct and complementary roles of the arms and legs in coordinated movement, illustrating how the body adapts its motor patterns in response to different physical challenges.

Here are some examples of differential learning strategies for running:

- Varying Surfaces: Train on different surfaces such as grass, sand, track, or gravel. Each surface changes the biomechanics of running, encouraging the patient to adapt their technique accordingly.
- Changing Speeds: Incorporate intervals of varying speeds. For example, alternate between sprinting, jogging, and walking. This variation helps the patient develop better control and efficiency at different paces.
- Obstacle Courses: Create a running course with obstacles such as cones, hurdles, or agility ladders. Navigating these obstacles requires the patient to adjust their stride, speed, and direction, enhancing their adaptability.
- Altered Footwear: Use different types of shoes (e.g., minimalist shoes, trail shoes, racing flats) during training. Each type of shoe can affect running mechanics, prompting the patient to adjust their form and technique.
- Incorporating Drills: Include specific running drills that focus on different aspects of running, such as high knees, butt kicks, or lateral shuffles. These drills can improve overall movement patterns and muscle activation.
- Environmental Changes: Run in different weather conditions (e.g., against the wind, rain, heat) to help the athlete learn to adjust their running strategy based on environmental factors.

This can progress to sprinting. For example, when sprinting upstairs, the body's natural mechanics often involve a high knee lift and a forceful drive of the legs, with the arms swinging in opposition to maintain balance and propel the runner forward. Under differential learning principles, an athlete may be encouraged to modify their sprinting mechanics by consciously altering the height of their knee drive or the angle of their arm swing to explore different ways of generating forward momentum. These changes, although initially challenging, allow the athlete's neuromuscular system to adapt, finding the most effective and efficient way to execute the movement. Variations like sprinting upstairs with exaggerated arm movements or focusing on explosive knee lifts can disrupt habitual patterns, stimulating muscle recruitment and coordination in new ways, thereby improving overall sprinting performance. When sprinting down stairs, the primary goal is often to decelerate and control the body's descent, which places significant demand on eccentric muscle actions. Differential learning could involve training in different conditions, such as sprinting downstairs while varying the angle of descent or adding resistance like sleds or weighted vests. Such variability can help athletes adapt their stride length, foot placement, and arm swing to manage the forces involved in descending stairs at high speeds. For instance, an athlete might alternate between sprinting downstairs in a more upright posture or a slightly forward-leaning position, training the body to respond to different postural adjustments that can enhance stability and control during the descent.

6.3.4 Jumping

Jumping is a fundamental motor skill that athletes frequently struggle with after ACLR. During the execution of jumps, athletes often transfer the load from the injured knee to the hip and/or ankle to compensate for weaknesses and limitations (Kotsifaki et al. 2021). In the case of double-legged jumps, a common compensation strategy involves shifting the load from the injured extremity to the uninjured extremity. While this strategy may initially help athletes navigate the challenges of jumping post-ACLR in the form of a local minimum in a potential landscape, it can have significant implications. The reliance on the uninjured extremity for load transfer can hinder the restoration of strength in the injured extremity, leading to increased asymmetries and imbalances in muscle development. Moreover, this compensation pattern is associated with an increased risk of a second ACL injury, as it fails to address the underlying issues and limitations in the rehabilitated limb. It is crucial for clinicians and athletes to recognize and address these compensation strategies to ensure comprehensive rehabilitation and reduce the likelihood of re-injury post-ACLR. In addition, this frequently leads to an overload of the healthy leg, which can lead to earlier fatigue with the same consequences for the other leg.

It has been shown that in-season differential training led to technical adaptations and increased spike-jump height in elite female players (Fuchs et al. 2020). The differential training program allowed players to experience a range of adaptability and to adjust toward an individual optimum in technical components of performance determinants (Fuchs et al. 2020) (Table 6.1).

See Fig. 6.1.

Table 6.1 Examples of how differential learning can be applied to practicing a double-legged jump task

Variations of the double-legged jump task	Change of environment	Change of athlete
Jump as far as you can. While you are jumping: Before jumping, 2–3 bunny hops, skipping both legs, skipping left leg, skipping right leg, high knees, left high knee, right high knee, butt kicks both legs, butt kicks left leg, butt kicks right leg, zig-zag, shuffle to left, shuffle to right Make a full turn to left, to right before you jump While jumping, keep arms across the chest, behind back, raise left arm, raise right arm, circles both arms, circle left arm, circle right arm Move your head to left, to right Close left eye, close right eye While landing, one arm in front of and the other arm behind you Land with a very wide stance or with a very narrow stance Land on toes while landing	Exercises in dark Exercises on sand With shoes or without shoes In an environment with loud music or noise from audience in stadium In a virtual reality environment	Perform exercises with fatigue Perform exercises without fatigue Perform exercises with weighted vest

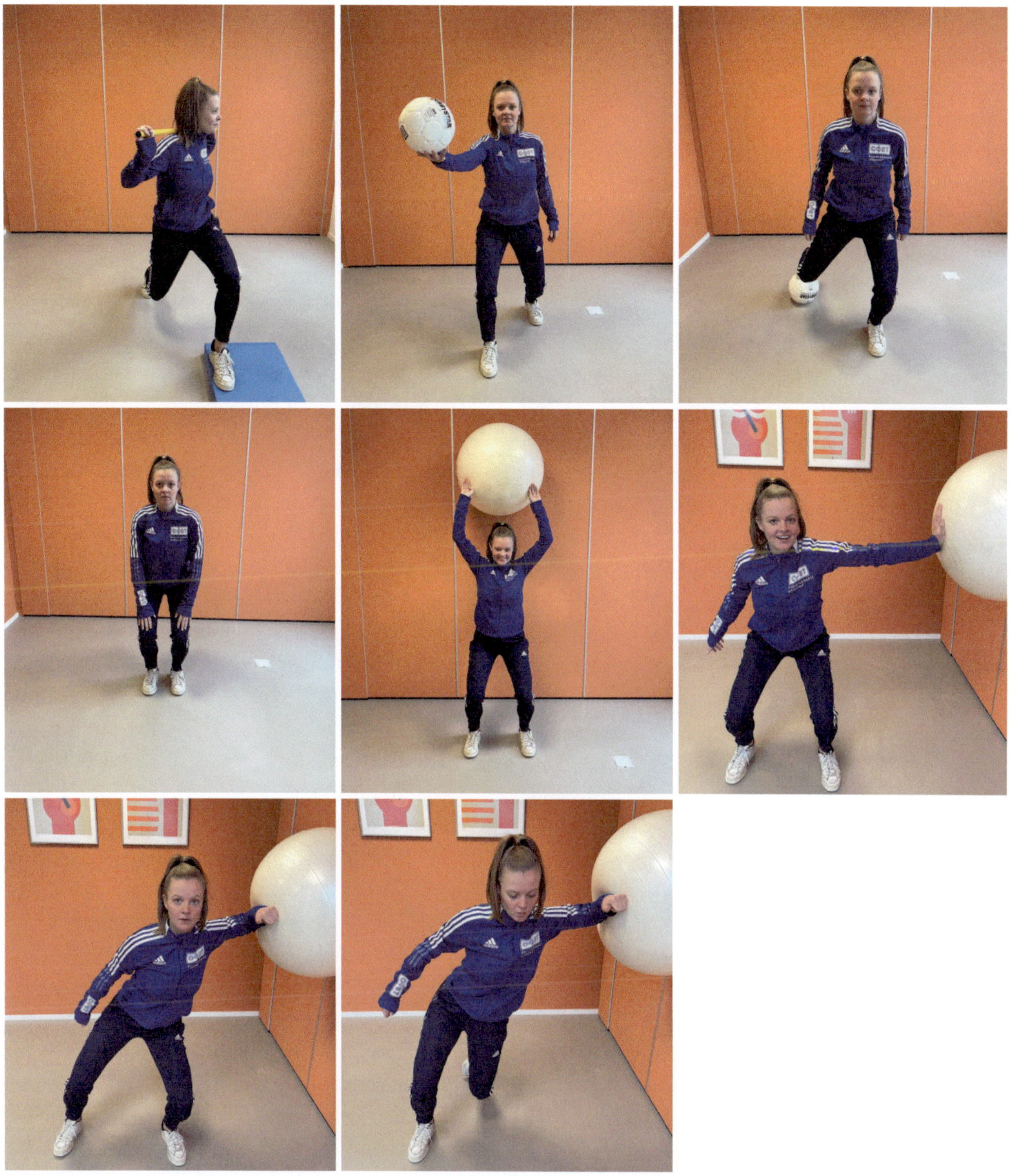

Fig. 6.1 The figure demonstrates various examples of differential learning applied to squats and lunges, including changes in stance width (narrow, wide, shoulder-width), asymmetrical stance (offset foot positioning), upper body adjustments (forward lean, lateral tilt, trunk rotation), overhead targets (reaching upward, asymmetrical arm positions), and head rotation (looking sideways, upward, or downward). These intentional movement variations encourage motor exploration, improve coordination, and enhance adaptability in lower-body exercises

6.4 Summary and Outlook

In conclusion, there is a growing body of evidence supporting the integration of differential learning (DL) principles into the motor learning domain, particularly in ACL rehabilitation. The incorporation of DL, with its emphasis on variability and individualized learning processes, holds promise for revolutionizing the approach to athlete recovery post-ACL reconstruction. The implementation of random practice strategies not only enhances motivation by introducing unpredictability into training sessions but also increases athlete engagement throughout the rehabilitation process. Furthermore, DL offers the potential for improved adaptability to dynamic changes on the field, addressing a potential limitation of current rehabilitation protocols. By integrating DL into ACL rehabilitation programs, clinicians and athletes can foster a more versatile and resilient approach to skill development and recovery. This shift toward embracing variability, creativity, and adaptability through DL methodology signifies a progressive step in optimizing rehabilitation outcomes and enhancing athletic performance post-injury. As further research continues to underscore the benefits of DL in ACL rehabilitation, its adoption into standard practice has the potential to revolutionize the traditional rehabilitation paradigm and empower athletes to reach new heights of success in their sporting endeavors. Nonetheless, many questions are unsolved and need more research, e.g., finding the individual optimum variations and how they are changing by mood or fatigue or circadian rhythms.

Questions

1. Which of the following sports has the highest relative risk (RR) for ACL injuries in female athletes?
   A. Volleyball
   B. Basketball
   C. Tennis
   D. Baseball
2. What is the primary biomechanical function of the anterior cruciate ligament (ACL)?
   A. To facilitate knee extension
   B. To resist anterior tibial translation and control rotational stability
   C. To support quadriceps contraction
   D. To increase knee valgus during movement
3. Which of the following is an intrinsic risk factor for ACL injuries?
   A. Playing on artificial turf
   B. Wearing shoes with a high friction coefficient
   C. Wider pelvis and increased quadriceps (Q) angle in females
   D. Sudden changes in weather conditions
4. What is a key limitation of traditional rehabilitation approaches after ACL reconstruction (ACLR)?
   A. They focus too much on movement variability.
   B. They emphasize only strength and range of motion.
   C. They prioritize external focus over internal focus.
   D. They encourage unstructured and chaotic training.
5. What is a primary concern with instructions that promote an internal focus of attention in ACL rehabilitation?
   A. They enhance automaticity in movement.
   B. They improve external feedback processing.
   C. They may reduce movement fluidity and naturalness.
   D. They eliminate movement variability.
6. Which of the following best describes the principle of differential learning in ACL rehabilitation?
   A. Practicing the same movement repeatedly to perfect technique
   B. Using varied and unpredictable movement patterns to enhance adaptation
   C. Eliminating movement errors to achieve ideal performance
   D. Restricting practice to low-intensity exercises for safety

7. How does differential learning contribute to postural stability after ACLR?
   A. By eliminating movement variability to improve balance
   B. By challenging the neuromuscular system with variability and unpredictability
   C. By reinforcing a single ideal movement strategy
   D. By focusing solely on strengthening the quadriceps
8. What has research suggested about gait patterns after ACLR?
   A. Gait abnormalities typically resolve within a few months.
   B. Individuals with ACLR show increased movement variability compared to healthy individuals.
   C. Altered gait patterns can persist for up to 5 years post-surgery.
   D. Traditional gait training eliminates all biomechanical deficits.
9. What is a major biomechanical issue observed in running after ACLR?
   A. Increased knee flexion and internal knee extension moment
   B. Decreased knee flexion motion and internal knee extension moment
   C. Enhanced knee valgus control and stability
   D. Reduced reliance on compensatory mechanisms
10. Why is movement variability considered beneficial in ACL rehabilitation?
    A. It helps individuals develop a more adaptable motor repertoire.
    B. It ensures movements are identical each time.
    C. It prevents neuromuscular adaptation.
    D. It reduces the need for motor learning principles.

References

Andrade R, Pereira R, Van Cingel R, Staal JB, Espregueira-Mendes J (2019) How should clinicians rehabilitate patients after ACL reconstruction? A systematic review of clinical practice guidelines (CPGs) with a focus on quality appraisal (AGREE II). Br J Sports Med 54:512–519. https://doi.org/10.1136/bjsports-2018-100310

Bartlett R, Wheat J, Robins M (2007) Is movement variability important for sports biomechanists? Sports Biomech 6(2):224–243. https://doi.org/10.1080/14763140701322994

Bram JT, Magee LC, Mehta NN, Patel NM, Ganley TJ (2021) Anterior cruciate ligament injury incidence in adolescent athletes: a systematic review and meta-analysis. Am J Sports Med 49(7):1962–1972. https://doi.org/10.1177/0363546520959619

Buckthorpe M (2019) Optimising the late-stage rehabilitation and return-to-sport training and testing process after ACL reconstruction. Sports Med 49(7):1043–1058. https://doi.org/10.1007/s40279-019-01102-z

Buckthorpe M, Della Villa F (2020) Optimising the 'mid-stage' training and testing process after ACL reconstruction. Sports Med 50(4):657–678. https://doi.org/10.1007/s40279-019-01222-6

Buckthorpe M, Gokeler A, Herrington L, Hughes M, Grassi A, Wadey R et al (2023) Optimising the early-stage rehabilitation process post-ACL reconstruction. Sports Med 54:49. https://doi.org/10.1007/s40279-023-01934-w

Chia L, De Oliveira Silva D, Whalan M, McKay MJ, Sullivan J, Fuller CW, Pappas E (2022) Non-contact anterior cruciate ligament injury epidemiology in team-ball sports: a systematic review with meta-analysis by sex, age, sport, participation level, and exposure type. Sports Med 52(10):2447–2467. https://doi.org/10.1007/s40279-022-01697-w

Della Villa F, Buckthorpe M, Grassi A, Nabiuzzi A, Tosarelli F, Zaffagnini S, Della Villa S (2020) Systematic video analysis of ACL injuries in professional male football (soccer): injury mechanisms, situational patterns and biomechanics study on 134 consecutive cases. Br J Sports Med 54(23):1423–1432. https://doi.org/10.1136/bjsports-2019-101247

Dowling AV, Corazza S, Chaudhari AM, Andriacchi TP (2010) Shoe-surface friction influences movement strategies during a sidestep cutting task: implications for anterior cruciate ligament injury risk. Am J Sports Med 38(3):478–485. https://doi.org/10.1177/0363546509348374

Failla MJ, Logerstedt DS, Grindem H, Axe MJ, Risberg MA, Engebretsen L et al (2016) Does extended preoperative rehabilitation influence outcomes 2 years after ACL reconstruction? Am J Sports Med 44(10):2608–2614. https://doi.org/10.1177/0363546516652594

Frank TD, Michelbrink M, Beckmann H, Schöllhorn WI (2008) A quantitative dynamical systems approach to differential learning: self-organization principle and order parameter equations. Biol Cybern 98(1):19–31. https://doi.org/10.1007/s00422-007-0193-x

Fu FH, Bennett CH, Lattermann C, Ma CB (1999) Current trends in anterior cruciate ligament reconstruction. Part 1: biology and biomechanics of reconstruction.

Am J Sports Med 27(6):821–830. https://doi.org/10.1177/03635465990270062501
Fuchs PX, Fusco A, Bell JW, von Duvillard SP, Cortis C, Wagner H (2020) Effect of differential training on female volleyball spike-jump technique and performance. Int J Sports Physiol Perform 15(7):1019–1025. https://doi.org/10.1123/ijspp.2019-0488
Ghanati HA, Letafatkar A, Shojaedin S, Hadadnezhad M, Schöllhorn WI (2022) Comparing the effects of differential learning, self-controlled feedback, and external focus of attention training on biomechanical risk factors of anterior cruciate ligament (ACL) in athletes: a randomized controlled trial. Int J Environ Res Public Health 19(16). https://doi.org/10.3390/ijerph191610052
Gholami F, Letafatkar A, Moghadas Tabrizi Y, Gokeler A, Rossettini G, Ghanati HA, Schöllhorn WI (2023) Comparing the effects of differential and visuo-motor training on functional performance, biomechanical, and psychological factors in athletes after acl reconstruction: a randomized controlled trial. J Clin Med 12(8):2845. https://doi.org/10.3390/jcm12082845
Goerger BM, Marshall SW, Beutler AI, Blackburn JT, Wilckens JH, Padua DA (2015) Anterior cruciate ligament injury alters preinjury lower extremity biomechanics in the injured and uninjured leg: the JUMP-ACL study. Br J Sports Med 49(3):188–195. https://doi.org/10.1136/bjsports-2013-092982
Gokeler A, Benjaminse A et al (2013) Return of normal gait as an outcome measurement in ACL-reconstructed patients. A systematic review. Int J Sports Phys Ther 8(4):441–451
Gokeler A, Dingenen B, Hewett TE (2022a) Rehabilitation and return to sport testing after anterior cruciate ligament reconstruction: where are we in 2022? Arthrosc Sports Med Rehabil 4(1):e77–e82. https://doi.org/10.1016/j.asmr.2021.10.025
Gokeler A, Grassi A, Hoogeslag R, van Houten A, Bolling C, Buckthorpe M et al (2022b) Return to sports after ACL injury 5 years from now: 10 things we must do. J Exp Orthop 9(1):73. https://doi.org/10.1186/s40634-022-00514-7
Gokeler A et al (2023) Motor learning principles during rehabilitation after anterior cruciate ligament injury. Arthroskopie 36:1–7. https://doi.org/10.1007/s00142-023-00606-1
Gornitzky AL, Lott A, Yellin JL, Fabricant PD, Lawrence JT, Ganley TJ (2016) Sport-Specific Yearly Risk and Incidence of Anterior Cruciate Ligament Tears in High School Athletes: A Systematic Review and Meta-analysis. Am J Sports Med 44(10):2716–2723. https://doi.org/10.1177/0363546515617742
Hogervorst T, Brand RA (1998) Mechanoreceptors in joint function. J Bone Joint Surg Am 80(9):1365–1378. https://doi.org/10.2106/00004623-199809000-00018
Johnston PT, McClelland JA, Webster KE (2018) Lower limb biomechanics during single-leg landings following anterior cruciate ligament reconstruction: a systematic review and meta-analysis. Sports Med 48(9):2103–2126. https://doi.org/10.1007/s40279-018-0942-0
Knurr KA, Kliethermes SA, Stiffler-Joachim MR, Cobian DG, Baer GS, Heiderscheit BC (2021) Running biomechanics before injury and 1 year after anterior cruciate ligament reconstruction in division I collegiate athletes. Am J Sports Med 49(10):2607–2614. https://doi.org/10.1177/03635465211026665
Kotsifaki A, Korakakis V, Graham-Smith P, Sideris V, Whiteley R (2021) Vertical and horizontal hop performance: contributions of the hip, knee, and ankle. Sports Health Multidiscipl Appr 13(2):128–135. https://doi.org/10.1177/1941738120976363
Lehmann T, Büchel D, Mouton C, Gokeler A, Seil R, Baumeister J (2021) Functional cortical connectivity related to postural control in patients six weeks after anterior cruciate ligament reconstruction. Front Hum Neurosci 15(July):1–11. https://doi.org/10.3389/fnhum.2021.655116
Mancino F, Gabr A, Plastow R, Haddad FS (2023) Anterior cruciate ligament injuries in female athletes. Bone Joint J 105-B(10):1033–1037. https://doi.org/10.1302/0301-620X.105B10.BJJ-2023-0881.R1
Mohammadi Orangi B, Yaali R, Bahram A, Aghdasi MT, van der Kamp J, Vanrenterghem J, Jones PA (2021) Motor learning methods that induce high practice variability reduce kinematic and kinetic risk factors of non-contact ACL injury. Hum Mov Sci 78(April):102805. https://doi.org/10.1016/j.humov.2021.102805
Moraiti CO, Stergiou N, Vasiliadis HS, Motsis E, Georgoulis A (2010) Anterior cruciate ligament reconstruction results in alterations in gait variability. Gait Posture 32(2):169–175. https://doi.org/10.1016/j.gaitpost.2010.04.008
Pairot-de-Fontenay B, Willy RW, Elias ARC, Mizner RL, Dubé M-O, Roy J-S (2019) Running biomechanics in individuals with anterior cruciate ligament reconstruction: a systematic review. Sports Med 49(9):1411–1424. https://doi.org/10.1007/s40279-019-01120-x
Pasanen K, Parkkari J, Rossi L, Kannus P (2008) Artificial playing surface increases the injury risk in pivoting indoor sports: A prospective one-season follow-up study in Finnish female floorball. Br J Sports Med 42(3):194–197. https://doi.org/10.1136/bjsm.2007.038596
Piskin D, Benjaminse A, Dimitrakis P, Gokeler A (2022) Neurocognitive and neurophysiological functions related to ACL injury: a framework for neurocognitive approaches in rehabilitation and return-to-sports tests. Sports Health Multidiscipl Appr 14(4):549–555. https://doi.org/10.1177/19417381211029265
Rigg JD, Panagodage Perera NK, Toohey LA, Cooke J, Hughes D (2023) Anterior cruciate ligament injury occurrence, return to sport and subsequent injury in the Australian High Performance Sports System: A 5-year retrospective analysis. Phys Ther Sport 64:140–146. https://doi.org/10.1016/j.ptsp.2023.10.001

Risberg MA, Holm I (2009) The long-term effect of 2 postoperative rehabilitation programs after anterior cruciate ligament reconstruction a randomized controlled clinical trial with 2 years of follow-up. Am J Sports Med 37(10):1958–1966. https://doi.org/10.1177/0363546509335196

Ross AG, Agresta B, McKay M, Pappas E, Cheng T, Peek K (2023) Financial burden of anterior cruciate ligament reconstructions in football (soccer) players: an Australian cost of injury study. Inj Prev 29(6):474–481. https://doi.org/10.1136/ip-2023-044885

Saber B, Bridger D, Agrawal K, D. (2024) A critical analysis of the factors contributing to anterior cruciate ligament injuries in female athletes. J Orthop Sports Med 6(4):203–209. https://doi.org/10.26502/josm.511500163

Sandon A, Kvist J, Hedevik H, Forssblad M (2025) Return to competition after ACL reconstruction: factors influencing rates and timing in Swedish football players. Knee Surg Sports Traumatol Arthrosc 33:1–12. https://doi.org/10.1002/ksa.12579

Schöllhorn WI (2000) Applications of systems dynamic principles to technique and strength training. Acta Acad Estonia 8:25–37

Tassignon B, Verschueren J, Baeyens J-P, Benjaminse A, Gokeler A, Serrien B, Clijsen R (2021) An exploratory meta-analytic review on the empirical evidence of differential learning as an enhanced motor learning method. Front Psychol 12(May). https://doi.org/10.3389/fpsyg.2021.533033

Tortoli E, Gokeler A, Tak I, Pellicciari L, Norte G (2024) Is visual reliance increased in athletes after acl injury? A scoping review. Sports Med 0123456789:2531. https://doi.org/10.1007/s40279-024-02085-2

Webster KE, Hewett TE (2022) Anterior cruciate ligament injury and knee osteoarthritis: an umbrella systematic review and meta-analysis. Clin J Sport Med 32(2):145–152. https://doi.org/10.1097/JSM.0000000000000894

Wiggins AJ, Grandhi RK, Schneider DK, Stanfield D, Webster KE, Myer GD (2016) Risk of secondary injury in younger athletes after anterior cruciate ligament reconstruction: a systematic review and meta-analysis. Am J Sports Med 44(7):1861–1876. https://doi.org/10.1177/0363546515621554

Wulf G, Lewthwaite R (2016) Optimizing performance through intrinsic motivation and attention for learning: The OPTIMAL theory of motor learning. Psychon Bull Rev 23(5):1382–1414. https://doi.org/10.3758/s13423-015-0999-9

Wulf G, Prinz W (2001) Directing attention to movement effects enhances learning: a review. Psychon Bull Rev 8(4):648–660. https://doi.org/10.3758/BF03196201

Zantop T, Petersen W, Sekiya JK, Musahl V, Fu FH (2006) Anterior cruciate ligament anatomy and function relating to anatomical reconstruction. Knee Surg Sports Traumatol Arthrosc 14(10):982–992. https://doi.org/10.1007/s00167-006-0076-z

7 Differential Learning and Falling Prevention: Learning to Balance

Delvydas Velička, Vidmantas Zaveckas, Agnė Slapšinskaitė-Dackevičienė, and Wolfgang I. Schöllhorn

It takes a child 1 year to acquire independent movement and 10 years to acquire independent mobility. An old person can lose both in a day.

–Professor Bernard Isaacs (British Geriatrician) (1924–1995)

7.1 Balance Problems in Society

A fall is defined as an unexpected and involuntary descent to the ground, floor, or a lower-level surface. Falls can result from slipping, tripping, or losing balance, whether on the ground or from a height (Montero-Odasso et al. 2022a, b). While falling at a younger age is often part of the learning process, in older adults, it can be life-threatening.

Falls among older adults are a major public health concern, particularly for vulnerable groups such as those with chronic illnesses, motor impairments, or cognitive disorders (Ambrose et al. 2023). According to the World Health Organization (WHO), falls are the second leading cause of accidental deaths worldwide, with the highest fatality rates occurring in lower-income countries. This highlights how fall-related risks vary depending on economic status, regional factors, and access to healthcare (Yoshida 2007). The financial burden is also significant, with the WHO estimating that fall-related healthcare costs amount to approximately €400 billion annually, covering hospitalization, rehabilitation, and long-term care (Harvey et al. 2024).

Falls are a leading cause of severe health complications among older adults, particularly bone fractures, which can have life-threatening consequences. One of the most concerning injuries is a femoral neck fracture, which significantly increases the risk of mortality within the first year following the fall (Harvey et al. 2024). Additionally, head injuries sustained during falls can lead to neurological damage and long-term functional decline (Zemek and Babl 2022).

Beyond physical consequences, falls also have a profound psychological impact. Many older

D. Velička (✉) · V. Zaveckas
Department of Sports Medicine, Faculty of Nursing, Medical Academy,
Lithuanian University of Health Sciences, Kaunas, Lithuania

A. Slapšinskaitė-Dackevičienė
Department of Sports Medicine, Faculty of Nursing, Medical Academy, Lithuanian University of Health Sciences, Kaunas, Lithuania

Faculty of Public Health, Health Research Institute, Medical Academy, Lithuanian University of Health Sciences, Kaunas, Lithuania

W. I. Schöllhorn
Institute for Sport Science, Johannes Gutenberg-University, Mainz, Germany

W. I. Schöllhorn, A. Slapšinskaitė-Dackevičienė (eds.), *Differential Learning in Physiotherapy*,
https://doi.org/10.1007/978-3-031-98787-8_7

adults develop a fear of falling again, leading to reduced physical activity and increased social isolation (Xu and Ma 2020).

Preventing falls requires a multifaceted approach addressing both individual and environmental factors. Physical activity programs that focus on balance, muscle strength, and mobility—such as Tai Chi, yoga, and physiotherapy—significantly reduce fall incidence among older adults (Xu and Ma 2020). This chapter explores the role of physical activity in prevention, offering detailed guidance on designing programs using differential learning (DL).

In addition to exercise, environmental modifications are crucial. Measures such as proper lighting, handrails, grab bars, non-slip flooring, and smart home technologies (e.g., motion-sensor lighting, fall detection systems) enhance safety. Community-based awareness campaigns further reduce risks by promoting vision checks, medication reviews, and appropriate footwear (Xu and Ma 2020).

Finally, policy-level interventions, including funding for fall prevention programs and geriatric training for healthcare professionals, are essential for widespread implementation. A combined approach at the individual, community, and policy levels can significantly reduce fall rates, improving public health and reducing healthcare costs.

7.2 Symptoms and Diagnosis of Balance

Balance control deficits contribute to increased fall risk and can be assessed through motoric tests and biomechanical diagnostics. Three primary diagnostic approaches exist: static balance, dynamic balance, and response to disturbances, with assessment methods also applicable for training.

Static balance evaluation involves standing on a force platform to measure the center of gravity's horizontal displacement. Medio-lateral and anterior-posterior sway areas indicate balance performance, where smaller sway requires rapid postural adaptation—an essential component of balance training (da Silva et al. 2018).

Dynamic balance assessment utilizes motoric tests on varied surfaces, from balance beams to slacklines, progressively reducing stability from double-leg stances to single-leg challenges. Interactive tools, such as digital balance boards and therapy spinning tops, facilitate dynamic training by integrating movement adaptation principles (Lacroix et al. 2016).

The third approach examines response to perturbations, where subjects experience sudden disturbances via mechanical pulls, direct pushes, or treadmill interruptions while walking. Recovery time to equilibrium serves as a key measure of balance control (Janura et al. 2020).

This progression mirrors the principle of second-order cybernetics, where the nervous system must continuously recalibrate movement patterns to match task difficulty. By manipulating exercise complexity—from stable, predictable conditions to highly variable and reactive environments—balance training fosters neuroplasticity, adaptability, and real-world resilience.

Beyond their diagnostic role, these approaches can be utilized as physiotherapeutic interventions by progressively increasing sensory input and motor variability. By systematically integrating these methods, balance training can be optimized to enhance neuromuscular control, postural stability, and fall prevention, particularly in clinical and rehabilitation settings.

7.2.1 Sensory Variability ("Noise")

Sensory variability arises from fluctuations in sensory input processing, which can impact an individual's perception of their body's position and movement. In conditions like developmental coordination disorder (DCD), excessive neural noise disrupts sensory inputs, leading to challenges in movement prediction and control. This heightened variability manifests as inconsistent motor performance and reliance on feedback mechanisms, resulting in slower and more effortful movements. Therapeutic approaches that incorporate structured sensory experiences can help recalibrate the sensory system, promoting optimal variability and improving motor function (Smits-Engelsman and Wilson 2013).

7.2.2 Motor Variability ("Noise")

Motor variability refers to the natural fluctuations in motor output during repeated movements. While some degree of variability is inherent and necessary for adaptability, excessive motor noise can hinder precise control. Research indicates that motor performance variability decreases with practice but is never eliminated due to inherent motor noise.

7.3 Sensorimotor Foundations of Balance Control

The complex process of regulating balance relies on the integration and coordination of several sensorimotor control regions, such as the brain, spinal cord, peripheral nervous system, and muscles. These components collectively maintain postural stability, enable seamless coordination of voluntary and reflexive motor actions, and adapt movements in response to outside disturbances/perturbations (Brumagne et al. 2019). Table 7.1 is relevant to the balance chapter as it provides a comprehensive summary of the sensorimotor control regions and their specific functions.

When these sensorimotor systems interact optimally and flexibly, they provide the necessary coordination and adaptability to maintain postural stability in various contexts. However, impairments in these regions—such as muscle weakness, delayed reaction times, and sensory conflicts—can significantly compromise balance, particularly among older adults.

These factors are interrelated and have profound implications for fall prevention strategies (Yang et al. 2023).

Table 7.1 Sensorimotor control regions and functions (Brumagne et al. 2019)

Region	Specific areas	Functions
Planning and initiation of voluntary movement	Primary somatosensory cortex, posterior parietal cortex, primary motor cortex, supplementary motor cortex, premotor cortex, prefrontal cortex	Initiation and coordination of voluntary movements, including postural regulation
Cerebellum	Sensory-motor integration and learning areas	Integration of sensory information for motor learning and refinement of movements
Basal ganglia and associated structures	Basal ganglia, vestibular nuclei, reticular formation	Regulation of basic movements, posture, and motor control
Spinal cord	Spinal networks, reflex mechanisms	Control of involuntary reflexes and connections with peripheral motor neurons for movement
Peripheral nervous system	Neural networks and sensory signals	Transmission of sensory information to the central nervous system and distribution of motor impulses
Muscles	Skeletal muscles	Execution of movements through muscle contractions, the final implementation of motor commands

Muscle Weakness Lower limb muscle strength parameters, especially in the quadriceps and calf muscles, play a critical role in maintaining stability (Moreland et al. 2004). Weakness in these muscles impairs the body's ability to recover from perturbations, increasing the risk of falls. Research by Sturnieks et al. (2008) demonstrated a strong correlation between reduced leg strength and a higher likelihood of falls among the elderly.

It does not just seem to be about maximum strength. The increase in force per unit time (force rate), in particular, has an influence on what happens.

Gollhofer conducted studies demonstrating that simply standing on one leg on a solid surface led to greater improvements in balance parameters than any weightlifting exercise. This finding provides a compelling explanation for the effectiveness of Tai Chi in fall prevention, as the practice involves numerous single-leg stances. Furthermore, these results suggest that encouraging older adults to incorporate more single-leg activities into their daily routines at home could be beneficial (Gollhofer 2004).

Delayed Reaction Times Efficient neuromuscular responses are critical for restoring balance following unexpected perturbations. However, aging and neurological conditions such as Parkinson's disease are associated with prolonged reaction times, thereby diminishing the likelihood of successful postural recovery. Lord et al. (2001) highlighted that slower reaction times are a significant predictor of falls in the elderly population.

Sensory Conflicts and Cognitive Load Maintaining balance relies on the efficient integration of sensory input and motor responses. However, cognitive distractions or multitasking can disrupt this process, leading to impaired postural control. Additionally, sensory conflicts, such as navigating in low-light conditions or uneven surfaces, further compromise stability. Yogev-Seligmann et al. (2008) explored the impact of dual-task interference on gait and balance, emphasizing its role in increasing instability among older adults.

Overall, the sensorimotor system can be seen as a dynamic and complex network operating across multiple time scales. Fluctuations propagate through different levels and manifest as variability, influencing movement planning and execution. This variability arises from basal ganglia circuits, the premotor cortex, and motor unit recruitment properties, impacting both motor control and adaptability (Churchland et al. 2006; Jones et al. 2002; Olveczky et al. 2005; van Beers et al. 2004).

7.3.1 Identifying Gait Abnormalities as Indicators of Balance Issues or the Possibility of Learning Balance

This section delves into the dual nature of gait abnormalities—how they can serve as both symptoms of impairment and potential sources of corrective adaptation. By identifying specific gait deviations and understanding their implications, we can explore novel, variance-enhancing strategies to optimize balance, stability, and mobility. The goal is not merely to "fix" movement but to expand the body's capacity to adapt, transforming gait challenges into a dynamic process of learning and self-organization.

Gait variations, such as stride length asymmetry, reduced arm swing, or increased lateral sway, often signal balance deficits (Hausdorff et al. 1995). These deviations may arise from imbalances in strength, coordination, or neurological function, influencing movement stability.

In the context of dynamic systems, the human body constantly adjusts to fluctuations in movement and posture, introducing an element of variability or "noise" into the motor control process. Abnormal gait patterns—such as stride length asymmetry, reduced arm swing, or side-to-side swaying—disrupt the natural flow of movement and introduce unpredictability into an individual's motor control by increased stiffness. One possible mechanism of these impairments in older adults is an increase in lower extremity muscle co-contraction. Muscle co-contraction is the simultaneous activation of agonist and antagonist muscle groups (Busse et al. 2006). Relatively high lower limb co-contraction may explain some of the mobility impairments associated with the conduct of executive tasks in older adults (Lo et al. 2017). Older adults with gait disturbances compensate with higher muscle co-activation, leading to increased limb stiffness and reduced adaptability in response to perturbations (Shkuratova et al. 2004). In a healthy system, variability in movement is not just random noise but an essential component of adaptive motor control. Research shows that the nervous system utilizes a controlled degree of variability to maintain flexibility and adaptability in motor tasks (Stergiou and Decker 2011). This principle aligns with stochastic resonance, where small fluctuations in motor patterns help refine movement and improve stability (Collins et al. 1995). However, excessive variability, as seen in gait abnormalities, can signal a breakdown in motor control, often leading to compensatory stiffness or rigidity.

This variability can be seen as "noise" that challenges the body's ability to maintain stability and adapt effectively. However, Nashner's groundbreaking research (Nashner 1973; Nashner 1976; Nashner 1983) suggests that this so-called noise is not merely a disruption but a key component of motor learning and postural control. The human body relies on a complex interplay between the vestibular, somatosensory, and visual systems to regulate balance and movement (Nashner 1973). These systems continuously process sensory inputs to adjust posture and gait in response to environmental demands. Nashner's studies on postural reflexes (Nashner 1976) demonstrated that movement variability is integral to adaptive motor control, as reflex responses are not rigid but rather dynamically adjusted based on sensory conditions.

His famous "moving platform" experiments (Nashner 1983) further revealed that postural control is based on adaptive strategies that shift depending on the reliability of sensory input. The force platform was manipulated so that the center of pressure was always in the same position above the force platform. Paradoxically, instead of maintaining balance, all participants fell within seconds—a striking demonstration that variability is not just an error in movement control but an essential requirement for balance and adaptability.

This means that when gait variations occur—such as a widened stance—it may serve as a compensatory mechanism to reduce fall risk, though it also introduces fluctuations into overall movement patterns. Similarly, gait abnormalities like festinating gait or difficulty halting movement create an added layer of unpredictability, demanding continuous motor adjustments to restore equilibrium. When sensory information is conflicting or unreliable, the nervous system compensates by increasing stiffness or modifying postural strategies to maintain stability.

Ultimately, Nashner's research challenges the conventional view of variability as a flaw in motor function. Instead, it highlights the idea that motor "noise" is an essential part of the body's ability to adapt, recalibrate, and fine-tune movement control in response to an ever-changing environment.

Recent research continues to underscore the critical role of variability in postural control and motor adaptation. For instance, a study examining postural control in older adults found that increased variability in the center of pressure (COP) is associated with greater low-frequency oscillations, suggesting that such variability may reflect adaptive mechanisms in response to aging-related changes in balance control (Delmas et al. 2021). These findings align with Nashner's earlier work, reinforcing the concept that variability is not merely a source of error but an essential feature of the motor control system, enabling effective adaptation to both internal and external perturbations.

For instance, a widened stance may force the body to compensate for balance difficulties, adding an element of fluctuation in the overall movement pattern. Similarly, gait abnormalities such as festinating gait or difficulty halting movement create additional unpredictability, requiring constant motor adjustments. These fluctuations in movement patterns push the body's proprioceptive and motor systems to react to and adapt to the variability in muscle strength, coordination, and overall stability. Research indicates that increased variability in proprioceptive acuity is associated with enhanced implicit motor adaptation. For instance, studies have found that individuals with greater proprioceptive variability exhibit more significant implicit adaptation, suggesting that the nervous system utilizes this variability to recalibrate motor outputs effectively (Tsay et al. 2021). However, age-related increases in proprioceptive variability may disrupt the integration of predicted and actual sensory feedback, leading to impaired visuomotor adaptation in older adults (Lei and Wang 2018). Gait abnormalities disrupt the natural balance between movement variability and stability, forcing the nervous system to adopt rigid, compensatory strategies to maintain control. This increased stiffness reduces adaptability, making movement less efficient and increasing the risk of instability and falls. Interventions with adaptive noise variability, enhancing motor flexibility rather than suppressing movement fluctuations. Besides extensive descriptions and re-interpretations of the variance phenomena in movement (Davids et al. 2006), the differential learning approach (Schöllhorn 2000) was instigated to consider noise as an active instrument ("order from noise") by enhancing the existing variance in movements by means of stochastic perturbations within the frame of stochastic resonance.

By including such "noisy" conditions into balance training, practitioners can improve the body's adaptability to sudden changes and unanticipated shifts in posture. This can be particularly useful for enhancing balance control in individuals with gait abnormalities, as they work to adapt to these real-world-like challenges and improve both reactive and anticipatory balance responses.

7.3.2 Gait Abnormalities as Symptoms or Potential Noise in Movement Variation

Walking may seem effortless, yet it relies on a complex interplay of motor control, balance, and neuromuscular adaptation. Each step exhibits subtle variations in length, rhythm, and force—an inherent variability that enables adaptation to changing terrains and unexpected disturbances. In a healthy system, this variability enhances movement fluidity, but gait abnormalities can disrupt it, increasing instability and fall risk.

Gait abnormalities are key indicators of motor control deficits, muscle weakness, or neurological conditions. Understanding these deviations (see below) is crucial for distinguishing pathological movement patterns from normal variations in motor performance.

Variable Stride Length: A noticeable difference in stride length between the left and right legs can point to imbalances in strength or motor control, which directly affect stability (Alexander 1996).

Shuffling Gait: A gait pattern in which the feet barely leave the ground, which disinhibits the risk of falling, often signals muscle weakness or incoordination (Soylu et al. 2021).

Reduced Arm Swing: Limited movement of the arms during walking indicates challenges in upper body coordination, affecting overall balance and stability (Meyns et al. 2013).

Widened Stance: A larger-than-usual distance between the feet while walking may reflect an individual's attempt to increase stability to compensate for balance difficulties (Nonnekes et al. 2018).

Festinating Gait: Small, rapid steps, commonly observed in Parkinson's disease, highlight impairments in balance and coordination (Welter et al. 2012).

Toe-Walking or Shuffling: Walking on tiptoes or dragging the feet can suggest muscle weakness or neurological conditions that interfere with proper foot lift (Kanko et al. 2021).

Trendelenburg Gait: Excessive pelvic tilt to one side during walking often points to weakness in the hip abductor muscles (Paavilainen et al. 1993).

Side-to-Side Swaying: Rocking from side to side during walking or an inability to maintain a straight path suggests underlying balance issues. Hip Rocking: Excessive lateral movement of the hips while walking can be attributed to muscle weakness or joint dysfunction (Kouvidis et al. 2009).

Difficulty Initiating or Halting Movement: Challenges in starting to walk or stopping abruptly may indicate motor planning or coordination deficits, impacting balance control (Horak 1997).

Arm Swing Imbalance: A significant difference in the swing of the left and right arms reflects uneven muscle strength or coordination, further compromising balance (Kanko et al. 2021).

Changes in Walking Speed: Sudden or erratic shifts in walking pace may indicate balance disorders or other health conditions requiring evaluation (Shkuratova et al. 2004).

Rather than viewing gait deviations solely as dysfunctions to be corrected, DL suggests they may serve as valuable stimuli for motor adaptation. Traditional physiotherapy often categorizes movement variability as error, but within the DL framework, these variations can drive neuroplasticity and enhance functional restoration. By embracing rather than suppressing movement irregularities, rehabilitation can leverage natural fluctuations to refine motor control and resilience.

Could it be that what we perceive as gait abnormalities are not merely dysfunctions but adaptive responses—signals of the body's attempt to reorganize movement strategies? If movement variability is an essential component of learning, then how do we differentiate between pathological deviation and functional adaptation? Should interventions aim to correct these variations entirely, or could they be strategically utilized to enhance motor control and stability? Understanding this fine balance could redefine how we approach gait rehabilitation—not by eliminating variability, but by optimizing it.

7.3.3 Balance Learning Strategy

Efficient locomotion requires precise coordination of body control, balance, and muscle activation to transition smoothly between static and dynamic states. Stability depends on controlled weight shifts, as improper distribution can lead to instability and falls (Buckley et al. 2024). The nervous system integrates balance and locomotion through hierarchical pathways, though the exact mechanisms remain under investigation (Chvatal and Ting 2013).

Muscle synergies simplify movement coordination by activating predefined patterns suited to biomechanical demands such as single-leg support and postural recovery (Chvatal and Ting 2013). These synergies enhance movement efficiency, reduce cognitive load, and improve injury prevention. Core stability is fundamental for postural control, ensuring efficient force transmission between the upper and lower body (Moosaei Saein et al. 2024). A strong and coordinated core enhances balance, adaptability, and injury resilience (Richardson et al. 1999). Fatigue of these muscles impairs dynamic stability, increasing fall risk (Davidson et al. 2004; Ozmen and Aydogmus 2016).

Leg strength, proprioception, and joint mobility are critical for balance control. Weak muscles lead to instability, shorter or uneven steps, and joint misalignment, elevating fall risk (Gao et al. 2023; Laughton et al. 2003; Bertschi et al. 2022). Balance corrections occur via rapid neuromuscular integration of gravitational, inertial, and ground reaction forces (Winter 1995; Horak 2006). Reflex pathways provide immediate adjustments, while cortical processes fine-tune responses for long-term adaptation (Taube et al. 2008; Dietz 2002). Age-related declines in motor unit firing rates and rate of force development impair postural stability, reducing the ability to recover from perturbations (Christie and Kamen 2010; Izquierdo et al. 1999; Pijnappels et al. 2005).

Joint mobility affects weight transfer and balance control, particularly in the ankle, where restricted plantar flexion is associated with impaired postural stability (Sung and Kim 2018). While reduced mobility can enhance tension for certain sports, excessive stiffness limits adaptability to uneven surfaces, increasing fall risk (Ferrucci et al. 2014).

Locomotion and balance are interdependent, requiring coordinated muscle activation and neural control (Gupta and Agarwal 2022). Muscle synergies operate proactively and reactively, integrating central gait patterns, brainstem balance control, and corticospinal pathways (Chvatal and Ting 2013). These mechanisms allow for stability across different motor tasks, from walking to grasping (D'Avella et al. 2006; Hamed and Schieber 2007). Rehabilitation should balance stability training with exposure to unpredictable conditions to enhance adaptive motor responses and functional resilience.

7.4 Balance Therapy

7.4.1 History

Balance training has become an integral component of multidisciplinary health and sports practices, encompassing athlete fitness, injury prevention, neurological rehabilitation, and overall health enhancement. While its modern applications are diverse, the origins of balance-related practices date back to ancient civilizations. Yoga, practiced for over 3000 years BCE, was initially a discipline for physical and mental well-being, later integrated into healthcare for posture and balance control (Yatham et al. 2023). Similarly, Tai Chi, developed as a Chinese martial art, was adapted for wellness and rehabilitation, with research confirming its effectiveness in reducing fall risk among older adults (Hallisy 2018).

During the nineteenth century, European and North American physical education emphasized military preparedness rather than rehabilitation. German gymnastics pioneer Friedrich Ludwig Jahn promoted Turnen to strengthen youth for service, prioritizing discipline and strength over balance (Shephard 2018). Similarly, Pehr Henrik Ling's Swedish gymnastics system influenced military and educational training but lacked a rehabilitative focus (Ljunggren 2024). It was not until the mid-twentieth century that balance therapy became a structured component of medical rehabilitation, particularly for patients with neurological or orthopedic disorders. Vestibular rehabilitation emerged as a targeted intervention for postural instability and dizziness, with studies confirming its benefits for stroke recovery and Parkinson's disease management (Klatt 2015).

Advancements in rehabilitation methodologies further refined balance therapy. Proprioceptive neuromuscular facilitation (PNF) enhanced motor function and postural control by integrating sensory feedback mechanisms (Cabanas-Valdés et al. 2021). By the late twentieth and early twenty-first centuries, balance therapy expanded into sports medicine and preventive healthcare. Research highlights that athletes engaging in balance training exhibit lower injury rates, particularly in the ankle and knee joints, while dynamic stability exercises have become essential for athletic conditioning (Horak 2006). Technological innovations, including balance boards, stability balls, and sensory platforms, further personalize rehabilitation programs, improving training outcomes (Behm and Anderson 2006).

The integration of virtual reality and wearable technology in balance therapy over the past two decades has enabled precise assessment and real-time therapy adaptation, benefiting older adults at high risk of falls and athletes recovering from injuries (Goble et al. 2017). Modern balance therapy is now a multidisciplinary field, incorporating neurology, physiotherapy, sports medicine, and digital technology to enhance accessibility and treatment efficacy. As the field evolved, its application diversified, extending beyond rehabilitation to sports science, where balance training is employed to improve coordination, dynamic stability, and muscle control.

Despite their interconnected nature, balance therapy and balance training serve distinct purposes. Balance therapy primarily focuses on restoring proprioception and postural stability in patients recovering from neurological and orthopedic conditions. In contrast, balance training aims to optimize movement efficiency and reduce injury risk in athletic performance. Given these distinctions, the following section provides a comparative analysis (Table 7.2), delineating their key differences in medical, sports, and health-related contexts.

Table 7.2 Differences between balance therapy and balance training

Criterion	Balance therapy	Balance training	Common scientific disciplines
Purpose	Designed for medical and rehabilitation purposes—to treat or mitigate balance disorders	Aimed at enhancing sports performance, preventing injuries, and improving functional capacity	Motor control science, neuroplasticity, and biomechanics
Target group	Individuals with vestibular disorders, neurological, or orthopedic conditions (e.g., stroke, Parkinson's disease, traumatic brain injuries)	Healthy individuals, athletes, and older adults, aiming to improve coordination and strength	Human movement science and sensorimotor integration
Application area	Used in medical and rehabilitation settings such as neurology, orthopedic therapy, and vestibular rehabilitation	Applied in sports training, senior fitness programs, and general health improvement	Kinesiology and exercise physiology
Methods: sensory stimulation	Vestibular rehabilitation (gaze stabilization, habituation exercises) and proprioceptive reeducation (joint position training, sensory cueing)	Proprioceptive enhancement drills (unstable surface training, barefoot exercises) and visual-motor coordination drills (target tracking, reaction-based training)	Neuroscience and sensorimotor adaptation
Methods: motor control training	Functional movement therapy (task-specific exercises, postural adjustments) and neuromuscular reeducation (reflex integration, biofeedback training)	Dynamic balance exercises (single-leg stance, agility drills) and core stability training (plank variations, rotational movements)	Motor learning and postural control science
Methods: strength and stability	Physiotherapeutic strength training (targeted muscle activation, resistance exercises for stability)	Functional strength training (weighted balance exercises, plyometric drills)	Muscle physiology, strength, and conditioning science
Differential learning: practical application	Instead of rigid, repetitive movements, DL introduces controlled variability, forcing the nervous system to adapt by embracing unpredictability. For balance therapy, this means challenging patients with ever-changing stimuli, fostering neuroplasticity and motor learning in ways that conventional training cannot	In sports and functional training, DL disrupts the movement autopilot, breaking stagnation and enhancing resilience. By exposing athletes to constantly shifting conditions, DL cultivates superior adaptability, because in real life and competition, no two movements are ever the same	Nonlinear dynamics, variability-based motor learning, and self-organization in motor control
Differential learning: the necessity of proper dosing	In therapy, DL must be precisely dosed to stimulate neuroplasticity without overwhelming the patient. Too little variation fails to create an adaptive response, while too much can lead to disorientation and increased fall risk. Gradual exposure to "noise" through progressive changes in movement tasks is key to maintaining a safe yet effective learning environment	In training, DL dosing is critical to prevent excessive fatigue and neurological overload. If the level of unpredictability is too low, learning stagnates; if it is too high, movement efficiency deteriorates. The correct "noise" dosage depends on the athlete's skill level, fatigue state, and cognitive load tolerance, ensuring optimal adaptation rather than system breakdown	Training load management, neurophysiology of adaptation, stress-response theory

(continued)

Table 7.2 (continued)

Criterion	Balance therapy	Balance training	Common scientific disciplines
Individualization	Highly individualized based on the patient's medical condition, neurological deficits, and functional limitations. Adjustments are made based on clinical assessment and recovery progress	Tailored to the athlete's or individual's fitness level, sport-specific demands, and performance goals. Progressions are based on adaptive responses and strength development	Personalized medicine, exercise prescription, and adaptation theory
Scientific basis	Based on medical and physiotherapy research, evidence-based medicine, and clinical trials	Rooted in sports science, biomechanics, and athletic training research	Biomechanics, rehabilitation science, and exercise science

7.4.2 Classical Approaches to Balance Training

Classical balance training methods, such as yoga, Qi Gong, and Tai Chi, are widely used among older adults to improve mobility and reduce the risk of falls (Liu-Ambrose et al. 2019). These practices strengthen lower limb muscles, enhance proprioception, and improve sensory integration abilities. Additionally, home-based Qi meditation helps develop body awareness and coordination (Dejvajara et al. 2022).

Artificial intelligence (AI) complements traditional methods by providing objective biomechanical analysis and personalized training programs. Wearable sensors and computer vision systems assess posture stability in real time and offer individualized recommendations, while AI algorithms can detect motor impairments before they develop into more serious balance issues (Meng et al. 2022).

Virtual reality (VR) and augmented reality (AR) training simulate real-world balance challenges, improving vestibular function and motor skills (Huang et al. 2024). Furthermore, AI analyzes long-term movement patterns and predicts fall risk, enabling preventive measures before significant motor impairments occur (Huang et al. 2024).

Recent studies suggest that AI-based programs can be nearly as effective as traditional physiotherapy sessions (Meng et al. 2022). To ensure accessibility, AI solutions are designed to meet the needs of older adults, incorporating intuitive user interfaces and easy-to-use applications.

Classical balance training methods, such as yoga, Qi Gong, and Tai Chi, are widely used among older adults to improve mobility and reduce the risk of falls (Liu-Ambrose et al. 2019). These practices strengthen lower limb muscles, enhance proprioception, and improve sensory integration abilities. Additionally, home-based Qi meditation helps develop body awareness and coordination (Dejvajara et al. 2022).

7.5 Balance Training Based on DL

This chapter part explores the role of DL in balance training, with a specific focus on its impact on heart physiology—electrocardiographic (ECG) parameter interactions. The chapter is divided into two main sections: static balance training with perturbation tasks and dynamic balance training with coordination tasks. By examining these varying conditions, this chapter highlights the potential of DL in enhancing both motor adaptability and cardiovascular function through movement variability.

7.5.1 Static Balance with Perturbation Task: Reflection on ECG Parameters Interactions

DL, which is based on movement variability, has long been recognized for its ability to enhance motor system adaptability without relying on mechanical repetition. Its application in balance training continues to provide empirical support for the DL approach within therapeutic and athletic contexts. The study of static balance with a perturbation task involved healthy male participants ($n = 13$) who performed two balance tasks while standing on the LIBRA balancing platform. The *first task* required participants to stand still without additional disturbances, aiming to assess their initial ability to maintain balance under stable conditions. The *second task* was more complex—participants had to perform squats under constantly changing conditions. For the first time, they were required to execute these exercises while simultaneously juggling two tennis balls. This dual-task challenge further increased the difficulty of the exercise, demanding higher levels of coordination and motor control. This situation aligned well with DL, as the motor system was continuously forced to adapt to changing conditions rather than relying on repetitive, mechanical movement patterns (Veličká et al. 2016). Participants' ECG was recorded both at rest and during the tasks. The main ECG parameters analyzed included RR intervals, JT intervals, and RR and JT interactions (Fig. 7.1).

As seen in Fig. 7.1, the study demonstrated that DL tasks, particularly squatting while juggling tennis balls, reduced the interactions between cardiac regulatory and metabolic mechanisms (RR and JT interactions), which may be linked to long-term adaptation processes. Even low-intensity exercises performed under variable conditions with augmented noise levels may significantly influence the cardiovascular system (Veličká et al. 2016).

These findings align with previous research exploring the interactions between movement variability and physiological responses. For example, studies on different forms of rhythmic exercise suggest that variation in movement patterns can optimize physiological adaptation. A study on rope skipping with different time intervals for variations of jumping technique points in the same direction (John et al. 2022). Varying between repetitive rope skipping, changing every 20 s, 10 s, and every 1 s revealed an optimal interaction between heart (HRV parameters) and brain (EEG parameters) at changes every 10 s, indicating an optimum tendency of variation. Increased interaction between the heart and brain points toward faster general adaptations and is associated with faster recovery after physical stress (John et al. 2022).

7.5.2 Effects of Dynamic Balance Training with Coordinative Tasks on ECG Parameter Interactions

DL has garnered increasing attention for its promising role in motor skill acquisition and

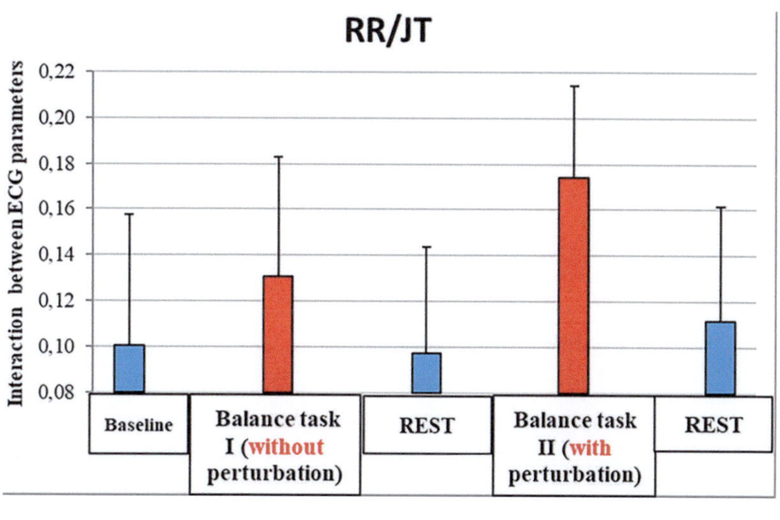

Fig. 7.1 Changes in interactions between ECG parameters (RR and JT) during static balance without and with perturbation

rehabilitation. In their 2005 study, Michelbrink and Schöllhorn utilized random walk analysis to assess the impact of DL on balance control, demonstrating that DL not only facilitates immediate improvements but also creates long-term adaptations in the motor system. These sustained benefits were not previously observed in externally guided (Villa et al. 2025; Needle and Howard 2024) or stimulation-based training methods (Carè et al. 2024) or external stimulation methods, such as vibrating insoles (Collins and Priplata 2003), highlighting DL's potential to enhance motor learning beyond conventional approaches.

Recent research has expanded beyond the effects of DL on balance, exploring its broader physiological impact. Velička (2020) examined heart-rate parameter interactions through ECG during both learned and unfamiliar unpredictable coordination tasks during treadmill walking (Table 7.3). Specifically, the ECG was recorded continuously, with the RR and JT intervals, as well as the duration of the QRS complex, measured for analysis. These parameters were subsequently examined as digital time series. It is posited that if a digital time series, or a pair of such series, encapsulates relevant information about the studied subject, this information can be expressed through mathematical relationships/associations/interactions (Maass and Timmer 2008).

Table 7.3 Order of coordination tasks on the treadmill

	List of coordination exercises on the treadmill
1	Arms extended to the sides
2	Wrist rotation backward
3	Elbow rotation backward
4	Shoulder rotation backward
5	Arm rotation: both arms simultaneously
6	Arm rotation: one arm following the other
7	Arm rotation: one arm forward, the other backward
8	Reaching up and down with arms
9	Arm rotation to the sides
10	Lifting clasped hands behind the back, up and down
11	Spinning around one's axis
12	Spinning around one's axis with shoulder lifting and lowering
13	Stretching arms and spreading fingers

Further, this study aimed to examine how dynamic interactions between ECG parameters shift during unpredictable coordination tasks, grouping individuals into three performance levels: sedentary individuals, physically active individuals (training two to four times per week), and elite athletes (members of the Lithuanian national team; Velička 2020).

Among the three groups, only the physically active individuals were familiar with coordination tasks, as these were a regular part of their training routine. Due to this learning experience, the tasks were considered "known" for this group. In contrast, the sedentary individuals and elite athletes performed these tasks for the first time, making them "unknown" for these participants. All groups performed the coordination tasks presented in Table 7.3 on a treadmill, altering trunk and arm movements every 30 s, as displayed on a tablet screen.

The study comprised three ECG recording phases: 5 min of standing (points 1–2), 10 min of walking with DL-based tasks (points 3–4), and 5 min of standing for recovery (points 5–6) (Fig. 7.2). Data analysis showed that elite athletes' responses during the unpredictable coordination tasks were highly similar to those of sedentary individuals, with weakened relationships/associations/interactions between ECG parameters at the start.

In contrast, physically active individuals who were familiar with coordination tasks showed a stronger initial correlation. Even though, as fatigue sets in, individual characteristics also influence the dynamic interactions and changes, leading to a weakening. These findings underscore the notion that fluctuations introduced by unpredictable coordination tasks, such as changes in body posture and arm movements, affect the muscle and CNS systems, with their impact observable via the heart's response. This creates a triadic relationship between the muscle, heart, and CNS—each adapting and interacting in response to the task's demands in a dynamic balance context.

Specifically, the data showed that the physical fluctuations inherent in unpredictable coordination tasks affect both the muscle (through move-

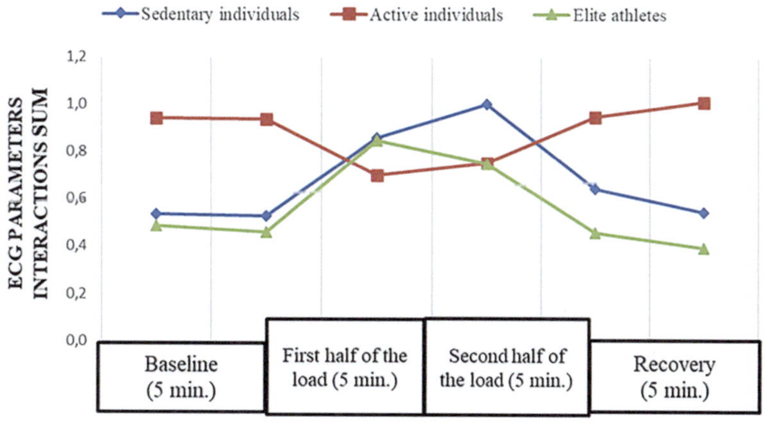

Fig. 7.2 Fluctuations in ECG parameters interactions across investigation phases in three performance levels groups during coordination tasks in a dynamic balance context—walking on a treadmill

ment variation) and the CNS (via motor control and adaptation). These fluctuations are captured in real-time through ECG measurements, revealing how the heart reflects these shifts. The findings suggest that unfamiliar tasks with added coordination challenges and movement variability—unlike standard exercise protocols—lead to a reduction in the correlation between ECG parameters, regardless of fitness level (Velička 2020). To further interpret these results, prior research on motor adaptation, balance control, and sensory noise suggests that the body adapts quickly to environmental changes through sensorimotor feedback and that unpredictable disturbances may enhance motor learning and adaptation. Previous research has demonstrated that unpredictable disturbances, like those in DL tasks, enhance motor learning and adaptation by stimulating sensorimotor feedback mechanisms (Horak and Macpherson 2011; Shadmehr et al. 2010). These disturbances foster an environment where the body can adapt more efficiently to changing conditions, offering a broader spectrum of benefits for both motor learning and cardiovascular health.

To sum up, the study highlights the profound impact of DL on both motor learning and cardiovascular health, emphasizing the role of sensorimotor feedback mechanisms in driving adaptation. The fluctuation and variability inherent in DL tasks simulate real-world conditions, challenging the body to continually adjust to shifting demands. This not only enhances the motor system's ability to learn and adapt to new movements but also triggers physiological changes that improve cardiovascular function, regardless of the individual's trainability level. The dual impact on motor skills and cardiovascular level suggests that DL can provide a holistic approach to rehabilitation, making it a powerful tool for improving overall physical performance and well-being. This reflective insight encourages further exploration of how environmental variability can be harnessed to optimize therapy outcomes across both motor and physiological domains.

As we explore the interactions between organisms and their environments, it is essential to consider how specific movement patterns—like walking and changing direction—play a role in postural control, especially in older adults. Research shows that older adults rely less on head-on-trunk rotation and more on trunk-on-pelvis rotation compared to younger adults. In this context, the decline in segmental spinal mobility contributes to postural instability during turning, which challenges balance. To counter these changes, foot movements serve a critical compensatory role, enhancing postural control and adaptability (Baird and Van Emmerik 2009). This raises an important question: How can gait be modeled using varying foot and lower extremity positions, angles, speeds, and accelerations through the DL methodology to better adapt to dynamic environmental conditions and improve balance during movement?

7.6 Future Clinical Applications Based on Differential Learning Principles

7.6.1 Sling Exercise for Therapy and Prevention

One method that aligns well with the DL principle of additional noise is Neurac© (Neuromuscular Activation), implemented using the Redcord equipment system. Neurac© focuses on testing and treating neuromuscular control with an emphasis on pain relief and optimizing body movement function through coordinated activation of both local and global muscle groups (ref). Neuromuscular control, a key aspect of the sensorimotor system, governs how the body controls movement and responds to external stimuli. The use of the closed kinematic chain and the instability created by the ropes and slings in the Redcord system increases muscle activation not only in agonist and antagonistic muscles but also in the core, promoting more balanced and efficient movement patterns.

Stabilization exercises within Neurac©—which focus on the co-contraction of deep core muscles and spinal stability—are integral in improving postural control (ref). Adding rope perturbations further enhances muscle activation, especially in relation to the muscle spindle system, which is vital for proprioception (Lundy-Ekman 2007). Interestingly, these spindle characteristics remain relatively unchanged in intrinsic muscles, even as age-related osteoligamentous changes occur (Boyd-Clark et al. 2002), which is crucial for maintaining effective proprioceptive regulation among older adults.

Furthermore, combining sling treatment with vibration significantly affects larger trunk muscles, which is beneficial in improving stability and muscle coordination (Choi and Kang 2013). This variability in treatment, including different vibration perturbations, allows physiotherapists to monitor individual patient responses and tailor interventions accordingly. The Neurac© method enables load modification without aggravating external structures by adjusting the leverage system and support area, ensuring an optimal challenge for both the neurophysiological and biomechanical systems (Kirkesola 2009; Saliba et al. 2010).

The method's high applicability across various physiotherapy settings is further supported by its ability to achieve maximum load without overloading the spinal column or joint system (Zaveckas 2018). For patients with chronic conditions, such as chronic neck pain, studies have shown that Neurac© training significantly improves pain, function, balance, fatigability, and quality of life (Yun et al. 2015). The method's versatility is not only beneficial for older adults but also for patients with acute or chronic pain and even elite athletes, as it enhances the communication between the brain, movement receptors, and muscles as part of the broader sensorimotor system.

Ultimately, Neurac© offers sufficient freedom of movement, allowing for easy adaptation of the support area and suspension points, while integrating DL principles into personalized physiotherapy sessions. This dynamic and adaptable approach aligns perfectly with the need for variability in training to enhance motor control, balance, and overall functional capacity in real-world settings.

7.6.2 Supine Bridge with Variability: A Sensorimotor Challenge

The Supine Bridge exercise, performed using Redcord suspension equipment, is a key component of the Neurac© treatment approach, integrating differential learning principles to enhance neuromuscular control, gluteal activation, and spinal stabilization. The patient begins the exercise in a supine position on a mat, with both feet suspended in Redcord slings and knees bent at 90 degrees. The arms rest naturally by the sides to provide minimal support, allowing for greater core activation. To initiate the movement, the hips are lifted off the mat, forming a straight line from the shoulders to the knees, ensuring controlled core and gluteal engagement throughout the movement. To increase instability and neuromuscular engagement, the therapist may manually perturb the slings or apply controlled vibration to stimulate proprioceptive feedback. Exercise intensity is progressively adjusted by modifying sling height, resistance levels, lever arm, or adding perturbations, ensuring optimal neuromuscular engagement without compromising body stability. The movement is performed within a pain-free range, with modifications applied as needed to prevent discomfort and enhance proper movement mechanics.

As the patient develops greater stability and neuromuscular control, the following progression variation principles can be introduced. Decreasing elastic cord tension enhances resistance and muscle activation. Eccentric or isometric contractions focus on controlled lowering (eccentric) or static holds (isometric) to challenge muscular endurance. Reducing the base of support by placing hands on the chest or introducing a balance cushion beneath the scapulae introduces instability. Introducing oscillations in the slings or applying vibration through Redcord Stimula further stimulates the sensorimotor system. Incorporating lumbar lateral flexion, leg abduction, or controlled pelvic rotation increases movement complexity and adaptability.

Questions

1. What is the primary objective of integrating differential learning (DL) into balance training and falls prevention?
2. How do balance problems impact different segments of society, particularly among older adults?
3. Why are falls among older adults considered a major public health concern, and what factors contribute to their frequency?
4. What are the three primary diagnostic approaches used to assess balance deficits?
5. How do sensorimotor control regions contribute to maintaining balance, and what are their key functions?
6. What role does sensory and motor variability play in balance control, and how can they affect motor learning?
7. How do gait abnormalities serve as both symptoms of balance impairments and potential opportunities for learning balance?
8. What are the differences between balance therapy and balance training, and how are they applied in different contexts?
   A. Therapy is for athletes; training is only for hospital patients.
   B. Therapy targets elite performance, training targets fall risk.
   C. Balance therapy focuses on restoring lost function after pathology under clinical supervision, whereas balance training refines or enhances stability in healthy or athletic populations.
   D. Both terms mean exactly the same thing.
   E. Therapy and training are distinguished solely by equipment cost.
9. What are some classical approaches to balance training, and how do they improve stability and fall prevention?
   A. Wobble boards, single-leg stances, Tai Chi, and perturbation treadmills progressively challenge the postural system, leading to reduced sway and a lower incidence of falls.
   B. Only seated breathing exercises are used.
   C. Electrical muscle stimulation without standing practice.
   D. Daily marathon running at a fixed speed.
   E. Static sitting in a chair for 30 min.
10. How does differential learning (DL) differ from classical balance training methods, and what are its key advantages?
   A. DL relies exclusively on heavy resistance work.
   B. DL repeats one ideal posture until perfect.
   C. DL introduces systematically unpredictable perturbations in direction, amplitude, and timing, forcing self-organized adaptation and producing broader transfer to real-world balance tasks.
   D. DL eliminates all sensory input to focus on vision.
   E. DL is identical to classical methods but uses louder music.

11. How does DL-based balance training impact the cardiovascular system, and what evidence supports this interaction?
    A. It always causes dangerous tachycardia.
    B. It leaves heart dynamics unchanged because balance and cardiovascular control are unrelated.
    C. DL sessions acutely raise heart-rate variability and baro-reflex sensitivity, indicating beneficial autonomic engagement documented by simultaneous ECG recordings.
    D. It suppresses blood pressure regulation for hours.
    E. No study has ever measured cardiac effects during balance practice.
12. What are the implications of using perturbation-based balance training on ECG parameters and heart-brain interactions?
    A. It produces complete heart block in most participants.
    B. It shows mild, transient increases in QT variability that parallel heightened cortical arousal, suggesting tighter heart-brain coupling during adaptive postural control.
    C. It eliminates all variability in RR intervals.
    D. It guarantees perfect synchrony between alpha waves and heartbeat.
    E. It has no measurable physiological effects.
13. What role do unpredictable coordination tasks play in enhancing balance control and adaptation?
    A. They distract the performer and worsen balance.
    B. They provide irrelevant entertainment value only.
    C. They enlarge the repertoire of postural solutions by forcing constant recalibration, thereby speeding adaptation to unexpected real-world perturbations.
    D. They reduce reaction speed by overloading attention.
    E. They have no influence on sensorimotor learning.
14. How can sling exercises and the Neurac© method be used for therapy and fall prevention?
    A. By locking the body rigidly to suppress all sway.
    B. By suspending limbs in ropes and elastic slings to create multi-planar instability, activating deep stabilizers and training reactive balance in a controlled yet variable environment.
    C. By eliminating gravity through underwater practice.
    D. By replacing standing work with seated meditation.
    E. By attaching weights to immobilize the center of mass.
15. What are some future clinical applications of DL-based balance training, and how might they improve rehabilitation and injury prevention?
    A. Fully automated VR perturbation systems and wearable feedback sensors could deliver individualized, variability-rich programs at home, shortening rehab times and reducing fall rates in high-risk populations.
    B. Daily use of rigid casts to prevent any joint movement.
    C. Replacing therapists with static instruction posters.
    D. Eliminating technology to focus only on verbal cues.
    E. Standardized one-size-fits-all protocols for every patient.

References

Alexander NB (1996) Gait disorders in older adults. J Am Geriatr Soc 44(4):434–451. https://doi.org/10.1111/j.1532-5415.1996.tb06417.x

Ambrose AF, Cruz L, Paul G (2023) Falls and fall prevention in older adults: causes, consequences, and intervention strategies. Clin Geriatr Med 39(1):1–14. https://doi.org/10.1016/j.cger.2022.08.001

Baird JL, Van Emmerik RE (2009 Dec) Young and older adults use different strategies to perform a standing turning task. Clin Biomech (Bristol) 24(10):826–832. https://doi.org/10.1016/j.clinbiomech.2009.08.006

Behm DG, Anderson KG (2006) The role of instability with resistance training. J Strength Cond Res 20(3):716–722. https://doi.org/10.1519/R-18435.1

Bertschi D, Kiss CM, Beerli N, Mauthner O, Kressig RW (2022) Impact of sarcopenia on daily functioning: a cross-sectional study among older inpatients. Aging Clin Exp Res 34:2041–2046. https://doi.org/10.1007/s40520-022-02147-4

Boyd-Clark LC, Briggs CA, Galea MP (2002) Muscle spindle distribution, morphology, and density in longus colli and multifidus muscles of the cervical spine. Spine 27(7):694–701. https://doi.org/10.1097/00007632-200204010-00005

Brumagne S, Diers M, Danneels L, Moseley GL, Hodges PW (2019) Neuroplasticity of sensorimotor control in low back pain. J Orthop Sports Phys Ther 49(6):402–414. https://doi.org/10.2519/jospt.2019.8489

Buckley JG, Frost SS, Hartley S, Rodacki ALF, Barrett BT (2024) Moving from stable standing to single-limb stance or an up-on-the-toes position: the importance of vision to dynamic balance control. PLoS One 19(7):e0307365. https://doi.org/10.1371/journal.pone.0307365

Busse ME, Wiles CM, van Deursen RW (2006) Co-activation: its association with weakness and specific neurological pathology. J Neuroeng Rehabil 3(1):26. https://doi.org/10.1186/1743-0003-3-26

Cabanas-Valdés R, Boix-Sala L, Coll-Cantí S (2021) Effects of core exercises in improving dynamic sitting balance, gait, and functional rehabilitation for subacute stroke patients (CORE-trial): study protocol for a randomized controlled trial. Int J Environ Res Public Health 18(12):6615. https://doi.org/10.3390/ijerph18126615

Carè M, Chiappalone M, Cota VR (2024) Personalized strategies of neurostimulation: from static biomarkers to dynamic closed-loop assessment of neural function. Front Neurosci 18. https://doi.org/10.3389/fnins.2024.1363128

Choi Y, Kang H (2013) The effects of sling exercise using vibration on trunk muscle activities of healthy adults. J Phys Ther Sci 25(10):1291–1294. https://doi.org/10.1589/jpts.25.1291

Christie A, Kamen G (2010) Short-term training adaptations in maximal motor unit firing rates and afterhyperpolarization duration. Muscle Nerve 41:651–660. https://doi.org/10.1002/mus.21539

Churchland MM, Afshar A, Shenoy KV (2006) A central source of movement variability. Neuron 52(6):1085–1096. https://doi.org/10.1016/j.neuron.2006.10.034

Chvatal SA, Ting LH (2013) Common muscle synergies for balance and locomotion. Front Comput Neurosci 7:48. https://doi.org/10.3389/fncom.2013.00048

Collins JJ, Chow CC, Imhoff TT (1995) Aperiodic stochastic resonance in excitable systems. Phys Rev E Stat Phys Plasmas Fluids Relat Interdiscip Topics 52(4):R3321–R3324. https://doi.org/10.1103/physreve.52.r3321

da Silva RA, Bilodeau M, Parreira RB, Teixeira DC, Amorim CF (2018) One-legged stance sway of older adults with and without falls. PLoS One 13(9):e0203887. https://doi.org/10.1371/journal.pone.0203887

Davids K, Bennett S, Newell KM (2006) Movement system variability. Human Kinetics, Champaign

D'Avella A, Portone A, Fernandez L, Lacquaniti F (2006) Control of fast-reaching movements by muscle synergy combinations. Journal of Neuroscience 26(30):7791–810. https://doi.org/10.1523/JNEUROSCI.0830-06.2006

Davidson BS, Madigan ML, Nussbaum MA (2004) Effects of lumbar extensor fatigue and fatigue rate on postural sway. Eur J Appl Physiol 93(1):183–189. https://doi.org/10.1007/s00421-004-1195-1

Dejvajara D, Aungkasuraphan R, Palee P, Phimphasak C (2022) Effects of home-based nine-square step exercises for fall prevention in Thai community-dwelling older adults during a COVID-19 lockdown: a pilot randomized controlled trial. Int J Environ Res Public Health 19(17):10514. https://doi.org/10.3390/ijerph191710514

Delmas S, Watanabe T, Yacoubi B, Christou EA (2021) Age-associated increase in postural variability relate to greater low-frequency center of pressure oscillations. Gait Posture 85:103–109. https://doi.org/10.1016/j.gaitpost.2020.12.019

Dietz V (2002) Proprioception and locomotor disorders. Nat Rev Neurosci 3(10):781–790. https://doi.org/10.1038/nrn939

Ferrucci L, Baroni M, Ranchelli A, Lauretani F, Maggio M, Mecocci P (2014) Interaction between bone and muscle in older persons with mobility limitations. Curr Pharm Des 20(19):3178–3197. https://doi.org/10.2174/1381612820666140317103544

Gao H, Zhao Y, Zhao L, Wang Z, Yan K, Gao B (2023) The role of oxidative stress in multiple exercise-regulated bone homeostasis. Aging Disease 14:1555–1582. https://doi.org/10.14336/AD.2023.0102

Goble DJ, Alhasan H, Hood V, Mainwaring F (2017) The effect of visual biofeedback on balance in the elderly population: a systematic review. Clin Interv Aging 12:1385–1394. https://doi.org/10.2147/CIA.S127023

Gollhofer A, Taube W (2004) Sensorimotor training. In: Komi PV (ed) Strength and power in sport, 2nd edn. Blackwell Science, Oxford, pp 399–411.

Gupta R, Agarwal R (2022) Human muscle synergy recruitment and variability assessment for walking speed prediction module design. IETE J Res. https://doi.org/10.1080/03772063.2022.2101555

Hallisy KM (2018) Tai Chi beyond balance and fall prevention: health benefits and its potential role in combatting social isolation in the aging population. Curr Geriatr Rep 7(2):57–66. https://doi.org/10.1007/s13670-018-0233-5

Hamed SB, Schieber MH (2007) Decoding M1 neurons during multiple finger movements. J Neurophysiol 98:327. https://doi.org/10.1152/jn.00760.2006

Harvey NC, Curtis EM, McEvoy C (2024) Impact of dementia and mild cognitive impairment on bone health in older people. Aging Clin Exp Res 37(1):5. https://doi.org/10.1007/s40520-024-02871-y

Hausdorff JM, Peng CK, Ladin Z, Wei JY, Goldberger AL (1995) Is walking a random walk? Evidence for long-range correlations in stride interval of human gait. J Appl Physiol 78(1):349–358. https://doi.org/10.1152/jappl.1995.78.1.349

Horak FB (1997) Clinical assessment of balance disorders. Gait Posture 6(1):76–84. https://doi.org/10.1016/S0966-6362(97)00018-0

Horak FB (2006) Postural orientation and equilibrium: what do we need to know about neural control of balance to prevent falls? Age Ageing 35(Suppl_2):ii7–ii11. https://doi.org/10.1093/ageing/afl077

Horak FB, Macpherson JM (2011) Postural orientation and equilibrium. In: Kandel ER, Schwartz JH, Jessell TM, Siegelbaum SA, Hudspeth AJ (eds) Principles of Neural Science, 5th edn. McGraw-Hill, New York, pp 935–947.

Huang R et al (2024) The effect of Tai Chi (Bafa Wubu) training and artificial intelligence-based movement-precision feedback on the mental and physical outcomes of elderly. Sensors (Basel) 24(19). https://doi.org/10.3390/s24196485

Izquierdo M, Aguado X, Gonzalez R, Lopez JL, Häkkinen K (1999) Maximal and explosive force production capacity and balance performance in men of different ages. Eur J Appl Physiol Occup Physiol 79:260–267. https://doi.org/10.1007/s004210050504

Janura M, Zahálka F, Svoboda Z, Janurová E (2020) Postural stability after treadmill and overground walking in young and elderly. Gait Posture 80:84–89. https://doi.org/10.1016/j.gaitpost.2020.05.014

John AT, Barthel A, Wind J, Rizzi N, Schöllhorn WI (2022) Acute effects of various movement noise in differential learning of rope skipping on brain and heart recovery analyzed by means of multiscale fuzzy measure entropy. Front Behav Neurosci 16:816334. https://doi.org/10.3389/fnbeh.2022.816334

Jones KE, Hamilton AF, Wolpert DM (2002) Sources of signal-dependent noise during isometric force production. J Neurophysiol 88(3):1533–1544. https://doi.org/10.1152/jn.2002.88.3.1533

Kanko RM, Laende EK, Strutzenberger G, Brown M, Selbie WS, DePaul V et al (2021) Assessment of spatiotemporal gait parameters using a deep learning algorithm-based markerless motion capture system. J Biomech 122:110414. https://doi.org/10.1016/j.jbiomech.2021.110414

Kirkesola G (2009) Neurac –a new treatment method for long-term musculoskeletal pain. J Fysioterapeuten 76:16–25

Klatt B (2015) The effect of vibrotactile feedback during balance and vestibular rehabilitation on functional balance outcomes. University of Pittsburgh

Kouvidis GK, Sommers MB, Giannoudis PV, Katonis PG, Bottlang M (2009) Comparison of migration behavior between single and dual lag screw implants for intertrochanteric fracture fixation. J Orthop Surg Res 4(1):16. https://doi.org/10.1186/1749-799X-4-16

Lacroix A, Kressig RW, Muehlbauer T, Gschwind YJ, Pfenninger B, Granacher U (2016) Effects of a supervised versus an unsupervised combined balance and strength training program on balance and muscle power in healthy older adults: a randomized controlled trial. Gerontology 62(3):275–288. https://doi.org/10.1159/000442087

Laughton CA, Slavin M, Katdare K, Nolan L, Bean JF, Kerrigan DC (2003) Aging, muscle activity, and balance control: physiologic changes associated with balance impairment. Gait Posture 18(2):101–108. https://doi.org/10.1016/S0966-6362(02)00200-X

Lei Y, Wang J (2018) The effect of proprioceptive acuity variability on motor adaptation in older adults. Exp Brain Res 236(2):599–608. https://doi.org/10.1007/s00221-017-5150-x

Liu-Ambrose T, Davis JC, Hsu CL (2019) Exercise to prevent falls in older adults with cognitive impairment. In: Falls and cognition in older persons. Springer, pp 243–258. https://doi.org/10.1007/978-3-030-24233-6_16

Ljunggren J (2024) A Swedish invention that conquered the world. In: A political history of sport in Sweden. Springer. https://doi.org/10.1007/978-3-031-46185-9_3

Lo J, Lo OY, Olson EA et al (2017) Functional implications of muscle co-contraction during gait in advanced age. Gait Posture 53:110–114. https://doi.org/10.1016/j.gaitpost.2017.01.010

Lord SR, Sherrington C, Menz HB (2001) Falls in older people: risk factors and strategies for prevention. J Am Geriatr Soc 49(12):1546–1552. https://doi.org/10.1046/j.1532-5415.2001.49156.x

Lundy-Ekman L (2007) Neuroscience fundamentals for rehabilitation, 3rd edn. Saunders, p 144

Meng D, Guo H, Liang S, Tian Z, Wang R, Yang G, Wang Z (2022) Effectiveness of a hybrid exercise program on the physical abilities of frail elderly and explainable artificial-intelligence-based clinical assistance. Int J Environ Res Public Health 19(12):6988. https://doi.org/10.3390/ijerph19126988

Meyns P, Bruijn SM, Duysens J (2013 Sep) The how and why of arm swing during human walking. Gait Posture 38(4):555–562. https://doi.org/10.1016/j.gaitpost.2013.02.006

Montero-Odasso M, Van Der Velde N et al (2022a) New horizons in falls prevention and management for older adults: a global initiative. Age Ageing 50(5):1499–1512. https://doi.org/10.1093/ageing/afab234

Montero-Odasso M, Van Der Velde N, Martin FC, Petrovic M, Tan MP, Ryg J, Aguilar-Navarro S, Alexander NB, Becker C, Blain H, Bourke R, Cameron ID, Camicioli R, Clemson L, Close J, Delbaere K, Duan L, Duque G, Dyer SM et al (2022b) World guidelines for falls prevention and management for older adults: a global initiative. Age Ageing 51(9). https://doi.org/10.1093/ageing/afac205

Moosaei Saein A, Kahrizi S, Boozari S (2024) Effects of unstable load and unstable surface ontrunk muscles activation and postural control in healthy subjects. J Biomech 173:112257. https://doi.org/10.1016/j.jbiomech.2024.112257

Moreland JD, Richardson JA, Goldsmith CH, Clase CM (2004) Muscle weakness and falls in older adults: a systematic review and meta-analysis. J Am Geriatr Soc 52(7):1121–1129. https://doi.org/10.1111/j.1532-5415.2004.52310.x

Nashner LM (1973) Vestibular and reflex control of normal standing. In: Stein RB, Pearson KG, Smith RS, Redford JB (eds) Control of posture and locomotion. Plenum Press, New York, pp 291–308

Nashner LM (1976) Adapting reflexes controlling the human posture. Exp Brain Res 26(1):59–72. https://doi.org/10.1007/BF00235249

Nashner LM (1983) Analysis of movement control in man using the movable platform. Adv Neurol 39:607–619

Needle AR, Howard JS (2024) Neural-targeted rehabilitation strategies to address neuroplasticity after joint injury. J Athl Train 59:1187. https://doi.org/10.4085/1062-6050-0215.23

Nonnekes J, Goselink RJM, Růžička E, Fasano A, Nutt JG, Bloem BR (2018) Neurological disorders of gait, balance and posture: a sign-based approach. Nat Rev Neurol 14(3):183–189. https://doi.org/10.1038/nrneurol.2017.178

Olveczky BP, Andalman AS, Fee MS (2005) Vocal experimentation in the juvenile songbird requires a basal ganglia circuit. PLoS Biol 3(5):e153. https://doi.org/10.1371/journal.pbio.0030153

Ozmen T, Aydogmus M (2016) Effect of core strength training on dynamic balance and agility in adolescent badminton players. J Bodyw Mov Ther 20(3):565–570. https://doi.org/10.1016/j.jbmt.2015.12.006

Paavilainen T, Hoikka V, Paavolainen P (1993) Cementless total hip arthroplasty for congenitally dislocated or dysplastic hips: technique for replacement with a straight femoral component. Clin Orthop Relat Res 297:71–81

Pijnappels M, Bobbert MF, van Dieën JH (2005) Control of support limb muscles in recovery after tripping in young and older subjects. Exp Brain Res 160:326–333. https://doi.org/10.1007/s00221-004-2014-y

Priplata AA, Niemi JB, Harry JD, Lipsitz LA, Collins JJ (2003) Vibrating insoles and balance control in elderly people. The Lancet 362(9390):1123–4. https://doi.org/10.1016/S0140-6736(03)14470-4

Richardson C, Jull G, Hodges P, Hides J, Panjabi MM (1999) Therapeutic exercise for spinal segmental stabilization in low back pain: Scientific basis and clinical approach. Churchill Livingstone

Saliba SA, Croy T, Guthrie R et al (2010) Differences in transverse abdominis activation with stable and unstable bridging exercises in individuals with low back pain. N Am J Sports Phys Ther 5:63–73

Schöllhorn WI (2000) Applications of systems dynamic principles to technique and strength training. Acta Acad Olympiquae Estoniae 8:67–85

Shadmehr R, Smith MA, Krakauer JW (2010) Error correction, sensory prediction, and adaptation in motor control. Annual Review of Neuroscience 33:89–108. https://doi.org/10.1146/annurev-neuro-060909-153135

Shephard RJ (2018) A history of health & fitness: Implications for education and sport. Springer

Shkuratova N, Morris ME, Huxham F (2004 Apr) Effects of age on balance control during walking. Arch Phys Med Rehabil 85(4):582–588. https://doi.org/10.1016/j.apmr.2003.06.021

Smits-Engelsman BC, Wilson PH (2013) Noise, variability, and motor performance in developmental coordination disorder. Dev Med Child Neurol 55(Suppl 4):69–72. https://doi.org/10.1111/dmcn.12311

Soylu G, Cakmak G, Yalvac Y, Yakaryilmaz FD, Ozturk ZA (2021) Relationship between age-related postural hyperkyphosis and sarcopenia. Curr Aging Sci 14(2):133–138. https://doi.org/10.2174/1874609814666210514103304

Stergiou N, Decker LM (2011) Human movement variability, nonlinear dynamics, and pathology: is there a connection? Hum Mov Sci 30(5):869–888. https://doi.org/10.1016/j.humov.2011.06.002

Sturnieks DL, St George R, Lord SR (2008) Balance disorders in the elderly. Clin Biomech 23(5):563–570. https://doi.org/10.1016/j.clinbiomech.2007.12.002

Sung ES, Kim JH (2018) Relationship between ankle range of motion and Biodex Balance System in females and males. J Exerc Rehabil 14(1):133–137. Published 2018 Feb 26. https://doi.org/10.12965/jer.35146.573

Taube W, Gruber M, Beck S, Faist M, Gollhofer A, Schubert M (2008) Cortical and spinal adaptations induced by balance training: correlation between stance stability and corticospinal activation. Eur J Neurosci 27(1):200–208. https://doi.org/10.1111/j.1460-9568.2007.05983.x

Tsay JS, Kim HE, Parvin DE, Stover AR, Ivry RB (2021) Individual differences in proprioception predict the extent of implicit sensorimotor adaptation. J Neurophysiol 125(4):1307–1321. https://doi.org/10.1152/jn.00585.2020

van Beers RJ, Haggard P, Wolpert DM (2004) The role of execution noise in movement variability. J Neurophysiol 91(2):1050–1063. https://doi.org/10.1152/jn.00652.2003

Velička D (2020) The effects of high-intensity interval training, occlusive training, and aerobic exercise sessions supplemented with differential learning tasks on the cardiovascular system of men: Doctoral dissertation (M 005, Medicine and Health Sciences, Nursing). Lithuanian Sports University

Velička D, Bernotienė G, Poderienė K, Vainoras A, Poderys J (2016) Differential training tasks trigger the decrease of concatenation between cardiovascular parameters. Baltic J Sport Health Sci 4(103):38–44

Villa S, Eliyah FJ, Weiss Y, Welsch R, Kosch T (2025) *Understanding* the influence of electrical muscle stimulation on motor learning: enhancing motor learning or disrupting natural progression? In: Thomas Kosch research archive. Springer

Welter ML, Lau B, Karachi C, Grabli D (2012) Normal and pathological gait: what we learn from Parkinson's disease. J Neurol Neurosurg Psychiatry 83(10):979–986. https://doi.org/10.1136/jnnp-2012-302263

Winter DA (1995) Human balance and posture control during standing and walking. Gait Posture 3(4):193–214. https://doi.org/10.1016/0966-6362(96)82849-9

Xu B, Ma L (2020) Falls and fall-related consequences among older people living in long-term care facilities in a megacity of China. Gerontology 66(6):523–531. https://doi.org/10.1159/000510469

Yang F et al (2023) A systematic review of perturbation-based balance training on reducing fall risk among individuals with stroke. Clin Biomech (Bristol, Avon) 109:106078. https://doi.org/10.1016/j.clinbiomech.2023.106078

Yatham P, Chintamaneni S, Stumbar S (2023) Lessons from India: a narrative review of integrating yoga within the US healthcare system. Cureus 15:e43466. https://doi.org/10.7759/cureus.38249

Yogev-Seligmann G, Hausdorff JM, Giladi N (2008) The role of executive function and attention in gait. Neuropsychologia 46(3):642–655. https://doi.org/10.1016/j.neuropsychologia.2008.01.002

Yoshida S (2007) A global report on falls prevention: epidemiology of falls. World Health Organization (WHO). Retrieved from https://promenaid.com/wp--content/uploads/2023/03/WHO-Study-Epidemiology-of-falls-in-older-age.pdf

Yun S, Kim YL, Lee SM (2015) The effect of neurac training in patients with chronic neck pain. J Phys Ther Sci 27(5):1303–1307. https://doi.org/10.1589/jpts.27.1303

Zaveckas V (2018) Neuromuscular activation (Neurac) method in treatment, physical wellness, and sport. In The 4th international scientific-practical conference "Exercise for Health and Rehabilitation" (p. XX). Lithuanian University of Health Sciences, Institute of Sports & Lithuanian Federation of Sports Medicine

Zemek R, Babl F (2022) Traumatic brain injury: progress and challenges in prevention, clinical care, and research. Lancet Neurol 21(11):1004–1060. https://doi.org/10.1016/S1474-4422(22)00309-X

HIIT: Considered as Various Fluctuations for Adaptive Processes in the Metabolism

8

Agnė Slapšinskaitė-Dackevičienė

8.1 What Is HIIT?

8.1.1 Evolution of Training Methods: From Classical Structures to Modern HIIT

The evolution of HIIT can be viewed as a refinement of the classical training structures developed in the Soviet Union and East Germany (GDR). These earlier systems, which emphasized periodization, endurance, and interval training, laid the foundation for modern training practices. The Soviet and GDR regimes were known for their scientifically driven approach to physical conditioning, personalizing training as early as the 1950s and reaching a fully developed concept by the 1970s (Girginov 2004; Krüger 2002; Matveyev 1981; Ozolin 1970).

The classical systems focused on four key training methods: the endurance method, extensive interval method, intensive interval method, and competition method (Matveyev 1964). These methods, rooted primarily in metabolic training, sought to improve both aerobic and anaerobic capacities. For example, the endurance method emphasized long, sustained efforts to build stamina, while the intensive interval method introduced high-intensity intervals to push an athlete's anaerobic threshold. The competition method prepared athletes for the mental and physical rigors of real competitive environments, simulating the demands of peak performance. HIIT, emerging from these traditions, offers a more differentiated and adaptable version of the intensive interval and competition methods. It was first popularized by Dr. Izumi Tabata, who famously tested the method on casual students rather than professional athletes, demonstrating its wide applicability across different fitness levels (Tabata 2019, 2022; Tabata et al. 1997). HIIT refines classical approaches by allowing for precise manipulation of variables such as interval intensity, duration, recovery periods, and exercise types.

Moreover, it is worth mentioning that circuit weight training (CWT) was an early approach to structured exercise aimed at improving overall fitness before HIIT gained prominence. It was designed as an efficient method to enhance multiple components of fitness, including muscular strength, cardiorespiratory endurance, and body composition (Wilmore et al. 1978). CWT sessions typically last 25–30 min and involve sequential resistance exercises with minimal rest (Gettman and Pollock 1981). A standard CWT protocol consists of three circuits of ten exer-

A. Slapšinskaitė-Dackevičienė (✉)
Department of Sports Medicine, Faculty of Nursing, Medical Academy, Lithuanian University of Health Sciences, Kaunas, Lithuania

Faculty of Public Health, Health Research Institute, Medical Academy, Lithuanian University of Health Sciences, Kaunas, Lithuania
e-mail: agne.slapsinskaite-dackeviciene@lsmu.lt

W. I. Schöllhorn, A. Slapšinskaitė-Dackevičienė (eds.), *Differential Learning in Physiotherapy*,
https://doi.org/10.1007/978-3-031-98787-8_8

cises, each performed for 30 s at 40% of one-repetition maximum (Gettman et al. 1982). Research has shown that CWT increases aerobic capacity by approximately 5%, compared to 15–25% in traditional aerobic programs, while also improving lean body mass (1–3.2 kg), reducing fat (0.8–2.9%), and enhancing strength (7–32%) (Gettman and Pollock 1981). In line, CWT alone leads to notable gains in VO_2 max (+12%), strength (+17%), and fat loss (−3.0%), and can be stated to be effective for enhancing overall fitness (Gettman et al. 1982). More recent research supports the efficacy of high-intensity circuit training (HICT), indicating that short-duration, high-intensity protocols can improve muscular endurance, with slight gender-specific improvements in muscle strength and aerobic fitness (Schmidt et al. 2015).

While classical training systems primarily emphasized metabolic pathways, particularly in endurance sports, CWT and modern HIIT apply more specific loads to different physiological structures, including muscles, tendons, the cardiovascular system, and the nervous system. This shift acknowledges that training adaptations extend beyond energy metabolism to encompass biomechanical and neuromuscular factors. For instance, HIIT can be tailored for rehabilitation, targeting specific muscle groups to enhance coordination and stability alongside metabolic benefits (Josyula and Alagesan 2024). In this way, HIIT represents not just an increase in intensity but a more comprehensive approach that accounts for the varying adaptation timescales of different body systems, promoting both performance enhancement and long-term physical integrity.

8.2 Different Forms of High-Intensity Training

High-intensity training most often represents a specific time-efficient exercise strategy to improve cardiorespiratory and metabolic performance (Buchheit and Laursen 2013; Gillen and Gibala 2014). It is characterized by brief and metabolically intense bouts of physical exertion interspersed with short periods of low-intensity recovery. HIIT manifests in various forms. According to Buchheit and Laursen, HIIT encompasses repeated short (<45 s) and long (2–4 min) high-intensity exercises, as well as short (≤10 s) repetitive sprint sequences or extended 20–30 s sprint interval sessions with transition periods (Buchheit and Laursen 2013). These diverse workouts, ranging from 5 to 40 min, are contingent upon an individual's current fitness level and the intensity of the activity, with the primary aim of enhancing cardiorespiratory and metabolic functions alongside overall physical fitness. HIIT trains the metabolic flexibility that is known as the ability to efficiently adapt metabolism by substrate sensing, trafficking, storage, and utilization, dependent on availability and requirement (Smith et al. 2018). HIIT's adaptability to different fitness levels and preferences is one of its key strengths.

HIIT is generally subcategorized into low—less than 15 min—and high-volume (greater than 15 min) HIIT based on the total time spent in active intervals (Sabag et al. 2022).

Tabata training originated from a study conducted by Japanese scientist Izumi Tabata in 1996 (Olson 2014). This study initiated a rethinking of the classical endurance training methods and can be considered the origin of HIIT. This particular regimen involves eight 20-s bouts of maximal effort interspersed with 10-s rest intervals, totaling 4 min. The participants in the original study were young males with an average age of 23 ± 1 years, most of whom were physically active. The study found that Tabata training improved aerobic capacity as much as moderate-intensity continuous training while also increasing anaerobic capacity by 28% (Olson 2014). This foundational pattern of 20 s of effort followed by 10 s of rest has since evolved into various regimens and exercises. For instance, even 12-week low-volume (<5 min) Tabata-style functional HIIT was highly effective for university female students to improve cardiorespiratory fitness, body fat, some cardiometabolic health outcomes, and habitual physical activity (Lu et al. 2023).

High-Intensity Functional Training (HIFT): An exercise modality that emphasizes functional, multi-joint movements that can be modified to any fitness level and elicit greater muscle recruitment than more traditional exercise (Feito et al. 2018). These movements are performed as quickly as possible based on individual capabilities. HIFT targets various physical characteristics, including cardiorespiratory endurance, muscle strength, speed, coordination, anaerobic power, agility, and flexibility (Feito et al. 2019). It has gained a lot of interest in the health sector.

Whole-body HIIT, also referred to as full-body training, integrates HIIT principles (i.e., short bursts of high-intensity exercise—defined as achieving ≥85% of Hrpeak) with bodyweight exercises, offering a comprehensive approach to HIIT (McRae et al. 2012). It is an effective way to engage multiple muscle groups and maximize calorie burn in a short period. These sessions involve repeated high-intensity exercises, where time to effort, time to recovery, and session duration are monitored. Exercise intensity is determined by the maximal number of movements achievable within a set time, making the sessions highly demanding (Machado et al. 2019).

HIIT promotes capillarization and metabolism linked to cardiorespiratory function through alternating high- and low-intensity intervals. Its various forms provide adaptable regimens for diverse fitness levels and objectives. Despite its effectiveness, a gap remains between HIIT's use in athletic training and its application in general fitness or rehabilitation. Athletes follow specialized HIIT protocols tailored to power, speed, or agility, whereas in public health, HIIT can drive rapid physiological adaptations independent of total energy expenditure (Biddle and Batterham 2015).

HIIT's rise underscores its dual role in performance and health promotion. Differential learning (DL), introduced by Schöllhorn (1999), emphasizes movement variability and adaptation through increased fluctuation. System dynamics principles used in DL have also been applied to metabolic regulation, though whether adaptations stem from the number or magnitude of fluctuations remains unclear (Bauer 2007; Kortmann and Schöllhorn 2006). Integrating these principles with HIIT research could enhance its effectiveness by targeting metabolic flexibility while also refining motor learning and skill acquisition.

8.3 HIIT: Variability in Intervention

HIIT, as previously mentioned, is characterized by alternating short bursts of high-intensity exercise—defined as achieving ≥85% of HRpeak or ≥80% of VO_2peak, or an equivalent measure—with recovery periods lasting ≤5 min (Martland et al. 2020) with recovery at 65% HRmax (Ramírez-Vélez et al. 2020). On a cycle ergometer, high intensity is typically defined as 80–150% of Wpeak (Morris et al. 2021). Alternatively, high intensity can also be assessed using perceived exertion, corresponding to a rating of 8 on the OMNI-Walk/Run scale (Follador et al. 2018). These variations in defining and measuring what is high intensity within HIIT protocols reflect the diversity in research approaches, emphasizing the importance of clear and consistent criteria to enhance the comparability and applicability of findings across studies. To address this, some of the key methodologies for measuring HR max within HIIT protocols will now be presented.

$$\text{HRmax} = 220 - \text{Age}$$

(Fox 1971)

$$\text{HRmax} = 206 - 0.7 \times \text{Age}$$

(Londeree and Moeschberger 1982)

$$\text{HRmax} = 207 - 0.7 \times \text{Age}$$

(Ekblom et al. 1973)

$$\text{HRmax} = 208 - 0.7 \times \text{Age}$$

(Tanaka et al. 2001)

$$\text{HRmax} = 211 - 0.64 \times \text{Age}$$

(Nes et al. 2013)

Individual Profile Considerations in HIIT HIIT protocols vary in stage duration, recovery type, and intensity, necessitating individualized program design. Factors such as circadian rhythm and fitness level differentiate beginners, intermediates, and advanced practitioners, primarily based on time to exhaustion. However, this categorization is only a preliminary step toward true individualization (Ammar et al. 2024; Horst et al. 2020). Recovery times, reflecting fitness and performance levels, further influence total session duration, highlighting the need for personalized HIIT adaptations.

Intensity and Duration as Determining Variables in HIIT Exercise intensity directly influences duration, determining individual strain. In HIIT sessions near VO_2max, higher intensity reduces the number of repetitions and necessitates longer recovery periods (Matveev 1965; Medbo and Tabata 1989). Structuring intervals based on Tmax (time to exhaustion at Vmax) optimizes endurance, with 50–75% of Tmax enabling sustained effort across repetitions. For individuals with lower initial fitness, high-repetition protocols can significantly improve VO_2max in a short time.

Several key variables (Fig. 8.1) in HIIT programs should be considered to optimize performance and recovery:

1. Intensity: The degree of exertion during exercises
2. Exercise selection (ES): The choice of exercises within the session
3. Stimulus time (ST): The duration constituting the training load indicator
4. Duration of sets (DS): The length of each set
5. Intervals between exercises (IBE): Time and frequency of rest between sets
6. Training time (TT): The overall length of the HIIT session
7. Recovery intensity and time (RI; RT): Factors influencing training load indicator

Optimizing Training Load and Metabolic Adaptations in Intervention Monitoring the training load throughout each HIIT session is paramount, with the total duration spanning from 4 to 32 min. Both internal (e.g., perceived effort) and external (e.g., HRmax, VO_2max) load monitoring methods can facilitate effective control. The success of the HIIT training protocols might be hindered by the aforementioned key variables in HIIT programs that could be the source of the variation/ "noise" in training that is pushing past these aerobic/anaerobic thresholds. It may further be incorporated to induce adaptations such as increased cardiovascular efficiency or improved lactate tolerance, augmenting the metabolic flexibility of both athlete and patient.

Crafting a HIIT training program demands expertise and a meticulous approach, particularly in monitoring variable loads during ses-

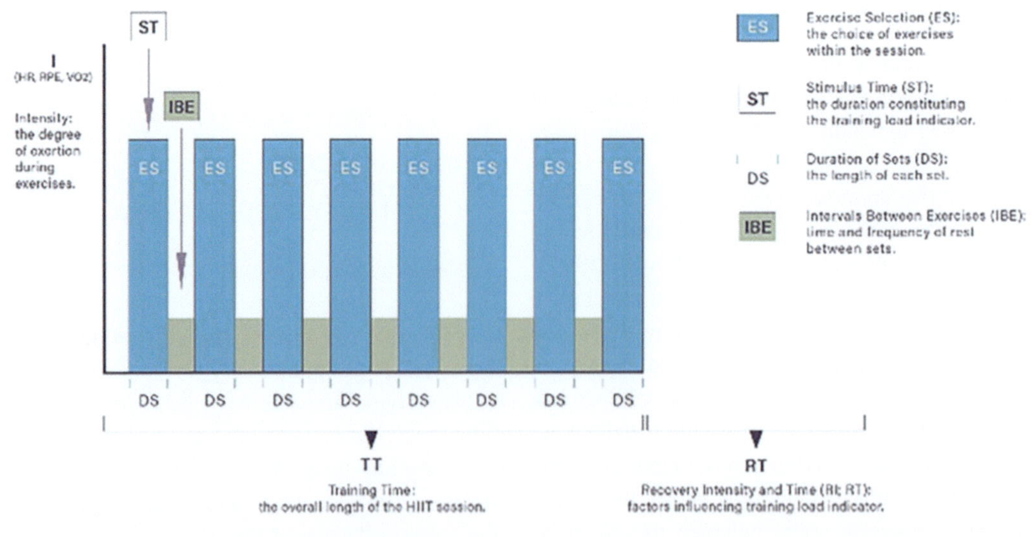

Fig. 8.1 Distribution of load of time on HIIT

sions (Buchheit and Laursen 2013). Considering the adaptive nature of HIIT, practitioners are advised to manipulate stimulus: *time variables, recovery durations,* and *exercise selection* in alignment with their individual profiles and to adapt the level of noise on the physiological system.

Enhancing metabolic flexibility requires an adaptive metabolic response to environmental demands, such as those imposed by HIIT (Smith et al. 2018). Optimizing HIIT necessitates a precise understanding of its variables and a personalized approach based on individual fitness levels and goals. Effective HIIT programming relies on strategic planning and continuous monitoring to maximize performance and overall well-being. Key to this process is inducing and optimizing physiological fluctuations in energy demand by carefully adjusting load variations and exercise selection.

8.4 Physiological Response to HIIT Training

Exercise-induced remodeling occurs at multiple levels, including the molecular level, enhancing fitness, optimizing energy processes, increasing muscle mass, and improving neuromuscular coordination, which benefits brain function. The physiological adaptations from HIIT result not only from intensity but also from the intrinsic nature of intermittent exercise, highlighting the need to understand its underlying mechanisms. The following sections will examine HIIT's effects on the cardiopulmonary system, metabolic health, inflammation, oxidative stress, skeletal muscles, mitochondrial function, and aerobic capacity.

Cardiopulmonary System HIIT has been shown to increase VO_2max in both sexes of older adults, highlighting its efficacy in enhancing cardiopulmonary function. Postexercise hypotension, mediated by various physiological mechanisms, contributes to improved blood pressure regulation and vascular function following HIIT sessions (Halliwill et al. 2014). These adaptations, including plasma volume expansion and angiogenesis, play pivotal roles in long-term improvements in cardiovascular health and fitness (Hopper et al. 1985).

Metabolic Health Regular physical training is well-documented to yield metabolic health benefits (Ito 2019). HIIT has emerged as an effective strategy comparable to moderate-intensity endurance training for improving metabolic health. Studies indicate that HIIT leads to reductions in body fat percentage and improvements in VO_2max without necessarily resulting in overall body weight loss. These findings support HIIT's role in enhancing metabolic parameters, particularly in sedentary individuals.

Inflammation and Oxidative Stress HIIT interventions are associated with shifts toward oxidative control in trained subjects, indicating a reduction in inflammation and oxidative stress. This shift toward a more oxidative state suggests improved metabolic regulation and cellular resilience, contributing to overall metabolic health (Lu et al. 2021).

Skeletal Muscles In response to HIIT, there are notable changes in protein expression within skeletal muscles, particularly related to antioxidant regulation and mitochondrial function. HIIT interventions have shown increases in MnSOD and SOD1 content, suggesting enhanced antioxidant capacity (Chrøis et al. 2020). Moreover, HIIT induces favorable adaptations in older individuals by increasing mitochondrial content, thereby potentially mitigating the progression of age-related sarcopenia and preserving muscle oxidative capacity.

Aerobic Capacity and Mitochondrial Health One of the most often mentioned benefits of HIIT is its ability to significantly improve aerobic capacity. For sedentary or recreationally active individuals (VO_2max under 55 ml/kg/min), it is often assumed that reaching VO_2max levels seen in elite athletes (above 60 ml/kg/min) requires years of training (Ekblom 1968; Hardman et al. 1986). Nonetheless, a study by

Hickson et al. (1977) demonstrated that just 10 weeks of consistent high-intensity exercise could increase VO_2max by an impressive 44% in untrained individuals. This regimen involved alternating high-intensity cycling and running sessions six days a week, leading to several participants reaching VO_2max levels comparable to those of highly trained athletes. This rapid improvement highlights the potential of HIIT to enhance aerobic fitness, especially in individuals with lower baseline fitness. Further, exercise training, including HIIT, contributes to improved mitochondrial health through mechanisms such as mitochondrial biogenesis and removal of dysfunctional mitochondria via mitophagy. These adaptations support the enhancement of aerobic capacity and overall metabolic function (Alizadeh Pahlavani et al. 2022). HIIT restores mitochondrial function through AMP-activated protein kinase-dependent biogenesis and mitophagy, optimizing cellular metabolism and performance (Sanchez-Padilla et al. 2014).

Mitochondria Function Many studies support the idea that deregulation of mitochondrial function underlies the onset of metabolic inflexibility (Smith et al. 2018), although a causal link between the two remains to be fully established (Gao et al. 2014). However, the increase reached through HIIT in mitochondrial density contributes to maintaining muscle oxidative capacity and potentially slowing down the progression of sarcopenia associated with aging (Søgaard et al. 2018). Moreover, mitochondrial bioenergetic function can be controlled through both acute changes, aimed to promptly modify activity, and longer-term transcriptional responses, aimed to regulate mitochondrial volume density (Smith et al. 2018). HIIT induces both qualitative and quantitative improvements in mitochondrial function by promoting biogenesis and enhancing mitochondrial quality control (Sorriento et al. 2021). This process repairs damaged mitochondria and stimulates the production of new ones, maintaining metabolic homeostasis. Mitochondria adapt to the energy demands of HIIT by increasing their capacity for ATP synthesis, metabolite sharing, and calcium handling (Spinelli and Haigis 2018). This adaptability makes HIIT a powerful tool for improving mitochondrial health and metabolic resilience, particularly in the face of aging and disease.

By leveraging these mitochondrial adaptations, HIIT not only supports metabolic flexibility but also offers a time-efficient and effective alternative to traditional endurance training. This is particularly relevant given the growing interest in exercise modalities that provide similar physiological benefits with reduced time and effort. Interval training modalities such as HIIT and sprint interval training (SIT) have gained significant popularity due to their ability to elicit comparable adaptations to endurance training, but in a fraction of the time and with reduced exercise volume (MacInnis and Gibala 2017; Memme et al. 2021). These high-intensity exercises recruit all motor units, promoting mitochondrial adaptations across all muscle fiber types, as shown in mixed fiber biopsy samples (MacInnis and Gibala 2017). The short, intense bouts of exercise characteristic of HIIT and SIT stimulate key signaling pathways that converge on PGC-1α, the master regulator of mitochondrial biogenesis, similarly to the adaptations seen in endurance training (Gibala et al. 2009; Little et al. 2011b). Furthermore, the rapid ATP hydrolysis and increased calcium (Ca^{2+}) release during high-intensity efforts enhance the activation of critical signaling kinases that are central to mitochondrial adaptation, which may explain why repeated HIIT and SIT sessions can increase mitochondrial content by 25–35% in as few as six to seven sessions (Egan et al. 2010; Gollnick et al. 1974; MacInnis and Gibala 2017).

Brain-Derived Neurotrophic Factor Brain-derived neurotrophic factor is assumed to be essential for brain plasticity, particularly in learning and memory (Bathina and Das 2015). BDNF also seems to be involved in energy regulation and osteogenesis (Camerino et al. 2016; Park et al. 2024). BDNF levels may be influenced by the type and intensity of an exercise program, along with an individual's physical performance and adaptation (Nofuji et al. 2012, 2008). Resting

BDNF levels have shown high variability, potentially due to individual differences or daily fluctuations in BDNF secretion (Begliuomini et al. 2008). BDNF is involved in the regulation of the circadian pacemaker in the central nervous system, with peak levels in the morning (08:00 h) that decline as the day progresses (Begliuomini et al. 2008). By 12:00 h, plasma BDNF levels are significantly lower compared to the early morning, suggesting that the observed fluctuations in BDNF may be partially due to the timing of blood sample collection (08:00 h–13:00 h) (Begliuomini et al. 2008). Taking this into account and scheduling therapy sessions earlier in the day, when BDNF levels are naturally higher, could potentially enhance the neuroplastic and therapeutic benefits.

Recently, a nine-week study of different high-intensity training methods (Fig. 8.2)—found that BDNF levels were significantly higher in the high-intensity power training (HIPT) group compared to the high-intensity endurance training (HIET) group ($p < 0.01$) (Murawska-Ciałowicz et al. 2021). These results suggest that postexercise BDNF levels are influenced by the type, intensity, and duration of the exercise performed. When BDNF levels are dependent on these variables, it could be linked to the variability or "*noise*" observed in DL systems, as exercise-induced neuroplasticity may contribute to differences in cognitive and neural processing outcomes.

Moreover, recent research highlights the cognitive benefits of exercise, particularly HIIT, for older adults (Blackmore et al. 2024). A six-month study comparing low-, moderate-, and high-intensity training found that only the HIIT group showed significant improvements in hippocampal function and paired associative learning (Blackmore et al. 2024). Strikingly, HIIT prevented age-related hippocampal volume loss and improved functional connectivity between neural networks, changes linked to increased BDNF and

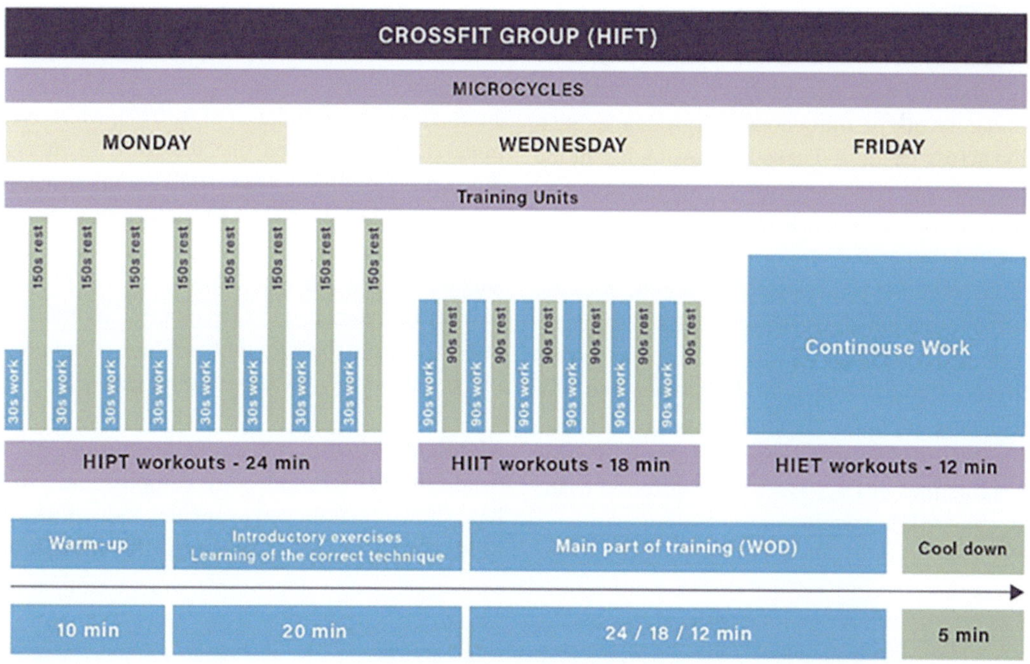

Fig. 8.2 Scheme of HIFT microcyles. (Adapted with a permission from Murawska-Ciałowicz et al. (2021). Note: *HIPT* high-intensity power training, *HIIT* high-intensity interval training, *HIET* high-intensity endurance training, *HIFT (cross fitness)* high-intensity interval training)

reduced cortisol. These findings emphasize the value of incorporating HIIT into therapeutic programs to enhance both physical and cognitive health in older adults.

Sex differences in HIIT responses have been observed, with studies indicating increased mass-specific mitochondrial respiratory capacity in males but not females (Chrøis et al. 2020). These variations may be influenced by differences in skeletal muscle metabolic properties. For instance, BDNF expression, affected by muscle fiber type and exercise intensity, showed increased mRNA levels in slow-twitch (soleus) muscles but decreased protein levels in fast-twitch (plantaris) muscles in rats after high-intensity training (Jiménez-Maldonado et al. 2016). While some studies report similar mitochondrial protein levels across genders, others suggest males experience greater reductions in body fat and improved insulin sensitivity, while females show increased VO_2max (Søgaard et al. 2018).

The delineation of plausible sex differences in response to HIIT underscores the complexity of most probably individualized adaptations to exercise stimuli (Horst et al. 2023). While some studies suggest a differential response between sexes, particularly in mitochondrial respiratory capacity and body composition changes, others indicate similar levels of mitochondrial protein expression across genders. These findings highlight the nuanced interplay between biological sex and exercise-induced adaptations, warranting further investigation of underlying mechanisms and optimized exercise prescription strategies. Moving forward, continued exploration of HIIT's mechanistic underpinnings and its applicability across diverse populations will be paramount for advancing our understanding of exercise physiology and refining interventions, especially once the principles of DL have been transferred to the theory of HIIT as well.

8.5 HIIT in Health and Rehabilitation

> Metabolic inflexibility is a hallmark of many age-related metabolic diseases but also plays a central role in, for instance, cancer and immune metabolism. (Smith et al. 2018)

Cardiovascular Diseases (CVD) CVDs, encompassing conditions like hypertension (Brito et al. 2018), poor glycemic control (Lee et al. 2020), dyslipidemia (Wallace et al. 1999), and obesity (Su et al. 2019), represent another area where HIIT holds promise. HIIT has demonstrated potent antihypertensive effects, with substantial acute reductions in blood pressure (Delgado-Floody et al. 2020). This reduction, if repeated regularly, can lead to significant reductions in cardiovascular and neurological risks for several hours during the day. HIIT can be a valuable tool for managing hypertension and improving cardiovascular health, particularly when tailored to individual fluctuations and appropriate noise levels in the intervention. Moreover, numerous HIIT protocols have been studied across various populations, including those with coronary artery disease, heart failure, chronic obstructive pulmonary disease, and metabolic syndrome, as summarized by Kessler et al. (2012). Moreover, meta-analysis revealed that the increase in cardiorespiratory fitness after HIIT is approximately double that achieved through moderate-intensity continuous training (Weston et al. 2014). The superior cardiovascular benefits of HIIT compared to moderate-intensity continuous training may stem from the variability or "*noise*" inherent in the fluctuating intensity of the exercise.

Metabolic Health When examining metabolic syndrome (MetS) and body composition, HIIT has shown significantly greater reductions in MetS components. For instance, HIIT resulted in a relative risk reduction of 0.5 (95% CI: 0.33–0.75, $p < 0.001$) for MetS, and improvements included decreases in waist circumference (−3 ± 5 cm vs. +1 ± 5 cm, $p = 0.01$) and fasting blood glucose (−25.8 ± 34.8 mg/dL vs. −3.9 ± 25.8 mg/dL, $p < 0.001$). The HIIT group also exhibited greater reductions in body fat mass (−2.1 ± 2.1 kg vs. 0 ± 2.2 kg, $p = 0.002$) and increases in lean body mass (0.9 ± 1.9 kg vs. -0.9 ± 3.2 kg, $p = 0.01$) compared to the moderate-intensity continuous training group (Dun et al. 2019). These enhanced reductions in MetS components and favorable body composition changes are likely due to the intensity variability, or "noise," inherent in HIIT, which promotes more dynamic metabolic and physiological adaptations.

These findings highlight HIIT's effectiveness in treating metabolic syndrome and improving insulin sensitivity, critical for reducing type 2 diabetes risk. A promising low-volume HIIT protocol for type 2 diabetes patients involves ten 1-min vigorous efforts at 90% of maximal aerobic capacity, with 1-min rest intervals. After just two weeks of training, three times a week, this regimen significantly lowered 24-h blood glucose levels in inactive individuals with type 2 diabetes (Little et al. 2011a). Plausibly, the fluctuations in exercise intensity, or "noise," improve metabolic flexibility and activate key pathways crucial for managing type 2 diabetes.

Inflammation and Oxidative Stress HIIT offers health benefits beyond physical fitness, with emerging evidence linking it to a reduced risk of certain cancers, such as breast and colon cancer. For example, acute high-intensity interval exercise (HIIE) has been shown to decrease colon cancer cell numbers in vitro and increase inflammatory cytokines immediately postexercise (Devin et al. 2019). However, this effect was transient, disappearing 120 min after exercise. These acute changes may influence colorectal cancer outcomes, potentially aiding in prevention or management. The transient reduction in cancer cells could be attributed to the "noise" from exercise-induced fluctuations in immune activity, cytokine levels, and metabolic stress, which may disrupt cancer cell proliferation and, with repeated bouts, enhance the body's protective mechanisms.

Skeletal Muscles For individuals with *Duchenne muscular dystrophy (DMD),* skeletal muscle fatigue poses a significant challenge, leading to a diminished ability to perform daily tasks and a marked decline in quality of life (Yamauchi et al. 2023). DMD, a genetic muscle-wasting disorder, manifests with progressive muscle weakness and heightened susceptibility to fatigue. In this context, isometric HIIT emerges as a recommended intervention. Isometric contractions, where the overall length of the muscle remains constant during contraction, are considered less damaging for dystrophic muscles. Studies have suggested isometric contractions as a feasible mode of exercise for patients with DMD, offering potential benefits in enhancing fatigue resistance and mitigating muscle pathology (Yamauchi et al. 2023). Incorporating specific, intentional fluctuations or variability into isometric HIIT protocols may optimize motor unit activation and enhance fatigue resistance in individuals with DMD.

Osteoarthritis, marked by joint pain and stiffness, often leads to physical inactivity (Roxburgh et al. 2023). About half of the patients report joint pain as the main barrier to exercise. Interval training, with controlled intensity variability, can help reduce pain by preventing repetitive strain and improving joint function, encouraging greater exercise participation. Additionally, HIIT interventions have shown significant potential in reducing the incidence of osteoarthritis and falls among older individuals. A notable single-arm trial involving 29 participants (mean age 63 ± 7 years; 66% women; 66% obese) assessed the effectiveness of HIIT on various health outcomes (Golightly et al. 2021). The intervention consisted of HIIT sessions conducted twice a week on a cycling ergometer or treadmill, including ten 1-min bouts at 90% of the participants' VO_2peak, interspersed with 1-min rest periods. Various assessments were conducted at baseline, 6 weeks, and 12 weeks to evaluate pain, function, and balance, utilizing tools such as the Western Ontario and McMaster Universities Osteoarthritis Index and the timed up-and-go test. The study achieved a 70% adherence rate with no reported adverse events. Notably, after 12 weeks, participants demonstrated significant improvements, including a decrease of 1.13 s in the 20-m fast-paced walk time (95% confidential intervals (CI): −1.61 to −0.64) and an increase of 2.6 stands in the 30-s chair stand (1.8–3.4). The structured intensity fluctuations in this HIIT protocol likely introduced additional "noise," potentially stimulating neuromuscular adaptations that improved balance, strength, and functional performance in older individuals.

The adaptability of HIIT protocols, in terms of intensity, duration, and work-to-rest ratios, allows for a bit more personalized approaches (HRmax, VO_2max, REP, etc.) that approach different fitness levels and objectives, whether focused on improving cardiovascular health, metabolic function, or even cancer prevention. Once again, restating the importance of dealing with metabolic inflexibility that is a hallmark of many age-related metabolic diseases but also plays a central role in, for instance, cancer and immune metabolism. The adaptability of HIIT protocols mirrors the concept of DL, which originally focused on enhancing adaptability in a coordinative sense but can also be applied to training metabolic flexibility. As mentioned, metabolic flexibility, the ability to efficiently switch between energy substrates, is critical in addressing age-related metabolic diseases, cancer, and immune dysfunction. This raises intriguing questions about the interplay between coordinative adaptability and metabolic flexibility—can one enhance the other, or how might they synergize when combined? For instance, John et al. explored brain-heart interactions after DL rope skipping, suggesting that integrating both coordinative and metabolic challenges could amplify adaptive responses.

In summary, HIIT has evolved from athletic conditioning to a valuable tool in rehabilitation, promoting physiological adaptations and fatigue resistance through intensity variation. By incorporating HIIT into rehabilitation, physiotherapists can enhance healing, function, and overall well-being in diverse clinical populations. HIIT also shows promise in mitigating age-related declines and addressing metabolic inflexibility, a key factor in age-related diseases, cancer, and immune dysfunction (Smith et al. 2018). As research on interval training's "noise" continues, its potential for improving health outcomes expands.

8.6 Why to Apply Differential Learning in Rehabilitation?

Differential learning (DL) is a motor learning model that enhances motor skills through variability and adaptability, widely used in sports to improve performance and control (Frank et al. 2008; Henz et al. 2018; Oftadeh et al. 2021). However, its application in rehabilitation remains underexplored. Schöllhorn et al. (2010) discuss DL's potential in prevention and rehabilitation, optimizing health outcomes through system fluctuations. In stroke rehabilitation, Repšaitė et al. (2015) show DL's ability to improve hand and arm function by introducing movement task variability. DL also aids in recovering fine motor control in focal hand dystonia (Rosset-Llobet and Fàbregas-Molas 2018) and improves spinal function and pain relief in elderly women with osteochondrosis (Vainauskas and Slapšinskaitė-Dackevičienė 2018). Additionally, DL reduces fall risk and enhances independence in the elderly (Karvelis and Slapšinskaitė Dackevičienė 2021), and it aids recovery after anterior cruciate ligament injury (Gokeler et al. 2023). These studies highlight DL's potential to enhance rehabilitation outcomes by promoting neuroplasticity, adaptability, and motor control recovery.

8.6.1 The Role of Exercise in Cognitive Rehabilitation and Neuroplasticity

While the potential of DL in rehabilitation is gaining recognition, the field continues to evolve, particularly in the context of cognitive health interventions. As the global population ages, addressing cognitive decline—particularly conditions such as dementia—becomes increasingly urgent. Emerging evidence suggests that various forms of exercise, especially HIIT, with its added noise due to intervals of load, may serve as effective interventions to mitigate cognitive decline and promote cognitive health in aging individuals. In the context of rehabilitation, incorporating HIIT with intentional variations in optimal load and technique, such as the approach used in rope skipping (John et al. 2022), may not only enhance physical recovery but also stimulate cognitive function by promoting optimal brain-heart interaction and is further expected to increase BDNF levels. An interesting question for future research is whether the HIIT methods are blunted by time. The different HIIT protocols may be combined in a kind of long-term application similar to periodization in high-performance sports. There is still a lack of research on the effects of repeated application of the same method. This also refers to the problem of whether a method has the same effect when the patient is coming to therapy again after one or more years. Observations in high-performance sport indicate that every method loses its effect over time, and that here, too, changes to the method bring advantages on a longer time scale.

In the context of healthy participants, research supports the idea that variations among different forms of HIIT can provide unique advantages, particularly in terms of brain-derived neurotrophic factor (BDNF) production (Murawska-Ciałowicz et al. 2021). The high-intensity functional training (HIFT; see Fig. 8.2 for microcycle) group, with significantly more coordinative tasks than the others, demonstrates how incorporating individual variability alongside diverse training modalities—such as high-intensity power training (HIPT), traditional HIIT, and high-intensity endurance training (HIET)—can influence BDNF levels. At stage 9 of a graded exercise test (GXT), BDNF levels were notably higher in the HIFT group (30%; $p < 0.05$) and the HIIT group (18%; $p < 0.05$), but no similar increase was observed in the HIET group (Murawska-Ciałowicz et al. 2021). Interestingly, after a Wingate Anaerobic Test (WAnT), BDNF concentrations decreased by 28% in the HIFT group, yet remained significantly higher than in the HIET group. These findings highlight the fact that BDNF responses differ depending on the type and intensity of exercise. It may suggest that the brain's adaptive capacity may be enhanced by *varying* training modalities. HIFT, in particular, appears to combine the benefits of multiple training forms, leading to a more significant and sustained increase in BDNF levels, which stand in line with DL and could have important implications for cognitive function, mental health, and neuroprotection. By incorporating different practices, HIFT not only optimizes physical performance but also supports brain health through enhanced BDNF secretion. These findings underscore the importance of variability in exercise programming for maximizing both physical and cognitive benefits and are in line with the differential learning approach.

There were several invitations to apply research of DL in rehabilitation since it recognizes that there is no single optimal solution for a given motor task (Vaz et al. 2017). This approach challenges the traditional notion that there is a "normal" or ideal movement pattern that all individuals should achieve. Instead, DL emphasizes the importance of exploring multiple task solutions that arise from the dynamic interaction between the individual and the task (i.e., HIIT). This perspective could be effectively applied to metabolism and HIIT, where the technique and path toward improvement are individualized, even though basic principles remain the same. Just as in movement techniques, where specificity in gait is emphasized (Carello et al. 1985; Turvey et al. 2012; Turvey et al. 2009), HIIT protocols should also account for individual metabolic responses and variations. This approach highlights the need for further research to explore the unique metabolic adaptations in different individuals, encouraging a more personalized approach to HIIT that could optimize outcomes for diverse populations and be translated into practical applications for individualized rehabilitation.

We once again state that movement variability is vital not only for developing flexible and adaptive motor behavior, suggesting that variability in practice can help individuals discover context-dependent performance strategies that are uniquely suited to their needs (Frank et al. 2008; Holt et al. 2010), but also for maintaining metabolic flexibility. Incorporating DL principles allows therapists to focus on enhancing an individual's adaptability and metabolic flexibility under varying conditions, rather than relying on standardized movement patterns. This approach supports a more personalized rehabilitation process while improving metabolic flexibility.

8.6.2 The Stochastic Resonance Principle in Physiotherapy

Stochastic resonance is a phenomenon where the presence of a certain level of "*noise*" or variability enhances the signal detection and processing capabilities of a system, rather than hindering it. This principle has been applied in the field of rehabilitation, particularly within the context of motor control (White et al. 2019) and recovery from pain (Washif et al. 2019). In physiotherapy, the idea is that introducing controlled levels of variability (or noise) into rehabilitation exercises can stimulate the nervous system and promote neuroplasticity, improving motor control and functional recovery. This approach contrasts with traditional rehabilitation models that often emphasize repetitive, standardized movements.

Stochastic resonance suggests that variability in movement patterns can lead to enhanced motor learning by challenging the system in a way that mimics natural fluctuations. This variability may take the form of changing movement speeds, altering task complexity, or introducing unpredictability in the training environment, all of which can enhance adaptability and recovery. In contrast to one-sided, therapist- or model-oriented approaches, DL in HIIT may offer a more personalized (i.e., circadian rhythms) and effective way to patient care, which is increasingly demanded in the rehabilitation context of the twenty-first century. The first step to improve the rehab is to adjust the fluctuating state in the client/patient (see Fig. 8.3). Let us explore how this patient-oriented DL approach could be incorporated into HIIT.

In Adjustment to the Stochastic Resonance It is crucial to understand the individual dynamics (either physiological, psychological, neuronal, circadian, sociological, etc.) during exercise. From our previous research, once studying the individual dynamics of pain (Slapsinskaite et al. 2015, 2017; Slapšinskaitė et al. 2018) as well as attention (Slapsinskaite et al. 2016), we came up with several notions related to the dynamics and spontaneous fluctuations. For instance: "*Attentional allocation toward pain results from the neural communication across the brain-wide network "connectome" which consists of pain-attention related circuits. Connectome is intrinsically dynamic and spontaneously fluctuating on multiple time-scales*" (Slapsinskaite et al. 2017). We came with the evidence that variation (switching) in painful locations (Idiosyncratic pain distribution patterns) during cycling seemed to increase time on task (Slapšinskaitė et al. 2018). These studies suggested qualitative changes from fluctuating to non-fluctuating perceived exertion shifts while cycling continuously at RPE = 15 and while running at 80% of maximal heart rate (Balagué et al. 2012). Understanding the nature of fluctuations can enhance therapeutic outcomes by aligning interventions with the dynamic nature of individual states, leading to more effective exercise strategies. It is important to understand that the fluctuation should be adjusted to the subjective information. The externally given fluctuations given by the therapist's sequence and duration of exercises should be adjusted to the athletes' response fluctuations. Only when both are adjusted to each other then optimal learning or metabolism adjustment happen. This dynamic nature of perception is in line with the ideas of Russian physiologist Ivan Sechenov (1829–1905), who emphasized the profound influence of activity on perception. Sechenov stated, "We do not hear but listen, we do not see but look," highlighting the active nature of our engagement with sensory input. The key to advancing exercise

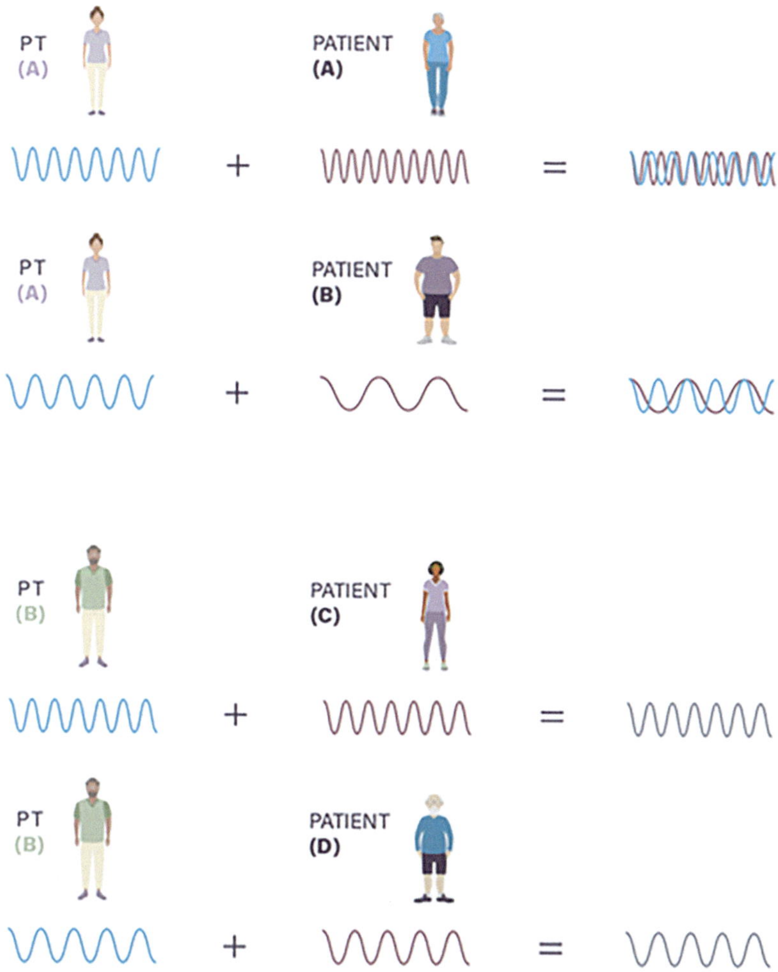

Fig. 8.3 Therapist-patient interaction model for optimizing variability in rehabilitation. (A). Novate PT (A) struggles to adjust to the fast fluctuations of patient A, resulting in noticeable dissonance in the therapy. Similarly, Novate PT (A) cannot adapt to the slower fluctuations of patient B, leading to further dissonance. In contrast, therapist B, with extensive experience, successfully adjusts to the noise of patient C, fostering a state of resonance. This positive outcome is mirrored in patient D, where therapist B is also able to adapt to the slower fluctuations effectively

strategies lies in appreciating the dynamic and fluctuating nature of human perception and exertion, among other bio-signals. By adjusting (reaching the stochastic resonance) from both the objective data of structured exercise and the subjective feedback from the body's sensory systems, we can develop more personalized, effective approaches that honor the complexity of individual experiences during physical activity.

Our brain is constantly monitoring movement patterns, particularly during the learning phase of new motor activities. Learning from differences (new/novelty exercises) or trying to keep the fluctuating state in clients or patients could encompass various aspects that can be used once determining the HIIT protocol of the session:

- Intensity: Referring to the level of exertion during exercises
- Exercise selection: Involving the selection of exercises within a session
- Stimulus time: Reflecting the duration constituting the training load indicator
- Duration of sets: Signifying the length of each set
- Intervals between exercises: Including the time and frequency of rest between sets
- Training duration: Denoting the overall length of the HIIT session

- Recovery intensity and time: Factors influencing the training load indicator

All these variables can be altered by noise, allowing for self-organization to find an individual's optimum and become more adjustable.

8.7 How Can HIIT Be Expanded by DL/SD Theory?

Keeping the Fluctuations Through the HIIT Protocol Variability One of the main issues in applying DL in PT is to emphasize a model for therapist-patient interaction that targets individual variability in a resonant manner between the therapist and the patient. Meaning that a physiotherapist provides an adequate noise level toward the HIIT session for the patient, making it possible to utilize maximally the inner capacities of the patient (not too much and not too little; optimal, see Fig. 8.4). Factors such as training load control, session length, weekly frequency, and exercise selection are all considered within this framework. Additionally, a basic guideline is proposed for developing a comprehensive HIIT program, utilizing an optimal approach for the patient. It is well known that engaging in more complex exercises requires greater energy expenditure and increased metabolic demands, thus influencing the dynamics of the training session, including the quality of movements and associated levels of fatigue.

Exercise selection emerges as a critical parameter in neuromuscular adaptation. While no definitive guidelines exist for selecting exercises in HIIT whole-body programs, considering the complexity of the motor task is suggested as a viable strategy when organizing the training session. According to the motor control perspective, exercises can be classified into two distinct groups: those with a unique movement pattern, such as jumping jack, and those with a combination of unique movements, exemplified by burpees. Therefore, integrating DL strategies into jumping jacks or burpees exercise selection can significantly expand the variety of movement patterns, optimizing neuromuscular adaptation through a more nuanced and flexible approach.

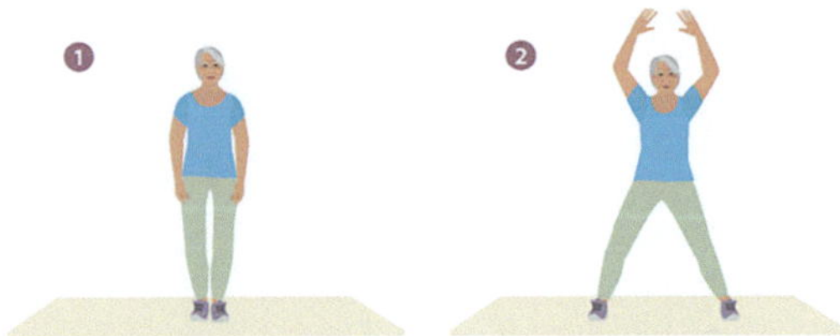

Fig. 8.4 The initial jumping jack exercise

This section of the book offers practical examples of applying DF principles within the construct of HIIT training.

Variations in Exercise
Because all the variations are intended to increase the fluctuation in the patient's body and mind, the variations are differentiated between internal (patient) and external (systemic environment) with being aware that both cannot be separated disjunctive, e.g., gravitational force is always a force between two bodies and expresses their relative attraction. The aim is that, by stimulating the body and mind in versatile ways, the adaptation processes in the patient should be initiated (Fig. 8.5).

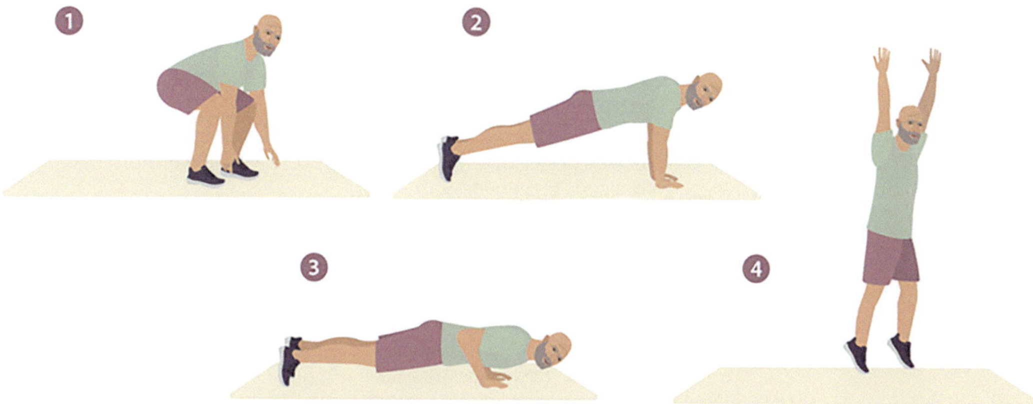

Fig. 8.5 The initial variation of the burpee exercise

Type of variation	Some examples
Variation provided by	Variations during the rehab are provided by PTs Variations during the rehab procedures are provided by the participant (the patient needs to create the variations)
Internal variation: variation in the body	Variation in the initial position (i.e., difference in the stance length, difference in the foot direction, using different heights—with knees bent, with arms bent) Varying in head position—chin in, chin out Performing the exercise without the neck (shoulders up) or with a very elongated neck Bent to one shoulder, bent to other shoulder (ear to the shoulder) Chest forward Changing the pelvis position—interior/exterior rotation, or moving the pelvis in a circle Jumping with just the toes
External variation: variation in sensorial input (visual, vestibular, proprioceptive)	Closing one eye Simultaneously blinking Making a circle with the head Moving the head up and down With and without eyes following the object in front Jumping on different surfaces
Internal variation: variation in the breathing	Adjust the breathing pattern to the rhythm of the exercise Breathe faster, shallower, deeper (abdominal breathing)
Internal variation: variation in the imagination	Jump on the floor as if it is hot as lava; perform several jumps in a row, flowing like water; be steady as a rock when doing a jumping jack Explode like a volcano when performing a jumping jack Jump like a kangaroo when performing several variations of jumping jacks
External variation: variation of the context	Variation in the beat of the music Active involvement of the subject in exercise performance and their motivation
Variation in the intensity	Variations in performance speed (i.e., different jump power) When the patient/client is performing the jumping jacks, the PT may ask them to change the speed—e.g., begin slowly and then accelerate, decelerate, alternate between slow, fast, and slower Variations in attention allocation (internal focus—e.g., focusing on specific calf muscles—vs. external focus—e.g., jumping as if lava is around) Changes in direction (rotating or moving around while performing jumping jacks)

(continued)

Type of variation	Some examples
Variation provided by	Variations during the rehab are provided by PTs Variations during the rehab procedures are provided by the participant (the patient needs to create the variations)
Internal variation: variation in the body	Variation in the initial position (i.e., difference in the stance length; difference in the foot direction; using different heights—with knees bent, with arms bent; shifting the weight to one side or the other) Variation in head position—chin in, chin out Performing the exercise without the neck (shoulders up) or with a very elongated neck Bent to one shoulder, bent to the other shoulder (ear to the shoulder) Chest forward during all 4 phases of the exercise Changing the pelvis position—interior/exterior rotation in all 4 phases of the exercise, or just the 1st and the 4th phases Varying the position of the hands in the 3rd phase of the exercise
External variation: variation in sensorial input (visual, vestibular, proprioceptive)	Closing one eye in all 4 phases of the exercise, or just in the 1st and 4th phases, or the 2nd and 3rd phases Simultaneously blinking in all 4 phases of the exercise, or just in the 1st and 4th phases, or the 2nd and 3rd phases Moving the neck up and down in all 4 phases of the exercise, or just in the 1st and the 4th phases, or the 2nd and 3rd phases With and without eyes following the object in front Jumping on different surfaces
Internal variation: variation in the breathing	Adjust the breathing pattern to the rhythm of the exercise, breathe faster, shallower, and deeper (abdominal breathing)
Internal variation: variation in the imagination	Perform burpees on the floor as if it is hot as lava; perform burpees in a flow like water; be steady as a rock when completing a burpee; imagine that you are melting while performing burpees; explode like a volcano once making burpees
External variation: variation of the context	Variation in the beat of the music Active involvement of the subject in exercise performance and their motivation
Variation in the intensity	Variations in performance speed (i.e., different burpee explosion power) While the patient/client is performing the burpees, the PT may ask them to change the speed—e.g., begin slowly and then accelerate, decelerate, or alternate between slow, fast, and slower tempos Variations in attention allocation (internal focus—focusing on the specific calf muscles—vs. external focus—jumping as if lava is around) Changes in the direction (rotating or moving around while performing burpees)

Examples of Application of Noise to PT Practice In a biological context, "noise" refers to random fluctuations in cellular and metabolic processes. Introducing controlled "noise" through exercise can aid rehabilitation, particularly for patients with metabolic diseases. For example, structured noise in rehabilitation exercises can improve insulin sensitivity and metabolic flexibility in conditions like type 2 diabetes or metabolic syndrome. This approach also benefits individuals with limited mobility, as it can stimulate metabolic processes and improve cellular function, even though subtle interventions like alternating pressure or performing HIIT in bed (Fig. 8.6).

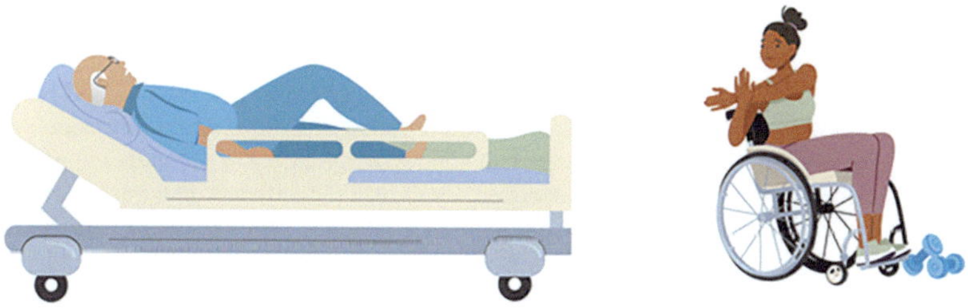

Fig. 8.6 The initial variation of the exercises in bed/wheelchair

Variations in Bed Exercises for Rehabilitation

Type of variation	Some examples
Variation provided by	Variations provided by the PT. PTs often introduce modifications to standard exercises to cater to patient needs and enhance the recovery process. These adjustments may include changes to arm lifts, leg raises, or pelvic tilts, each suited to the patient's goals and abilities Variations provided by the patient. Patients themselves can create slight variations in the exercises, promoting independence and awareness. For example, lifting the right arm slightly higher than the left, or moving the left leg with a wider arc, can engage different muscle groups and motor pathways, contributing to more comprehensive recovery
Internal variation: variation in the body	*Lying supine (on back)* Core squeeze: contract abdominal muscles as if bracing for impact, hold for 10 s, and then release Lift your legs and trace letters in the air (e.g., "A", "B", "C") using slow, controlled movements. For each letter or movement, try varying the duration of holding the letter (e.g., 3, 5, or 10 s) and the rest time in between (e.g., 5-s break, then repeat) Trace letters with your toes or fingers, holding each position for 3–5 s. Move in different directions and at different angles to improve dexterity and coordination Leg presses: press one leg down into the bed without moving it, creating resistance and activating thigh muscles Arm presses: gently push arms downward against the bed, focusing on shoulder engagement and chest activation Leg raises and holds: single-leg lift with knee bent: lift one leg with a bent knee while keeping the other leg grounded, hold, and then switch Double-leg lift with assistance: lift both legs slightly with a pillow or rolled towel under knees for stability, engaging core and thighs *Lying prone (on stomach)* With an external aim—watching TV in a prone position Back and shoulder activation: arm lifts (superman variation): lift arms slightly off the bed, keeping them straight or bent at the elbows, and hold for isometric contraction Leg lifts: alternately lift one leg off the bed, hold for 5–10 s, and switch, engaging glutes and lower back Full-body hold: lift chest slightly off the bed with arms to the side or under the shoulders for a brief hold and then release Glute squeeze: tighten gluteal muscles for 5–10 s, release, and repeat Scapular retraction: draw shoulder blades together and down, hold, and then release to engage upper back muscles. While lying on a rolling board, pull on the ropes in different directions. Hold the retraction, pull the ropes toward your body or away, and engage your shoulder blades for 5–10 s. Hold ropes in loops over the bed and move them in different directions (up, down, side to side) while keeping your shoulder blades pulled together and down. Hold for 5–10 s and release *Side-lying* Leg and arm exercises: leg lifts: lift top leg slightly up, hold for 5–10 s, and then release, focusing on gluteus medius and thigh muscles Arm reach: extend the top arm upward or outward, holding it in place to engage the shoulder. Move your fingers—spread them wide and then curl them gently—to engage smaller hand muscles Hip press: press hips gently into the bed, activating core and hip stabilizers Side bridge variation: with a slight lift of the trunk, hold a side bridge position with support from the lower arm

(continued)

Type of variation	Some examples
External variation: variation in sensorial input (visual, vestibular, proprioceptive)	Eye movements: exercises like closing one eye or moving the head up and down while performing the exercise in bed can enhance vestibular and proprioceptive balance PT is pointing a laser in different directions around the room. As you perform your exercise, follow the laser with your eyes. Or letters or numbers are projected on a wall or screen. As you do your exercise, try to read the letters or numbers in different directions Visual focus: engaging eyes to follow an object while lifting arms or legs in bed creates coordination between vision and movement
Internal variation: variation in the breathing	Breath synchronization with the exercise performed in bed: matching breathing patterns with exercise rhythm can improve respiratory control and muscle engagement Breath intensity adjustments to the exercise performed in bed: adjusting between shallow and deep breathing can have a calming effect on the nervous system. Remember, you can breathe through different pathways. Inhaling through the teeth: gently inhale through your teeth, allowing the air to pass between them with a soft, controlled sound Inhaling through the tongue (Ujjayi breathing): inhale through the tongue, making a soft sound in the back of the throat (similar to "ocean breath" in yoga, known as Ujjayi) Nostril breathing: Begin by closing the right nostril with your thumb and inhaling through the left nostril. Close the left nostril with your ring finger, and exhale through the right nostril. Alternative: switch sides, closing the left nostril and inhaling through the right and then closing the right nostril and exhaling through the left *Lying supine (on back)* Slow inhalation with arm raises: breathe in deeply through the nose, raising one or both arms above the chest, and then slowly exhale while lowering them Exhale on leg presses: perform a leg press into the bed while exhaling, tightening the core gently on each exhalation Deep abdominal breathing: focus on expanding the abdomen during inhalation, holding briefly, and then slowly exhaling through the mouth to engage deep abdominal muscles. Wiggle your toes gently during inhalation and relaxation to enhance lower-body awareness Paired breath holds with core activation: inhale, hold, and then squeeze core muscles. Take a deep breath, hold briefly, and then gently contract the core muscles while exhaling slowly to enhance core stability Alternating breath and muscle contraction: inhale deeply, press arms or legs against the bed during exhalation, and repeat with different limbs for a full-body activation. During each limb press, spread your fingers or toes wide and then relax them to include distal joint activation *Lying prone (on stomach)* Controlled breathing to activate the back muscles: alternate rhythmic breaths: 4-6-8 or 4-8-6. You can experiment with different breathing counts to increase the challenge and intensity of back muscle activation. As the rhythm lengthens (e.g., 4-8-6), you will feel a greater emphasis on breath control Long exhalations with arm/leg raises: inhale deeply and then slowly raise one arm or leg off the bed, exhaling completely to engage lower back muscles Abdominal bracing with breath holds: take a deep breath in, hold briefly, and then exhale slowly while bracing the abdomen and lower back Short breaths with upper body movements: "Sniff" Breathing for shoulder lifts: take three quick, shallow breaths in through the nose ("sniffs") while lifting shoulders slightly off the bed, and then exhale fully while lowering Back and chest coordination: focus on breathing into the lower back by expanding ribs outward, and then exhale while gently pressing the chest into the bed to activate stabilizers *Side-lying* Deep inhalation for side expansion: focus on expanding the ribcage on the side that is facing up. Inhale deeply, feeling the ribs expand, and then exhale to relax and engage the side core Paired breathing with leg lifts: inhale deeply, and then lift the top leg while exhaling, holding the leg position briefly before releasing it down Breathing and core activation with shoulder or hip movements: inhale for shoulder stabilization. With the bottom arm under the head, inhale deeply to stabilize the shoulder, and then exhale and gently lift the top arm or leg to engage core and hip muscles Side squeeze breathing: take a deep breath in and then exhale slowly while gently squeezing both sides of the ribcage, as if drawing them toward the center. While squeezing, rotate the wrists in small circles or wiggle your fingers and toes to incorporate distal joint movement

(continued)

Type of variation	Some examples
Internal variation: variation in the imagination	*Supine imagery exercises:* Floating in water: visualize being buoyant on water, using gentle leg and arm movements as if floating. Imagining water resistance can enhance the sense of movement and relaxation. Picture the subtle resistance of the water against your limbs as you make gentle movements. This resistance helps guide your movements, adding to the feeling of relaxation and ease Hint: as you float, let your body naturally sway in the water, feeling each arm or leg move with calm resistance, like you are gliding effortlessly Embryo position: picture yourself as an embryo, curled in a protective, nurturing space. Imagine a strong beam of energy emerging from your core, connecting to your limbs. As you gently move or stretch, feel this energy activating the muscles that provide you with stability, like a supportive force that helps you grow and rise. Focus on how your core feels as you move—like the center of your being radiating strength, supporting your arms or legs as if they are extensions of your body's energy Hedgehog position (curled and protected): imagine yourself as a hedgehog, curled into a ball for protection. The energy from your core connects to your limbs, offering stability as you brace against the world. As you expand, feel the core tighten and support every small movement, just like a hedgehog's protective armor that keeps it stable and safe. Visualize the strength of your core as your "armor," supporting and protecting your movements. When you move your arms or legs, they feel grounded and stable, like the hedgehog moving with confidence despite its small size Eagle position (open and expansive): picture yourself as an eagle soaring through the sky. The core acts as the central force, with the energy of your body extending into your limbs, providing balance and freedom in flight. As you stretch your arms or legs, feel the lift and stability, as if your core is the anchor that helps you glide through the air with ease and control Arm and leg movements with weightless imagery: visualize lifting arms and legs in space, creating the feeling of weightlessness as if supported by gentle waves *Prone imagery exercises:* Swimming stroke simulation: imagine doing a slow, controlled swimming stroke to engage back and shoulder muscles without actual movement Skydiving visualization: envision the sensation of being suspended in air; as patients raise their arms or legs, imagine pushing against an invisible surface Sand resistance: visualize pressing down on sand as if pushing arms and legs into the ground, creating an added sense of resistance. While pressing your arms, flex and extend your wrists, or gently spread and curl your fingers to engage the hand and forearm muscles. Similarly, while pressing your legs, flex your ankles (toes up) and then point your toes downward to activate the calves and foot muscles *Seated imagery exercises:* Rocking chair motion: imagine being on a gentle rocking chair, swaying back and forth with controlled trunk activation and leg movement. Simultaneously, move your wrists slightly or spread and curl your fingers Squeezing a balloon: visualize holding a balloon between the knees, squeezing gently for inner thigh engagement Climbing visualization: picture climbing stairs or a hill, lifting knees with a steady rhythm, focusing on the imagined sense of ascent and resistance *Wheelchair or rollator imagery:* Propelling through water: imagine moving through water while gripping handles, using controlled motions to propel forward with resistance Leaping over hurdles: picture lifting legs as if over hurdles, activating hip flexors, or as if marching in place with high steps. When lowering, press your toes downward Wind resistance: imagine a breeze while pushing against it with arms or legs, creating an added sense of force with each movement. As you push forward with your arms, rotate your wrists slightly and spread your fingers wide to simulate cutting through the air. When pulling back, curl your fingers into a loose fist to engage the forearm muscles
External variation: variation of the context	Music beats: different beats can motivate patients to vary movement speeds, adding an element of rhythmic noise while performing exercise in bed Personal motivation: engaging the patient's motivation can affect how actively they participate, impacting the recovery process once they are in bed

(continued)

Type of variation	Some examples
Variation in the intensity	Speed variations: alternating speeds during exercises—beginning slowly and then accelerating—can improve both fast and slow muscle fiber engagement Attention focus: patients can vary focus between internal (muscle feeling) and external (imagining hot/cold surfaces) to enhance neuromuscular control Internal focus: concentrate on the sensation of specific muscles as they engage. For arms, focus on how your wrist and finger movements feel—such as spreading your fingers or curling them into a fist—while performing a larger movement. For legs, notice the stretch or tension in your ankles and toes as you flex or point them during an exercise External focus (Imagining surfaces): picture touching hot or cold surfaces with your hands or feet. For hands, imagine brushing fingertips across an icy or warm surface, alternately spreading your fingers wide and then gently curling them. For feet, pretend to press your toes onto hot sand or cold tiles, engaging the toes and ankles in reaction Switching attention: alternate between focusing internally on how muscles feel and externally on imagined sensations or resistance. While shifting focus, integrate small movements like wrist rotations or ankle circles to deepen neuromuscular engagement Directional changes: rotating or moving in various directions, especially with movements like leg lifts in bed, engages multiple stabilizing muscles

Additional variation might come from the HIIT structure:

- Intensity: Referring to the level of exertion during exercises
- Exercise selection: Involving the selection of exercises within a session and applying the DL principles to a single exercise that is being performed
- Stimulus time: Reflecting the duration constituting the training load indicator
- Duration of sets: Signifying the length of each set
- Intervals between exercises: Including the time and frequency of rest between sets
- Training duration: Denoting the overall length of the HIIT session
- Recovery intensity and time: Factors influencing the training load indicator

HIIT's versatility allows for modification based on individual fitness levels and special conditions, with intensity set as a percentage of the maximum. It can be adapted to various exercise modes, from cycling to bed exercises. DL emphasizes frequent switching between intensity levels, which enhances both metabolic and neuromuscular adaptations. By crossing physiological thresholds, "noise" can activate specific energy systems, improving performance. Studies show that carefully applying intensity, interval timing, and recovery can restore functional capacity, enhance strength, and improve cardiovascular health in rehabilitation. When combined with DL, HIIT becomes a powerful tool for optimizing health and rehabilitation.

Questions

1. How can you improve your metabolic flexibility in daily life by incorporating different types of exercise, including HIIT?
2. When designing your own HIIT workout, how can you balance stimulus time, training time, and recovery intensity to match your fitness goals?
3. How can incorporating unique movement patterns and varied exercises in HIIT, as suggested by differential learning, enhance your strength, agility, and injury prevention?
4. Have you ever noticed how unexpected variations in movement improve learning and coordination during exercise? How can you apply this principle, using differential learning, to physiotherapy sessions for patients, especially those aiming to improve mobility?
5. How can you adapt physiotherapy exercises to match a patient's daily energy levels and recovery state, using principles of differential learning to improve metabolic flexibility and enhance movement patterns over time, rather than following a rigid routine?

6. Which of the following adaptations is associated with HIIT in skeletal muscles?
   A. Decrease in mitochondrial content
   B. Increased protein expression related to antioxidant regulation
   C. Reduced muscle mass
   D. Decreased neuromuscular coordination
7. Match the adaptation with its corresponding effect
   A. Mitochondrial health
   B. Cardiopulmonary system
   C. Metabolic health
      (i) Increases VO_2max and improves blood pressure regulation
      (ii) Enhances mitochondrial biogenesis and removal of dysfunctional mitochondria
      (iii) Reduces body fat percentage and increases muscle mass
8. What does the DL model emphasize in the context of motor learning?
   A. Consistency in exercise regimens
   B. Learning through stochastic perturbations
   C. Strict adherence to traditional training methods
   D. The importance of individual variability in training
9. In terms of exercise selection, which of the following is suggested for enhancing neuromuscular adaptation in HIIT programs?
   A. Focusing only on high-intensity exercises
   B. Including exercises with unique movement patterns and combinations of movements
   C. Using the same exercises in every session
   D. Avoiding complex exercises
10. What is a key principle behind the differential learning model in rehabilitation?
   A. Emphasizing uniformity in exercise performance
   B. Encouraging variability and adaptation through different motor tasks
   C. Focusing solely on the objective data of structured exercise
   D. Minimizing the subjective feedback from the body

References

Alizadeh Pahlavani H, Laher I, Knechtle B, Zouhal H (2022) Exercise and mitochondrial mechanisms in patients with sarcopenia. Front Physiol 13:1040381. https://doi.org/10.3389/fphys.2022.1040381. eCollection 2022

Ammar A, Simak ML, Salem A, Horst F, Schöllhorn WI (2024) Unveiling individuality in the early phase of motor learning: a machine learning approach for analysing weightlifting technique in novices. Front Bioeng Biotechnol 12:1426058. https://doi.org/10.3389/fbioe.2024.1426058

Balagué N, Hristovski R, Aragonés D, Tenenbaum G (2012) Nonlinear model of attention focus during accumulated effort. Psychol Sport Exerc 13(5):591–597. https://doi.org/10.1016/j.psychsport.2012.02.013

Bathina S, Das UN (2015) Brain-derived neurotrophic factor and its clinical implications. Arch Med Sci 11(6):1164–1178. https://doi.org/10.5114/aoms.2015.56342

Bauer G (2007) Veränderung von physiologischen und biomechanischen Parametern durch den Einsatz eines differentiellen Techniktrainings im Radsport. na

Begliuomini S, Lenzi E, Ninni F, Casarosa E, Merlini S, Pluchino N et al (2008) Plasma brain-derived neurotrophic factor daily variations in men: correlation with cortisol circadian rhythm. J Endocrinol 197(2):429. https://doi.org/10.1677/JOE-07-0376

Biddle SJH, Batterham AM (2015) High-intensity interval exercise training for public health: a big HIT or shall we HIT it on the head? Int J Behav Nutr Phys Act 12:1–8. https://doi.org/10.1186/s12966-015-0254-9

Blackmore DG, Schaumberg M, Ziaei M, Belford S, To XV, O'Keeffe I et al (2024) Long-term improvement in hippocampal-dependent learning ability in healthy, aged individuals following high intensity interval training. Aging Dis 16(3):1732–1754. https://doi.org/10.14336/AD.2024.0642

Brito LC, Fecchio RY, Peçanha T, Andrade-Lima A, Halliwill JR, Forjaz CLM (2018) Postexercise hypotension as a clinical tool: a "single brick" in the wall. J Am Soc Hypertens 12(12):e59–e64. https://doi.org/10.1016/j.jash.2018.10.006

Buchheit M, Laursen PB (2013) High-intensity interval training, solutions to the programming puzzle: Part I: cardiopulmonary emphasis. Sports Med 43(5):313–338. https://doi.org/10.1007/s40279-013-0029-x

Camerino C, Conte E, Cannone M, Caloiero R, Fonzino A, Tricarico D (2016) Nerve growth factor, brain-derived neurotrophic factor and osteocalcin gene relationship in energy regulation, bone homeostasis and reproductive organs analyzed by mRNA quantitative evaluation and linear correlation analysis. Front Physiol 7:456. https://doi.org/10.3389/fphys.2016.00456

Carello C, Turvey MT, Kugler PN (1985) The informational support for upright stance. Behavioral and Brain Sciences 8(1):151–152. https://doi.org/10.1017/S0140525X00020021

Chrøis KM, Dohlmann TL, Søgaard D, Hansen CV, Dela F, Helge JW, Larsen S (2020) Mitochondrial adaptations to high intensity interval training in older females and males. Eur J Sport Sci 20(1):135–145. https://doi.org/10.1080/17461391.2019.1615556

Delgado-Floody P, Izquierdo M, Ramirez-Velez R, Caamano-Navarrete F, Moris R, Jerez-Mayorga D et al (2020) Effect of high-intensity interval training on body composition, cardiorespiratory fitness, blood pressure, and substrate utilization during exercise among prehypertensive and hypertensive patients with excessive adiposity. Front Physiol 11:558910. https://doi.org/10.3389/fphys.2020.558910

Devin JL, Hill MM, Mourtzakis M, Quadrilatero J, Jenkins DG, Skinner TL (2019) Acute high intensity interval exercise reduces colon cancer cell growth. J Physiol 597(8):2177–2184. https://doi.org/10.1113/JP277648

Dun Y, Thomas RJ, Smith JR, Medina-Inojosa JR, Squires RW, Bonikowske AR et al (2019) High-intensity interval training improves metabolic syndrome and body composition in outpatient cardiac rehabilitation patients with myocardial infarction. Cardiovasc Diabetol 18:1–11. https://doi.org/10.1186/s12933-019-0907-0

Egan B, Carson BP, Garcia-Roves PM, Chibalin AV, Sarsfield FM, Barron N et al (2010) Exercise intensity-dependent regulation of peroxisome proliferator-activated receptor γ coactivator-1α mRNA abundance is associated with differential activation of upstream signalling kinases in human skeletal muscle. J Physiol 588(10):1779–1790. https://doi.org/10.1113/jphysiol.2010.188011

Ekblom B (1968) Effect of physical training on oxygen transport system in man

Ekblom B, Kilbom Å, Soltysiak J (1973) Physical training, bradycardia, and autonomic nervous system. Scand J Clin Lab Invest 32(3):251–256. https://doi.org/10.3109/00365517309082468

Feito Y, Heinrich KM, Butcher SJ, Poston WSC (2018) High-intensity functional training (HIFT): definition and research implications for improved fitness. Sports 6(3):76. https://doi.org/10.3390/sports6030076

Feito Y, Brown C, Olmos A (2019) A content analysis of the high-intensity functional training literature: a look at the past and directions for the future. Hum Mov 20(2):1–15. https://doi.org/10.5114/hm.2019.81020

Follador L, Alves RC, Ferreira SDS, Buzzachera CF, Andrade VFDS, Garcia EDS d A et al (2018) Physiological, perceptual, and affective responses to six high-intensity interval training protocols. Percept Mot Skills 125(2):329–350. https://doi.org/10.1177/0031512518754584

Fox SM III (1971) Physical activity and the prevention of coronary heart disease. Ann Clin Res 3:404–432

Frank TD, Michelbrink M, Beckmann H, Schöllhorn WI (2008) A quantitative dynamical systems approach to differential learning: self-organization principle and order parameter equations. Biol Cybern 98(1):19–31. https://doi.org/10.1007/s00422-007-0193-x

Gao AW, Cantó C, Houtkooper RH (2014) Mitochondrial response to nutrient availability and its role in metabolic disease. EMBO Mol Med 6(5):580–589. https://doi.org/10.1002/emmm.201303782

Gettman LR, Pollock ML (1981) Circuit weight training: a critical review of its physiological benefits. Phys Sportsmed 9(1):44–60. https://doi.org/10.1080/00913847.1981.11710988

Gettman LR, Ward P, Hagan RD, Monteiro AG, Alveno DA, Prado M et al (1982) A comparison of combined running and weight training with circuit weight training. J Sports Med Phys Fitness 14(4):229–234

Gibala MJ, McGee SL, Garnham AP, Howlett KF, Snow RJ, Hargreaves M (2009) Brief intense interval exercise activates AMPK and p38 MAPK signaling and increases the expression of PGC-1α in human skeletal muscle. J Appl Physiol 106:929. https://doi.org/10.1152/japplphysiol.90880.2008

Gillen JB, Gibala MJ (2014) Is high-intensity interval training a time-efficient exercise strategy to improve health and fitness? Appl Physiol Nutr Metab 39(3):409–412. https://doi.org/10.1139/apnm-2013-0187

Girginov V (2004) Totalitarian sport: Towards an understanding of its logic, practice and legacy. Totalitarian Mov Polit Relig 5(1):25–58. https://doi.org/10.1080/1469076042000223392

Gokeler A, Nijmeijer EM, Heuvelmans P, Tak I, Ramponi C, Benjaminse A (2023) Motor learning principles during rehabilitation after anterior cruciate ligament injury: Time to create an enriched environment to improve clinical outcome. Arthroskopie 36(3):164–170. https://doi.org/10.1007/s00142-023-00606-1

Golightly YM, Smith-Ryan AE, Blue MNM, Alvarez C, Allen KD, Nelson AE (2021) High-intensity interval training for knee osteoarthritis: a pilot study. ACR Open Rheumatol 3(10):723–732. https://doi.org/10.1002/acr2.11318

Gollnick PD, Piehl K, Saltin B (1974) Selective glycogen depletion pattern in human muscle fibres after exercise of varying intensity and at varying pedalling rates. J Physiol 241(1):45–57. https://doi.org/10.1113/jphysiol.1974.sp010639

Halliwill JR, Sieck DC, Romero SA, Buck TM, Ely MR (2014) Blood pressure regulation X: what happens when the muscle pump is lost? Post-exercise hypotension and syncope. Eur J Appl Physiol 114:561–578. https://doi.org/10.1007/s00421-013-2761-1

Hardman AE, Williams C, Wootton SA (1986) The influence of short-term endurance training on maximum oxygen uptake, submaximum endurance and the ability to perform brief, maximal exercise. J. Sports Sci 4:109–116. https://doi.org/10.1080/02640418608732106

Henz D, John A, Merz C, Schöllhorn WI (2018) Post-task effects on EEG brain activity differ for various differential learning and contextual interference protocols.

Front Hum Neurosci 12:19. https://doi.org/10.3389/fnhum.2018.00019

Hickson RC, Bomze HA, Holloszy JO (1977) Linear increase in aerobic power induced by a strenuous program of endurance exercise. J. Appl. Physiol 42:372–376. https://doi.org/10.1152/jappl.1977.42.3.372

Holt KG, Wagenaar RO, Saltzman E (2010) A dynamic systems: constraints approach to rehabilitation. Braz J Phys Ther 14:446–463. https://doi.org/10.1590/S1413-35552010000600002

Hopper K, Hollister W, Davey R, Semler A (1985) Release of galactosyltransferase from peritoneal macrophages during acute inflammation. Journal of cellular physiology 124(1):137–145. https://doi.org/10.1002/jcp.1041240122

Horst F, Hoitz F, Slijepcevic D, Schons N, Beckmann H, Nigg BM, Schöllhorn WI (2023) Identification of subject-specific responses to footwear during running. Scientific Reports 13(1):11284. https://doi.org/10.1038/s41598-023-38090-0

Horst F, Janssen D, Beckmann H, Schöllhorn WI (2020) Can individual movement characteristics across different throwing disciplines be identified in high-performance decathletes? Front Psychol 11:2262. https://doi.org/10.3389/fpsyg.2020.02262

Ito S (2019) High-intensity interval training for health benefits and care of cardiac diseases-the key to an efficient exercise protocol. World J Cardiol 11(7):171. https://doi.org/10.4330/wjc.v11.i7.171

Jiménez-Maldonado A, Cerna-Cortés J, Castro-Rodríguez EM, Montero SA, Muñiz J, Rodríguez-Hernández A et al (2016) Effects of moderate-and high-intensity chronic exercise on brain-derived neurotrophic factor expression in fast and slow muscles. Muscle Nerve 53(3):446–451. https://doi.org/10.1002/mus.24757

John AT, Barthel A, Wind J, Rizzi N, Schöllhorn WI (2022) Acute effects of various movement noise in differential learning of rope skipping on brain and heart recovery analyzed by means of multiscale fuzzy measure entropy. Front Behav Neurosci 16:816334. https://doi.org/10.3389/fnbeh.2022.816334

Josyula S, Alagesan J (2024) Comparative analysis of high-intensity interval training and traditional rehabilitation programs for accelerated recovery from musculoskeletal injuries. J Back Musculoskelet Rehabil 37(2):437–443. https://doi.org/10.3233/BMR-230146

Karvelis M, Slapšinskaitė Dackevičienė A (2021) Does physical exercises make a difference for risk of falling and independence of the elderly? In: The 7th international scientific conference "exercise for health and rehabilitation": the 3rd of December, 2021 Kaunas, Lithuania: book of abstracts/Lithuanian University of Health Sciences. Department of Sports Medicine, Lithuanian Federation of Sports Medicine, Kaunas

Kessler HS, Sisson SB, Short KR (2012) The potential for high-intensity interval training to reduce cardiometabolic disease risk. Sports Med 42(6):489–509. https://doi.org/10.2165/11630910-000000000-00000

Kortmann T, Schöllhorn WI (2006) Neue Ansätze der Bewegungswissenschaft als Grundlage für ein modernes Techniktraining im Rudern–Bewegungsstabilität durch Wiederholung oder durch Adaptation? Berichtsband Rudersymposium

Krüger A (2002) Strength through joy: the culture of consent under fascism, Nazism and Francoism. In: The international politics of sport in the twentieth century. Routledge, London, pp 77–99

Lee AS, Johnson NA, McGill MJ, Overland J, Luo C, Baker CJ et al (2020) Effect of high-intensity interval training on glycemic control in adults with type 1 diabetes and overweight or obesity: a randomized controlled trial with partial crossover. Diabetes Care 43(9):2281–2288. https://doi.org/10.2337/dc20-0342

Little JP, Gillen JB, Percival ME, Safdar A, Tarnopolsky MA, Punthakee Z et al (2011a) Low-volume high-intensity interval training reduces hyperglycemia and increases muscle mitochondrial capacity in patients with type 2 diabetes. J Appl Physiol 111(6):1554–1560. https://doi.org/10.1152/japplphysiol.00921.2011

Little JP, Safdar A, Bishop D, Tarnopolsky MA, Gibala MJ (2011b) An acute bout of high-intensity interval training increases the nuclear abundance of PGC-1α and activates mitochondrial biogenesis in human skeletal muscle. Am J Physiol Regul Integr Comp Physiol 300:R1303. https://doi.org/10.1152/ajpregu.00538.2010

Londeree BR, Moeschberger ML (1982) Effect of age and other factors on maximal heart rate. Res Q Exerc Sport 53(4):297–304. https://doi.org/10.1080/02701367.1982.10605252

Lu Y, Wiltshire HD, Baker JS, Wang Q (2021) Effects of high intensity exercise on oxidative stress and antioxidant status in untrained humans: a systematic review. Biology 10(12):1272. https://doi.org/10.3390/biology10121272

Lu Y, Wiltshire HD, Baker JS, Wang Q, Ying S (2023) The effect of Tabata-style functional high-intensity interval training on cardiometabolic health and physical activity in female university students. Front Physiol 14:1095315. https://doi.org/10.3389/fphys.2023.1095315

Machado AF, Baker JS, Figueira Junior AJ, Bocalini DS (2019) High-intensity interval training using whole-body exercises: training recommendations and methodological overview. Clin Physiol Funct Imaging 39(6):378–383. https://doi.org/10.1111/cpf.12433

MacInnis MJ, Gibala MJ (2017) Physiological adaptations to interval training and the role of exercise intensity. J Physiol 595(9):2915–2930. https://doi.org/10.1113/JP273196

Martland R, Mondelli V, Gaughran F, Stubbs B (2020) Can high intensity interval training improve health outcomes among people with mental illness? A systematic review and preliminary meta-analysis of inter-

vention studies across a range of mental illnesses. J Affect Disord 263:629–660. https://doi.org/10.1080/02640414.2019.1706829
Matveyev LP (1964) Problem of periodization the sport training. FiS Publisher, Moscu
Matveev LP (1965) Das Problem der Periodisierung des sportlichen Trainings. DSB/BAL
Matveev LP (1981) Fundamentals of sports training. Progress Publishers, Moscow
McRae G, Payne A, Zelt JGE, Scribbans TD, Jung ME, Little JP, Gurd BJ (2012) Extremely low volume, whole-body aerobic–resistance training improves aerobic fitness and muscular endurance in females. Appl Physiol Nutr Metab 37(6):1124–1131. https://doi.org/10.1139/h2012-093
Medbo JI, Tabata I (1989) Relative importance of aerobic and anaerobic energy release during short-lasting exhausting bicycle exercise. J Appl Physiol 67(5):1881–1886. https://doi.org/10.1152/jappl.1989.67.5.1881
Memme JM, Erlich AT, Phukan G, Hood DA (2021) Exercise and mitochondrial health. J Physiol 599(3):803–817. https://doi.org/10.1113/JP278853
Morris NR, Hill K, Walsh J, Sabapathy S (2021) Exercise & Sports Science Australia (ESSA) position statement on exercise and chronic obstructive pulmonary disease. J Sci Med Sport 24(1):52–59. https://doi.org/10.1016/j.jsams.2020.08.007
Murawska-Ciałowicz E, de Assis GG, Clemente FM, Feito Y, Stastny P, Zuwała-Jagiełło J et al (2021) Effect of four different forms of high intensity training on BDNF response to Wingate and Graded Exercise Test. Sci Rep 11(1):8599. https://doi.org/10.1038/s41598-021-88069-y
Nes BM, Janszky I, Wisløff U, Støylen A, Karlsen T (2013) Age-predicted maximal heart rate in healthy subjects: The HUNT Fitness Study. Scand J Med Sci Sports 23(6):697–704. https://doi.org/10.1111/j.1600-0838.2012.01445.x
Nofuji YU, Suwa M, Moriyama Y, Nakano H, Ichimiya A, Nishichi R et al (2008) Decreased serum brain-derived neurotrophic factor in trained men. Neurosci Lett 437(1):29–32. https://doi.org/10.1016/j.neulet.2008.03.057
Nofuji Y, Suwa M, Sasaki H, Ichimiya A, Nishichi R, Kumagai S (2012) Different circulating brain-derived neurotrophic factor responses to acute exercise between physically active and sedentary subjects. J Sports Sci Med 11(1):83. https://doi.org/10.3390/ijerph19010317
Oftadeh S, Bahram A, Yaali R, Ghadiri F, Schöllhorn WI (2021) External focus or differential learning: is there an additive effect on learning a futsal goal kick? Int J Environ Res Public Health 19(1):317. https://doi.org/10.3390/ijerph19010317
Olson M (2014) TABATA: it'sa HIIT! ACSMs Health Fit J 18(5):17–24. https://doi.org/10.1249/FIT.0000000000000065
Ozolin NG (1970) Sovremennaya sistema sportivnoy trenirovki [Modern system of sports training]. Physical Education and Sports Publication, Moscow
Park EJ, Truong V-L, Jeong W-S, Min W-K (2024) Brain-derived neurotrophic factor (BDNF) enhances osteogenesis and may improve bone microarchitecture in an ovariectomized rat model. Cells 13(6):518. https://doi.org/10.1016/j.jhep.2019.06.030
Ramírez-Vélez R, Tordecilla-Sanders A, Téllez-T LA, Camelo-Prieto D, Hernández-Quiñonez PA, Correa-Bautista JE et al (2020) Effect of moderate-versus high-intensity interval exercise training on heart rate variability parameters in inactive Latin-American adults: a randomized clinical trial. J Strength Cond Res 34(12):3403–3415. https://doi.org/10.1519/JSC.0000000000001833
Repšaitė V, Vainoras A, Berškienė K, Baltaduonienė D, Daunoravičienė A, Sendžikaitė E (2015) The effect of differential training-based occupational therapy on hand and arm function in patients after stroke: results of the pilot study. Neurol Neurochir Pol 49(3):150–155. https://doi.org/10.1016/j.pjnns.2015.04.001
Rosset-Llobet J, Fàbregas-Molas S (2018) Rehabilitation and plasticity of task-specific focal hand dystonia. In: Dressler D, Altenmüller E, Krauss JK (eds) Treatment of dystonia. Cambridge University Press, Cambridge, pp 256–260
Roxburgh BH, Campbell HA, Cotter JD, Reymann U, Williams MJA, Gwynne-Jones D, Thomas KN (2023) Acute and adaptive cardiovascular and metabolic effects of passive heat therapy or high-intensity interval training in patients with severe lower-limb osteoarthritis. Physiol Rep 11(11):e15699. https://doi.org/10.14814/phy2.15699
Sabag A, Little JP, Johnson NA (2022) Low-volume high-intensity interval training for cardiometabolic health. J Physiol 600(5):1013–1026. https://doi.org/10.1113/JP281210
Sanchez-Padilla J, Guzman JN, Ilijic E, Kondapalli J, Galtieri DJ, Yang B et al (2014) Mitochondrial oxidant stress in locus coeruleus is regulated by activity and nitric oxide synthase. Nat Neurosci 17(6):832–840. https://doi.org/10.1038/nn.3717
Schmidt D, Anderson K, Graff M, Strutz V (2015) The effect of high-intensity circuit training on physical fitness. J Sports Med Phys Fitness 56(5):534–540
Schöllhorn WI (1999) Individualität-ein vernachlässigter Parameter. Leistungssport 29(2):5–12.
Schöllhorn WI, Beckmann H, Davids K (2010) Exploiting system fluctuations. Differential training in physical prevention and rehabilitation programs for health and exercise. Medicina 46(6):365. https://doi.org/10.3390/medicina46060052
Slapsinskaite A, Razon S, Serre NB, Hristovski R, Tenenbaum G, Reddy H et al (2015) Local pain dynamics during constant exhaustive exercise. PLoS One 10(9):e0137895. https://doi.org/10.1371/journal.pone.0137895
Slapsinskaite A, García S, Razon S, Balagué N, Hristovski R, Tenenbaum G (2016) Cycling outdoors facilitates external thoughts and endurance. Psychol Sport Exerc 27:78–84. https://doi.org/10.1016/j.psychsport.2016.08.002

Slapsinskaite A, Hristovski R, Razon S, Balagué N, Tenenbaum G, Slapšinskaite A et al (2017) Metastable pain-attention dynamics during incremental exhaustive exercise. Front Psychol 7:1–9. https://doi.org/10.3389/fpsyg.2016.02054

Slapšinskaitė A, Razon S, Balagué N, Ščiupokas A, Hristovski R, Tenenbaum G (2018) Idiosyncratic pain patterns during exhaustive exercise. Glob J Health Sci 10(6):44. https://doi.org/10.5539/gjhs.v10n6p44

Smith RL, Soeters MR, Wüst RCI, Houtkooper RH (2018) Metabolic flexibility as an adaptation to energy resources and requirements in health and disease. Endocr Rev 39(4):489–517. https://doi.org/10.1210/er.2017-00211

Søgaard D, Lund MT, Scheuer CM, Dehlbaek MS, Dideriksen SG, Abildskov CV et al (2018) High-intensity interval training improves insulin sensitivity in older individuals. Acta Physiol 222(4):e13009. https://doi.org/10.1111/apha.13009

Sorriento D, Di Vaia E, Iaccarino G (2021) Physical exercise: a novel tool to protect mitochondrial health. Front Physiol 12:660068. https://doi.org/10.3389/fphys.2021.660068

Spinelli JB, Haigis MC (2018) The multifaceted contributions of mitochondria to cellular metabolism. Nat Cell Biol 20(7):745–754. https://doi.org/10.1038/s41556-018-0124-1

Su L, Fu J, Sun S, Zhao G, Cheng W, Dou C, Quan M (2019) Effects of HIIT and MICT on cardiovascular risk factors in adults with overweight and/or obesity: a meta-analysis. PLoS One 14(1):e0210644. https://doi.org/10.1371/journal.pone.0210644

Tabata I (2019) Tabata training: one of the most energetically effective high-intensity intermittent training methods. J Physiol Sci 69(4):559–572. https://doi.org/10.1007/s12576-019-00676-7

Tabata I (2022) Tabata training: the science and history of HIIT. Academic Press, London.

Tabata I, Irisawa K, Kouzaki M, Nishimura K, Ogita F, Miyachi M (1997) Metabolic profile of high intensity intermittent exercises. Med Sci Sports Exerc 29(3):390–395. https://doi.org/10.1097/00005768-199703000-00015

Tanaka H, Monahan KD, Seals DR (2001) Age-predicted maximal heart rate revisited. J Am Coll Cardiol 37(1):153–156. https://doi.org/10.1016/s0735-1097(00)01054-8

Turvey MT, Romaniak-Gross C, Isenhower RW, Arzamarski R, Harrison S, Carello C (2009) Human odometer is gait-symmetry specific. Proc R Soc B Biol Sci 276(1677):4309–4314. https://doi.org/10.1098/rspb.2009.1134

Turvey MT, Harrison SJ, Frank TD, Carello C (2012) Human odometry verifies the symmetry perspective on bipedal gaits. J Exp Psychol Hum Percept Perform 38(4):1014. https://doi.org/10.1037/a0027853

Vainauskas E, Slapšinskaitė-Dackevičienė A (2018) Repetitive or differential exercises are better for elderly women with lower back osteochondrosis? In: The 4th international scientific-practical conference "Exercise for health and rehabilitation": the 29th of November, 2018 Kaunas, Lithuania: book of abstracts/ Lithuanian University of Health Sciences. Institute of Sports, Lithuanian Federation of Sports, Kaunas

Vaz DV, Silva PL, Mancini MC, Carello C, Kinsella-Shaw J (2017) Towards an ecologically grounded functional practice in rehabilitation. Hum Mov Sci 52:117–132. https://doi.org/10.1016/j.humov.2017.01.010

Wallace JP, Bogle PG, King BA, Krasnoff JB, Jastremski CA (1999) The magnitude and duration of ambulatory blood pressure reduction following acute exercise. J Hum Hypertens 13(6):361–366. https://doi.org/10.1038/sj.jhh.1000797

Washif JA, Teichmann J, Kok L-Y, Schmidtbleicher D (2019) Using stochastic resonance and strength training as part of a rehabilitation programme for recurrent low back pain treatment: a case study. J Exercise Rehabil 15(1):139

Weston KS, Wisløff U, Coombes JS (2014) High-intensity interval training in patients with lifestyle-induced cardiometabolic disease: a systematic review and meta-analysis. Br J Sports Med 48(16):1227–1234. https://doi.org/10.1136/bjsports-2013-092576

White O, Babič J, Trenado C, Johannsen L, Goswami N (2019) The promise of stochastic resonance in falls prevention. Front Physiol 9:1865. https://doi.org/10.3389/fphys.2018.01865

Wilmore JH, Parr RB, Girandola RN, Ward P, Vodak PA, Barstow TJ et al (1978) Physiological alterations consequent to circuit weight training. Phys Sportsmed 9(2):115–120

Yamauchi N, Tamai K, Kimura I, Naito A, Tokuda N, Ashida Y et al (2023) High-intensity interval training in the form of isometric contraction improves fatigue resistance in dystrophin-deficient muscle. J Physiol 601(14):2917–2933. https://doi.org/10.1113/jp284532

Appendix: Questions and Answers: Solution

Chapter 1

1. **What are the two main assumptions in classical physiotherapy and training that the chapter critiques?**
   A universal, person- and time-independent "ideal" movement model can be applied to everyone.
   Such a model is best achieved by numerous repetitions and corrective copying of the supposed ideal.
2. **How does the concept of individuality in movement differ between "weak" and "strong" forms?**
   Weak individuality = everyday sense: no groups are found; movements look idiosyncratic but overlap; variability is often dismissed as "noise."
   Strong individuality = forensic standard: each person shows unique and reliably repeatable signatures that can identify them across time, a requirement now met by machine learning pattern recognition.
3. **Why do traditional statistical methods struggle to capture true individuality in motor behavior?**
   Classical analyses rely on group averages, linear models and a few discrete-time landmarks. Person-specific fluctuations are treated as error; intra- and inter-individual variance overlaps, so distinct signatures are blurred and individuality is effectively "averaged out."
4. **How does process-oriented analysis offer a more detailed view of movement variation than discrete-time approaches?**
   Process-oriented, time-continuous/topological methods track the whole waveform, revealing how both metrics and the underlying movement *shape* vary from trial to trial and across learning. Discretetime approaches capture only isolated points, so qualitative shifts in coordination remain hidden.
5. **What historical or cultural influences have shaped the belief in repetition as a foundation for learning?**
   The faith in repetition stems from military drill and obedience training (Sparta, Roman legions), classical pedagogy (Plato's advocacy of rote learning), and later industrial/behaviorist models that equated practice with laying deep "tracks." Phrases like the Roman maxim *Repetitio est mater studiorum* illustrate how these traditions canonized repetition in education, sport, and therapy.
6. **How do concepts like movement topology and movement metrics help explain qualitative changes in motor learning?**
   A. Both concepts only measure amplitude changes, so they cannot reveal qualitative differences.
   B. Topology captures changes in the *shape* or class of a movement, whereas metrics track size- or time-based adjustments; separating them makes true coordination shifts visible.

W. Schöllhorn, A. Slapšinskaitė-Dackevičienė (eds.), *Differential Learning in Physiotherapy*, https://doi.org/10.1007/978-3-031-98787-8

C. They are two ways of averaging group data to minimize variance.
D. Using them removes the need for time-continuous analysis.
E. They show that metrics are irrelevant for learning.

Correct answer: B. Topology captures changes in the *shape* or class of a movement, whereas metrics track size- or time-based adjustments; separating them makes true coordination shifts visible.

7. **Why might individuality in movement appear even at the beginning of the learning process?**
A. Group instruction quickly forces learners to diverge from each other.
B. Pattern-recognition studies of absolute beginners show stable, person-specific trajectories before much practice, implying anatomical-neuromotor uniqueness from the outset.
C. Early measurements are dominated by random error masquerading as individuality.
D. Novices share identical topologies, so individuality cannot be detected until later.
E. Equipment differences, not learners, create the first movement variations.

Correct answer: B. Pattern-recognition studies of absolute beginners show stable, person-specific trajectories before much practice, implying anatomicalneuromotor uniqueness from the outset.

8. **What challenges arise when trying to generalize therapeutic interventions based on group averages?**
A. Large between-person variability and tipping-point effects mean a protocol that helps the "average" can overshoot, stall, or backfire in many individuals.
B. Group averages guarantee that every patient will respond identically.
C. Averages reduce statistical power, making any intervention appear ineffective.
D. They eliminate ethical approval requirements, so studies become harder to publish.
E. Group data automatically account for all interaction effects among variables.

Correct answer: A. Large between-person variability and tipping-point effects mean a protocol that helps the "average" can overshoot, stall, or backfire in many individuals.

9. **How do epistemological concepts like uncertainty and nonlinearity affect how we interpret therapy outcomes?**
A. They indicate that classical physics provides an exact template for rehabilitation.
B. They prove that, with enough variables, perfect prediction of therapy success is possible.
C. They show causality in living systems is always linear and time reversible.
D. They justify ignoring individual differences because randomness cancels them out.
E. They remind us that outcomes are probabilistic and sensitive to small, often unmeasured factors, so predictions from any model remain tentative.

Correct answer: E. They remind us that outcomes are probabilistic and sensitive to small, often unmeasured factors, so predictions from any model remain tentative.

10. **How might a shift from repetition-based models to variability-based approaches change therapy or coaching practices?**
A. Treatment sessions would become shorter because variability removes the need for feedback.
B. Therapists would ask patients to stop practicing once a movement feels comfortable.
C. Coaches would focus exclusively on copying expert models with greater precision.
D. Practitioners would deliberately vary both metrics and topologies, treating individual differences as resources, thereby fostering adaptability instead of chasing a single "ideal" repetition.
E. Exercises would rely solely on machine-paced drills to enforce uniformity.

Correct answer: D. Practitioners would deliberately vary both metrics and topologies, treating individual differences as resources, thereby fostering adaptability instead of chasing a single "ideal" repetition.

Chapter 2

1. **What are the key philosophical and scientific differences between first- and second-order cybernetics?**
   First-order cybernetics views systems as objective and externally observable; the observer is separate from the system. Second-order cybernetics, in contrast, includes the observer within the system, recognizing that perception, context, and meaning shape understanding. In movement learning, this shift means learning is self-organized and context-dependent, not universally prescriptive.
2. **How does Differential Learning reinterpret variability and error within the learning process?**
   DL treats variability and error as integral to learning rather than obstacles. Purposeful variations ("noise") help the learner's system destabilize existing patterns and reorganize into new, more adaptive ones. Errors thus become opportunities for exploration and self-organization.
3. **In what ways does Differential Learning challenge repetition- and correction-based models of traditional motor learning?**
   DL opposes traditional models that focus on repeating ideal movements and minimizing deviations. It proposes that learners develop unique solutions through exploration and variability, leading to more robust and individualized motor skills.
4. **How is cybernetic feedback traditionally used in motor-learning theories and how does DL reinterpret it?**
   Traditional motor-learning theories use feedback loops to minimize errors and achieve a target model of movement. DL, however, emphasizes feedback as a means to stimulate change, allowing the learner to reorganize their own movement patterns without enforcing a fixed ideal.
5. **What is the significance of subjective information in the Differential Learning framework?**
   Subjective information represents the learner's internal perception, experience, and prior knowledge. DL uses this concept to tailor variability and learning conditions to each learner's individuality, rather than applying identical external conditions.
6. **How do the cerebellum, basal ganglia, and cerebral cortex contribute differently to movement control and learning?**
   A. All three act only as passive relays for spinal reflexes.
   B. Basal ganglia fine-tune eye movements, while cerebellum plans speech.
   C. Cerebral cortex stores vestibular reflexes and nothing else.
   D. Cerebellum times and smooths synergies, basal ganglia select/inhibit competing action "programs," and cerebral cortex plans and initiates voluntary movements.
   E. Each structure controls exactly one joint of the body.
   Correct answer: D. Cerebellum times and smooths synergies, basal ganglia select/inhibit competing action "programs", and cerebral cortex plans and initiates voluntary movements.
7. **What role do mirror neurons play in understanding movement and action in others?**
   A. They discharge only when we perform an action, never when we observe.
   B. They fire both when we execute an action and when we watch someone else do it, providing a neural basis for action understanding and imitation.
   C. They are vestibular cells that stabilize gaze during rotation.
   D. They inhibit cerebellar plasticity during repetitive drills.
   E. They create muscle twitches in the observer's limbs.
   Correct answer: B. They fire both when we execute an action and when we watch someone else do it, providing a neural basis for action understanding and imitation.

8. **How does cortical plasticity support learning even after developmental stages are complete?**
   A. Adult cortex becomes anatomically fixed and cannot change synapses.
   B. Neurons lose all dendritic spines once puberty ends.
   C. Training reduces BDNF levels, blocking new connections.
   D. Plasticity survives only in the spinal cord, not in the brain.
   E. Experience-dependent synaptic changes—e.g., neuronal growth modulated by BDNF—allow remapping and skill acquisition throughout life.

   Correct answer: E. Experience-dependent synaptic changes—e.g., neuronal growth modulated by BDNF—allow remapping and skill acquisition throughout life.
9. **Why is it problematic to treat perception and action as separate processes in movement science?**
   A. Neurophysiological evidence (e.g., readiness potentials, common-coding, mirror-neuron activations) shows tightly coupled, bidirectional loops, so splitting them ignores their integrated nature.
   B. Because perception stops once movement begins.
   C. Action pathways are located only in the spinal cord, perception only in the cortex.
   D. Separating them eliminates all neural noise, making learning impossible.
   E. It is not problematic; the two systems never interact.

   Correct answer: A. Neurophysiological evidence (e.g., readiness potentials, common-coding, mirror-neuron activations) shows tightly coupled, bidirectional loops, so splitting them ignores their integrated nature.
10. **How does the presented neurophysiological model support Differential Learning (DL) over repetition-based training?**
   A. It proves that eliminating variability accelerates synaptic growth.
   B. It shows vestibular dominance makes error-reduction essential.
   C. It emphasizes self-organizing plastic circuits driven by variable mechano-sensory input, aligning with DL's noise-rich, non-repetitive practice rather than uniform correction.
   D. It concludes that efference copies cancel all learning signals.
   E. It demonstrates that augmented external feedback is mandatory for change.

   Correct answer: C. It emphasizes self-organizing plastic circuits driven by variable mechano-sensory input, aligning with DL's noise-rich, non-repetitive practice rather than uniform correction.

Chapter 3

1. **What are the fundamental differences between traditional repetition-based training and the Differential Learning Approach?**

   Traditional approaches view skill acquisition as the gradual reduction of error toward a single "ideal" movement that must be rehearsed and corrected until it stabilizes. DL dismisses the notion of one best pattern: Every attempt is intentionally changed so that the neuromuscular system is bombarded with variable, sometimes "wrong" executions. The resulting noise destabilizes the old coordination, forces continuous self-organization, and yields an adaptable, rather than a uniform, solution.
2. **How does the concept of stochastic resonance contribute to motor learning and skill acquisition?**

   Stochastic resonance describes a nonlinear phenomenon in which an optimal level of random noise amplifies the detection of weak signals. In the motor domain, adding taskspecific fluctuations can elevate barely detectable proprioceptive cues above threshold, allowing the learner's nervous system to sense and exploit subtle information that would otherwise remain hidden.

3. **What role does movement variability play in enhancing adaptability and self-organization in motor learning?**
   Variation supplies the system with a rich search space of kinematic and kinetic possibilities. By exploring this space, the performer discovers multiple coordinative states and thereby becomes robust against perturbations. Variability is therefore not an error to be suppressed but a prerequisite for emergent stability and creative problem-solving.
4. **Which biomechanically based interventions lead to central nervous stimulation and self-organization?**
   Exercises that manipulate ground-reaction forces, joint torques, or segmental inertia (for example, changing shoe heel height, surface compliance, load distribution, or limb segmentation) create novel mechanoreceptive (beside all other sensory) input. Such altered afference travels via proprioceptive pathways to subcortical and cortical centers, provoking reorganization of internal models without the need for explicit instruction.
5. **What experimental evidence from sports supports the effectiveness of movement variability in learning and performance?**
   Empirical studies show that athletes who practiced sprint, hurdle sprint, shot put, basketball free throw, football goal shooting, volleyball perception and jumps or tennis serve with deliberately varied boundary conditions improved performance and transfer more than control groups who repeated the traditional textbook technique. Machine learning classifiers confirmed that successful athletes retained distinctive, non-average signatures rather than converging on a single "ideal" pattern.
6. **How can the stochastic resonance model be transferred to the training of endurance sports?**
   A. By adding white-noise audio during warm-up only.
   B. By periodically altering cadence, gradient, body-/extremity-posture, footwear hardness, etc., so that moderate biomechanical noise enhances proprioceptive sensitivity and aerobic efficiency.
   C. By holding speed constant and minimizing variability in stride.
   D. By replacing outdoor runs with treadmill sessions at fixed incline.
   E. By masking all sensory input with earplugs and blindfolds.
   Correct answer: B. By periodically altering cadence, gradient, body-/extremity-posture, footwear hardness, etc., so that moderate biomechanical noise enhances proprioceptive sensitivity and aerobic efficiency.
7. **In what ways can the principles of movement variability and self-organization be applied to physiotherapy and rehabilitation?**
   A. By prescribing one error-free movement and having the patient repeat it 200 times.
   B. By using robotic exoskeletons that lock joints into a single trajectory.
   C. By designing tasks that systematically vary load, direction and timing so the patient's nervous system explores alternative coordinations and selects the momentarily most functional.
   D. By eliminating any unpredictable surface or perturbation.
   E. By instructing the patient to observe but never perform the task.
   Correct answer: C. By designing tasks that systematically vary load, direction, and timing, so the patient's nervous system explores alternative coordinations and selects the momentarily most functional.
8. **What are the potential risks of too much or too little variability in training, and how can they be managed?**
   A. Excessive variability guarantees injury; zero variability guarantees mastery.
   B. Too little variability can lead to over-use syndromes and stagnation, whereas too much can cause chaos and inconsistent performance; regulating noise intensity and monitoring fatigue keeps variability in a beneficial window.
   C. High variability always improves motivation, so it carries no risk.

D. Low variability accelerates learning for all athletes.
E. Risks are irrelevant because the nervous system self-protects automatically.

Correct answer: B. Too little variability can lead to over-use syndromes and stagnation, whereas too much can cause chaos and inconsistent performance; regulating noise intensity and monitoring fatigue keeps variability in a beneficial window.

9. **How does the research presented in this chapter lay the groundwork for the application of DL in physiotherapy, as discussed in later chapters?**
   A. By proving that repetition is indispensable for neural recovery.
   B. By demonstrating that only visual feedback drives cortical change.
   C. By showing that spinal reflexes cannot be modified in adults.
   D. By documenting neurophysiological and biomechanical evidence that variable, noise-rich practice reorganizes central pathways, a principle later translated into patient-specific therapy protocols.
   E. By concluding that movement variability is detrimental to motor relearning.

   Correct answer: D. By documenting neurophysiological and biomechanical evidence that variable, noise-rich practice reorganizes central pathways, a principle later translated into patient-specific therapy protocols.

10. **How does DL challenge conventional assumptions about error correction and feedback in learning?**
   A. It requires continuous real-time verbal corrections from the coach.
   B. It replaces physical practice with mental imagery alone.
   C. It argues that external error correction can be counter-productive because amplified intrinsic variability already supplies sufficient information for self-optimization, reducing the need for augmented feedback.
   D. It keeps the traditional hierarchy but adds vibration to each joint.
   E. It views errors as pathological noise that must be eliminated immediately.

   Correct answer: C. It argues that external error correction can be counter-productive because amplified intrinsic variability already supplies sufficient information for selfoptimization, reducing the need for augmented feedback.

Chapter 4

1. **In what ways is the adaptability of a musician's motor system crucial for injury prevention and long-term performance?**

   Because it allows the system to respond effectively to internal or external changes, reducing the risk of injury and maintaining optimal function over time. A rigid system is more prone to dysfunction when demands increase or vary.

2. **How does focal dystonia illustrate the consequences of excessive rigidity in movement patterns?**

   Focal dystonia often arises in highly trained musicians whose neural systems cannot adapt to new demands. This rigidity impairs motor flexibility, leading to dysfunctional automatisms during performance.

3. **What are the key differences between traditional rehabilitation approaches and differential learning when addressing musician-related injuries?**

   Traditional approaches aim to restore or correct specific movements, often based on fixed models. In contrast, differential learning introduces variation and "noise" to promote self-organization and flexibility, helping the system find new, individualized solutions.

4. **Why has conventional music education emphasized imitating fixed models, and what are the potential drawbacks of this approach?**

   Because it assumes that the teacher's model is correct and efficient. However, this neglects individual variability and can reduce adaptability, increasing the risk of injury and limiting personal expression.

5. **How does the principle of self-organization in DL contrast with explicit technical correction in traditional pedagogy?**

   DL alters task constraints—different bow weights, fingerings, or body positions—so that intrinsic feedback and neural noise drive the emergence of a better pattern; traditional pedagogy diagnoses a fault and prescribes conscious technical fixes, keeping the teacher, not the system, in charge of change.

6. **How do sensory motor retuning (SMR) and differential learning (DL) complement each other when rehabilitating injured musicians?**

   A. SMR strengthens finger muscles, while DL focuses on rhythm and timing.
   B. SMR isolates healthy movement patterns; DL restores them through repetition.
   C. SMR alters perception and proprioception; DL introduces variability to enhance adaptability.
   D. SMR and DL are used sequentially: SMR before injury and DL after.
   E. SMR is cognitive therapy, while DL is purely physical.

   Correct answer: C. According to the text, SMR changes the proprioceptive perception of the task, helping to override dysfunctional automatisms. DL, on the other hand, induces fluctuations through variations that promote system reorganization and flexibility. Together, they target both perception and adaptability.

7. **Why may some musicians resist DL, and how can teachers ease its adoption?**

   A. Musicians resist DL because it discourages creativity, which teachers must accept.
   B. Musicians see DL as disorganized; teachers can convince them with scientific evidence.
   C. Musicians find DL boring; teachers should use humor to make it engaging.
   D. Musicians find DL uncomfortable due to unpredictability; teachers should clarify its purpose and guide creativity.
   E. Musicians are too experienced for DL; teachers should only apply it to beginners.

   Correct answer: D. Musicians often feel discomfort with the unpredictability and apparent "wrongness" of DL. Teachers can ease adoption by clearly explaining its purpose and encouraging the musician's creative input, which is often surprisingly limited during practice.

8. **How do instrument setup, posture, or practice routines affect neuromotor flexibility in musicians?**

   A. They have minimal impact if musicians warm up properly.
   B. Uniform routines build consistency, which always enhances flexibility.
   C. Repetition of fixed setups fosters accuracy and reduces stress.
   D. Lack of variability in posture and routines reduces flexibility and adaptability.
   E. Only incorrect posture affects flexibility, not practice routines.

   Correct answer: D. The text emphasizes that rigid, unchanging routines limit motor variability and reduce a musician's flexibility to adapt to different or evolving performance contexts, increasing injury risk. Varied practice supports a more adaptable neuromotor system.

9. **How can deliberate variability in practice enhance—rather than destabilize—performance consistency?**

   A. It increases conscious control of movements during concerts.
   B. It confuses the motor system temporarily, which weakens automatisms.
   C. It forces the body to abandon bad habits through constant correction.
   D. It trains the performer to focus more on the final sound than the movement.
   E. It builds flexible automatisms that are more resilient to change.

   Correct answer: E. DL works by creating instability that forces the motor system to reorganize, ultimately leading to more resilient and adaptable automatisms. This flexibility is essential for consistent performance under changing conditions.

10. **What is a practical way to integrate DL into a musician's daily routine without hindering technical progress?**
    A. Replace all scales with DL noise exercises and stop repertoire work entirely.
    B. Practice only random gestures for 2 months before returning to pieces.
    C. Begin each session with a 5-min block of systematic variations or practice a technique or part of a piece that is not improving as expected, to observe results. Then proceed to normal repertoire, gradually letting variability become an implicit habit.
    D. Avoid DL on concert days because it erases motor memory.
    E. Use DL only in physiotherapy clinics, never in the practice room.
    Correct answer: C. Experts encourage musicians to use short DL blocks—especially in technical or expressive areas that have stagnated—and then return to normal repertoire practice. Over time, the variability becomes an implicit part of their motor behavior.

Chapter 5

1. **How does differential learning (DL) differ from traditional occupational therapy methods in stroke rehabilitation?**
   A. DL encourages patients to perform tasks only according to specific fixed patterns, without changing the conditions.
   B. DL focuses on performing tasks under varying conditions, promoting brain plasticity and movement variability.
   C. Traditional occupational therapy typically involves tasks performed in a specific environment to reduce variability.
   D. DL uses only a particular physiological posture, preventing the patient from adapting their movement in different conditions.
   Correct answer: B. DL focuses on performing tasks under varying conditions, promoting brain plasticity and movement variability.
2. **Why is it important to introduce variations in tasks during differential learning-based occupational therapy?**
   A. Variations help maintain patient interest and motivation, as the tasks become more engaging.
   B. Variations help the brain adapt and reorganize, promoting better retention of motor skills and long-term functional improvements.
   C. Variations reduce therapy time, as patients achieve their goals more quickly.
   D. Variations are only necessary to ensure that patients perform tasks in different positions.
   Correct answer: B. Variations help the brain adapt and reorganize, promoting better retention of motor skills and long-term functional improvements.
3. **What is the reasoning behind limiting task repetitions to only two or three times in DLbased occupational therapy?**
   A. Repeating the same movement pattern multiple times can enhance muscle memory and motor skills without requiring adaptation.
   B. Repeating tasks too often is necessary for patients to fully master a skill, and limiting repetitions would hinder progress.
   C. Limiting repetitions encourages brain adaptation and plasticity, preventing patients from becoming too comfortable with a single movement, thus promoting better functional recovery.
   D. Task repetitions should be limited to ensure that patients experience sufficient rest to avoid fatigue and optimize recovery time.
   Correct answer: C. Limiting repetitions encourages brain adaptation and plasticity, preventing patients from becoming too comfortable with a single movement, thus promoting better functional recovery.

4. **How does differential learning promote longterm brain plasticity in stroke rehabilitation?**
   A. Introducing task variations forces the brain to adapt and reorganize, leading to better retention of motor skills and more sustainable functional improvements.
   B. Differential learning promotes brain plasticity by using only repetitive tasks.
   C. The brain is unable to adapt to different task variations, so no significant long-term plastic changes occur.
   D. Long-term changes in brain structure occur only when tasks are performed in exactly the same way every time.
   Correct answer: A. Introducing task variations forces the brain to adapt and reorganize, leading to better retention of motor skills and more sustainable functional improvements.
5. **What is the significance of performing tasks at varying body positions in differential learning-based occupational therapy?**
   A. It helps improve strength in a single, fixed position.
   B. It allows the therapist to evaluate the patient's ability to maintain a static posture.
   C. It encourages the patient to focus exclusively on one movement pattern.
   D. It challenges the body and the brain in different ways, enhancing motor learning and promoting functional adaptability.
   Correct answer: D. It challenges the body and the brain in different ways, enhancing motor learning and promoting functional adaptability.
6. **What role does trunk stability play in stroke rehabilitation, and how can DL help in this regard?**
   A. Trunk stability is important only for restoring balance, but it does not affect limb function.
   B. Trunk stability helps only with walking, but it is not necessary for other daily movements.
   C. Trunk stability is crucial as it provides the foundation for proper limb movement and balance in functional activities, and DL can assist by encouraging tasks in various body positions.
   D. Trunk stability is not important in rehabilitation, as the focus is solely on the upper limbs.
   Correct answer: C. Trunk stability is crucial as it provides the foundation for proper limb movement and balance in functional activities, and DL can assist by encouraging tasks in various body positions.
7. **How does the use of differential learning in stroke rehabilitation impact healthcare costs?**
   A. Differential learning can reduce healthcare costs by promoting faster and more sustainable recovery, reducing the duration of hospital stay and long-term care requirements.
   B. Differential learning may increase healthcare costs as the rehabilitation process takes longer.
   C. Differential learning has no impact on healthcare costs.
   D. Differential learning requires greater investment in rehabilitation technologies, thus increasing costs.
   Correct answer: A. Differential learning can reduce healthcare costs by promoting faster and more sustainable recovery, reducing the duration of hospital stay and long-term care requirements.

Chapter 6

1. **Which of the following sports has the highest relative risk (RR) for ACL injuries in female athletes?**
   A. Volleyball
   B. Basketball
   C. Tennis
   D. Baseball
   Correct answer: B. Basketball

2. **What is the primary biomechanical function of the anterior cruciate ligament (ACL)?**
   A. To facilitate knee extension
   B. To resist anterior tibial translation and control rotational stability
   C. To support quadriceps contraction
   D. To increase knee valgus during movement
   Correct answer: B. To resist anterior tibial translation and control rotational stability
3. **Which of the following is an intrinsic risk factor for ACL injuries?**
   A. Playing on artificial turf
   B. Wearing shoes with a high friction coefficient
   C. Wider pelvis and increased quadriceps (Q) angle in females
   D. Sudden changes in weather conditions
   Correct answer: C. Wider pelvis and increased quadriceps (Q) angle in females
   Here are seven multiple-choice questions based on the provided text, with correct answers indicated:
4. **What is a key limitation of traditional rehabilitation approaches after ACL reconstruction (ACLR)?**
   A. They focus too much on movement variability.
   B. They emphasize only strength and range of motion.
   C. They prioritize external focus over internal focus.
   D. They encourage unstructured and chaotic training.
   Correct answer: B. They emphasize only strength and range of motion.
5. **What is a primary concern with instructions that promote an internal focus of attention in ACL rehabilitation?**
   A. They enhance automaticity in movement.
   B. They improve external feedback processing.
   C. They may reduce movement fluidity and naturalness.
   D. They eliminate movement variability.
   Correct answer: C. They may reduce movement fluidity and naturalness.
6. **Which of the following best describes the principle of differential learning in ACL rehabilitation?**
   A. Practicing the same movement repeatedly to perfect technique
   B. Using varied and unpredictable movement patterns to enhance adaptation
   C. Eliminating movement errors to achieve ideal performance
   D. Restricting practice to low-intensity exercises for safety
   Correct answer: B. Using varied and unpredictable movement patterns to enhance adaptation
7. **How does differential learning contribute to postural stability after ACLR?**
   A. By eliminating movement variability to improve balance
   B. By challenging the neuromuscular system with variability and unpredictability
   C. By reinforcing a single ideal movement strategy
   D. By focusing solely on strengthening the quadriceps
   Correct answer: B. By challenging the neuromuscular system with variability and unpredictability
8. **What has research suggested about gait patterns after ACLR?**
   A. Gait abnormalities typically resolve within a few months.
   B. Individuals with ACLR show increased movement variability compared to healthy individuals.
   C. Altered gait patterns can persist for up to 5 years post-surgery.
   D. Traditional gait training eliminates all biomechanical deficits.
   Correct answer: C. Altered gait patterns can persist for up to 5 years post-surgery.
9. **What is a major biomechanical issue observed in running after ACLR?**
   A. Increased knee flexion and internal knee extension moment
   B. Decreased knee flexion motion and internal knee extension moment
   C. Enhanced knee valgus control and stability
   D. Reduced reliance on compensatory mechanisms

Correct answer: B. Decreased knee flexion motion and internal knee extension moment

10. **Why is movement variability considered beneficial in ACL rehabilitation?**
    A. It helps individuals develop a more adaptable motor repertoire.
    B. It ensures movements are identical each time.
    C. It prevents neuromuscular adaptation.
    D. It reduces the need for motor learning principles.
    Correct answer: A. It helps individuals develop a more adaptable motor repertoire.

Chapter 7

1. **What is the primary objective of integrating differential learning (DL) into balance training and falls prevention?**
   The central aim is to expose the postural control system to a broad spectrum of unpredictable perturbations so it can self-organize more flexible and robust balance strategies, thereby reducing the likelihood of falls in daily life.
2. **How do balance problems impact different segments of society, particularly among older adults?**
   Poor balance limits mobility in children with developmental delay, increases ankle-sprain risk in athletes, and in older adults leads to social isolation, loss of independence, and a sharply elevated incidence of injurious falls.
3. **Why are falls among older adults considered a major public health concern, and what factors contribute to their frequency?**
   Falls are the leading cause of injuryrelated death over age 65, drive billions in healthcare costs, and often trigger a downward spiral of inactivity. Contributing factors include sensory degradation (vision, vestibular), sarcopenia, polypharmacy, cognitive slowing, and environmental hazards.
4. **What are the three primary diagnostic approaches used to assess balance deficits?**
   The most common diagnostic tests for balance deficits fall into three categories: static, dynamic, and reactive balance.
5. **How do sensorimotor control regions contribute to maintaining balance, and what are their key functions?**
   The vestibular nuclei provide rapid headin-space information; the cerebellum calibrates timing and scaling of postural corrections; brainstem reticular circuits generate anticipatory muscle synergies; and cortical-basal-ganglia loops select context-appropriate balance strategies.
6. **What role does sensory and motor variability play in balance control, and how can they affect motor learning?**
   A moderate amount of variability supplies exploratory "noise" that lets the nervous system test alternate solutions; too little leads to rigidity and over-use, while too much becomes destabilizing. Well-calibrated variability, therefore, accelerates adaptation during training.
7. **How do gait abnormalities serve as both symptoms of balance impairments and potential opportunities for learning balance?**
   Altered stride length, wider base, or asymmetric step timing signal deficient postural control, yet these very deviations can be harnessed as targeted perturbations—by exaggerating or rhythmically varying them—to teach the system more effective balance responses.
8. **What are the differences between balance therapy and balance training, and how are they applied in different contexts?**
   A. Therapy is for athletes; training is only for hospital patients.
   B. Therapy targets elite performance, and training targets fall risk.
   C. Balance therapy focuses on restoring lost function after pathology under clinical supervision, whereas balance training refines or enhances stability in healthy or athletic populations.

D. Both terms mean exactly the same thing.
E. Therapy and training are distinguished solely by equipment cost.

Correct answer: C. Balance therapy focuses on restoring lost function after pathology under clinical supervision, whereas balance training refines or enhances stability in healthy or athletic populations.

9. **What are some classical approaches to balance training, and how do they improve stability and fall prevention?**
A. Wobble boards, single-leg stances, Tai Chi, and perturbation treadmills progressively challenge the postural system, leading to reduced sway and a lower incidence of falls.
B. Only seated breathing exercises are used.
C. Electrical muscle stimulation without standing practice.
D. Daily marathon running at a fixed speed.
E. Static sitting in a chair for 30 min.

Correct answer: A. Wobble boards, single-leg stances, Tai Chi, and perturbation treadmills progressively challenge the postural system, leading to reduced sway and a lower incidence of falls.

10. **How does differential learning (DL) differ from classical balance training methods, and what are its key advantages?**
A. DL relies exclusively on heavy resistance work.
B. DL repeats one ideal posture until perfect.
C. DL introduces systematically unpredictable perturbations in direction, amplitude, and timing, forcing self-organized adaptation and producing broader transfer to real-world balance tasks.
D. DL eliminates all sensory input to focus on vision.
E. DL is identical to classical methods but uses louder music.

Correct answer: C. DL introduces systematically unpredictable perturbations in direction, amplitude, and timing, forcing self-organized adaptation and producing broader transfer to real-world balance tasks.

11. **How does DL-based balance training impact the cardiovascular system, and what evidence supports this interaction?**
A. It always causes dangerous tachycardia.
B. It leaves heart dynamics unchanged because balance and cardiovascular control are unrelated.
C. DL sessions acutely raise heart rate variability and baro-reflex sensitivity, indicating beneficial autonomic engagement documented by simultaneous ECG recordings.
D. It suppresses blood pressure regulation for hours.
E. No study has ever measured cardiac effects during balance practice.

Correct answer: C. DL sessions acutely raise heart rate variability and baro-reflex sensitivity, indicating beneficial autonomic engagement documented by simultaneous ECG recordings.

12. **What are the implications of using perturbationbased balance training on ECG parameters and heart-brain interactions?**
A. It produces complete heart block in most participants.
B. It shows mild, transient increases in QT variability that parallel heightened cortical arousal, suggesting tighter heart-brain coupling during adaptive postural control.
C. It eliminates all variability in RR intervals.
D. It guarantees perfect synchrony between alpha waves and heartbeat.
E. It has no measurable physiological effects.

Correct answer: B. It shows mild, transient increases in QT variability that parallel heightened cortical arousal, suggesting tighter heart-brain coupling during adaptive postural control.

13. **What role do unpredictable coordination tasks play in enhancing balance control and adaptation?**
A. They distract the performer and worsen balance.

B. They provide irrelevant entertainment value only.
C. They enlarge the repertoire of postural solutions by forcing constant recalibration, thereby speeding adaptation to unexpected real-world perturbations.
D. They reduce reaction speed by overloading attention.
E. They have no influence on sensorimotor learning.

Correct answer: C. They enlarge the repertoire of postural solutions by forcing constant recalibration, thereby speeding adaptation to unexpected real-world perturbations.

14. **How can sling exercises and the Neurac© method be used for therapy and fall prevention?**
    A. By locking the body rigidly to suppress all sway.
    B. By suspending limbs in ropes and elastic slings to create multi-planar instability, activating deep stabilizers and training reactive balance in a controlled yet variable environment.
    C. By eliminating gravity through underwater practice.
    D. By replacing standing work with seated meditation.
    E. By attaching weights to immobilize the center of mass.

    Correct answer: B. By suspending limbs in ropes and elastic slings to create multi-planar instability, activating deep stabilizers and training reactive balance in a controlled yet variable environment.
15. **What are some future clinical applications of DL-based balance training, and how might they improve rehabilitation and injury prevention?**
    A. Fully automated VR perturbation systems and wearable feedback sensors could deliver individualized, variability-rich programs at home, shortening rehab times and reducing fall rates in high-risk populations.
    B. Daily use of rigid casts to prevent any joint movement.
    C. Replacing therapists with static instruction posters.
    D. Eliminating technology to focus only on verbal cues.
    E. Standardized one-size-fits-all protocols for every patient.

    Correct answer: A. Fully automated VR perturbation systems and wearable feedback sensors could deliver individualized, variabilityrich programs at home, shortening rehab times and reducing fall rates in high-risk populations.

Chapter 8

1. **How can you improve your metabolic flexibility in daily life by incorporating different types of exercises, including HIIT?**

    Short explanation. Metabolic flexibility refers to the body's ability to adapt energy metabolism based on demand and substrate availability. HIIT improves this flexibility by alternating high- and low-intensity intervals, enhancing both aerobic and anaerobic pathways. Through varied forms like Tabata, HIFT, and whole-body HIIT, it trains the body to efficiently regulate energy use, promoting better metabolic adaptation and overall performance.
2. **When designing your own HIIT workout, how can you balance stimulus time, training time, and recovery intensity to match your fitness goals?**

    Short explanation. Balancing stimulus time, training time, and recovery intensity in HIIT requires individualization based on fitness level, time to exhaustion, and recovery capacity. Higher intensities demand shorter work bouts and longer recovery, while moderate loads allow sustained effort. By adjusting these variables—stimulus time, total session duration, and recovery intensity—HIIT can be optimized to match personal goals, enhance metabolic flexibility, and improve overall performance.

3. **How can incorporating unique movement patterns and varied exercises in HIIT, as suggested by differential learning, enhance your strength, agility, and injury prevention?**

   Short explanation. Incorporating unique movement patterns and varied exercises in HIIT, as suggested by the Differential Learning approach, enhances strength, agility, and injury prevention by promoting variability and adaptability in movement. Differential Learning introduces controlled fluctuations, or "noise," that challenge the nervous system, stimulating neuroplasticity and improving motor control. When applied to HIIT, these fluctuations can be achieved by altering exercise type, tempo, coordination demands, or environmental conditions. Exercises such as jumping jacks or burpees, which combine multiple movement patterns, create higher neuromuscular demands and energy expenditure, driving deeper adaptive responses. In physiotherapy, this approach enables therapists to individualize sessions by adjusting the level of variability according to each patient's capacity, ensuring an optimal level of challenge that promotes progress without overload. As a result, integrating Differential Learning principles into HIIT enhances movement quality, coordination, and resilience, contributing to improved performance and reduced injury risk in both athletic and rehabilitative settings.

4. **Have you ever noticed how unexpected variations in movement improve learning and coordination during exercise? How can you apply this principle, using differential learning, to physiotherapy sessions for patients, especially those aiming to improve mobility?**

   Short explanation. A single answer cannot fully explain how unexpected variations improve learning and coordination because the effects depend on each individual's dynamic physiological, psychological, neuronal, and circadian states. In physiotherapy, Differential Learning can be applied by introducing controlled variability—such as changes in intensity, exercise selection, set duration, rest intervals, or total session length—while continuously monitoring the patient's responses. The externally applied fluctuations from the therapist should align with the patient's internal fluctuations to reach a stochastic resonance, optimizing motor learning, coordination, and mobility. By respecting the dynamic and fluctuating nature of perception and exertion, therapists can create personalized sessions that promote self-organization, adaptability, and more effective rehabilitation outcomes.

5. **How can you adapt physiotherapy exercises to match a patient's daily energy levels and recovery state, using principles of differential learning to improve metabolic flexibility and enhance movement patterns over time, rather than following a rigid routine?**

   Short explanation. This question is intended more for reflection and critical thinking rather than having a single "correct answer." It encourages considering how to tailor physiotherapy exercises to each patient's daily state, using Differential Learning principles to improve metabolic flexibility and movement patterns over time, rather than simply applying a rigid, one-size-fits-all routine.

6. **Which of the following adaptations is associated with HIIT in skeletal muscles?**
   A. Decrease in mitochondrial content
   B. Increased protein expression related to antioxidant regulation
   C. Reduced muscle mass
   D. Decreased neuromuscular coordination

   Correct answer: B. Increased protein expression related to antioxidant regulation

7. **Match the adaptation with its corresponding effect**
   A. Mitochondrial health
   B. Cardiopulmonary system

C. Metabolic health
   (i) Increases VO_2max and improves blood pressure regulation
   (ii) Enhances mitochondrial biogenesis and removal of dysfunctional mitochondria
   (iii) Reduces body fat percentage and increases muscle mass

Correct answers: A-(ii), B-(i), C-(iii)

8. **What does the DL model emphasize in the context of motor learning?**
   A. Consistency in exercise regimens
   B. Learning through stochastic perturbations
   C. Strict adherence to traditional training methods
   D. The importance of individual variability in training

   Correct answer: B. Learning through stochastic perturbations

9. **In terms of exercise selection, which of the following is suggested for enhancing neuromuscular adaptation in HIIT programs?**
   A. Focusing only on high-intensity exercises
   B. Including exercises with unique movement patterns and combinations of movements
   C. Using the same exercises in every session
   D. Avoiding complex exercises

   Correct answer: B. Including exercises with unique movement patterns and combinations of movements

10. **What is a key principle behind the differential learning model in rehabilitation?**
   A. Emphasizing uniformity in exercise performance
   B. Encouraging variability and adaptation through different motor tasks
   C. Focusing solely on the objective data of structured exercise
   D. Minimizing the subjective feedback from the body

   Correct answer: B. Encouraging variability and adaptation through different motor tasks

MIX
Papier aus verantwortungsvollen Quellen
Paper from responsible sources
FSC® C105338

If you have any concerns about our products,
you can contact us on
ProductSafety@springernature.com

In case Publisher is established outside the EU,
the EU authorized representative is:
Springer Nature Customer Service Center GmbH
Europaplatz 3, 69115 Heidelberg, Germany

Printed by Libri Plureos GmbH
in Hamburg, Germany